P9-DGY-407

worried
sick

Worried Sick

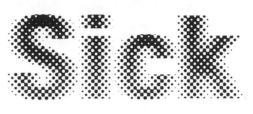

A Prescription for Health in an Overtreated America

Nortin M. Hadler, M.D.

The University of North Carolina Press
Chapel Hill

This book was published with the assistance of the
H. Eugene and Lillian Youngs Lehman Fund of the
University of North Carolina Press. A complete list
of books published with the assistance of the Lehman
Fund appears at the end of the book.

Designed by April Leidig-Higgins
Set in Minion by Copperline Book Services, Inc.
Manufactured in the United States of America

The paper in this book meets the guidelines for
permanence and durability of the Committee on
Production Guidelines for Book Longevity of the
Council on Library Resources.

Library of Congress Cataloging-in-Publication Data
Hadler, Nortin M.
Worried sick: a prescription for health in an
overtreated America / Nortin M. Hadler.
p.   cm.
Includes bibliographical references and index.
ISBN 978-0-8078-3187-8 (cloth: alk. paper)
    1. Medical care — United States.   2. Medical
policy — United States.   3. Older people — Medical
care — United States.   4. Medical care — Utilization
— United States.   5. Health care reform — United
States.   I. Title.
    [DNLM: 1. Delivery of Health Care — utilization
— United States — Popular Works.   2. Aging —
psychology — United States — Popular Works.
3. Health Policy — United States — Popular Works.
4. Health Promotion — United States — Popular works.
5. Unnecessary Procedures — utilization — United
States — Popular Works.   W 84 AA1 H131W   2008]
RA395.A3H332   2008
362.10973 — dc22   2007042147

A Caravan book. For more information, visit
www.caravanbooks.org.

cloth   12 11 10 09 08   5 4 3 2 1

To a generation of students
and generations of patients
for all they taught me,

and to
Carol S. Hadler,
who made the last forty-five
years full, fun, and complete

contents

tables

acknowledgment

Publishing books has been a major part of
my career, books written for physicians and
scholars who share my research interests.
Publishing books for a general audience is an
entirely different exercise, but I grew to relish
the process with *Worried Sick*. The reason
in part is the encouragement and support of
David Perry and his staff at UNC Press. What
a privilege to have such a resource on campus,
just a few blocks from my office.

worried
sick

Introduction

The social construction of health in the United States, and to a lesser degree elsewhere, has features that are counterproductive. We are becoming increasingly medicalized, made to think that all life's challenges demand clinical intervention, when the science dictates otherwise. We are at grave risk of what I call "Type II Medical Malpractice" — doctors doing the unnecessary, albeit very well (as opposed to Type I Medical Malpractice, which is doctors doing the necessary unacceptably poorly). Until the public at large comes to recognize the dangers of medicalization and Type II Medical Malpractice and decries both, there will be no pressure to reform an egregiously self-serving national medical enterprise. We will continue to condemn its costliness rather than its abysmal lack of cost-effectiveness.

My primary objective in writing *Worried Sick* is to provide readers with the perspectives and skills necessary to advocate for themselves in the contemporary health-care delivery system. I have spent over three decades honing the ability to communicate complex issues to patients, mostly in clinical settings. Lately, I have produced a series of essays on health-care matters for ABCNews.com that I've crafted for a very wide audience. While I can't do as well in print as I could face to face, responding to an individual's questions and challenges, I am confident that the message of this book will be loud and clear. I have written as if I were conversing with a patient rather than speaking to a colleague. Each chapter provides a fresh, often startling, even counterintuitive take on topics that we all hear about almost daily. All of these topics are darlings of the health journalists; each supports an industry. It requires an open mind to look at them critically and then to turn them inside out. I hope that I've eased readers into this exercise. If so, I will have transformed them into very sophisticated guardians of their own health.

However, I am very uncomfortable asking the reader simply to accept my arguments. I need to provide the detailed, rigorous support for the exercise. Hence, each chapter has a shadow chapter in the supplementary readings, which are much more than annotated bibliographies. The shadow chapters are more detailed, technical, and heavily referenced than their counterparts but are still designed to be instructional and accessible to the interested general readership while satisfying the most demanding of my peers. My intent is for all readers to feel the need to read the shadow chapter once the thrust of the main chapter is apparent. The shadow chapters highlight the many crucial papers published in the last few years.

I have a second agenda in writing *Worried Sick*, beyond teaching the reader how to make informed personal choices regarding his or her well-being. This book teaches how such a perspective translates into informing issues in health-care policy that are relevant to all of us. I am convinced that the major stumbling block to rational health care in the United States is not the entropy nurtured by the interests vested in the status quo but the social construction of health. Americans think their medicine is the "best," if only they could afford it. This book is the catwalk for the displaying of the medical emperor's new clothes. My patients, my students, my children and grandchildren, as well as yours, need to recognize and decry medicalization and Type II Medical Malpractice. Only then will physicians be able to cast off the shackles of the contemporary medical enterprise and be able to minister to the sick once again. Only then will rational health care be possible. I return to this prospect in chapter 14.

Desperately Well

This book is not written as a resource for people who are no longer well. It offers few insights into developing the courage to cope with particular diseases and the illnesses they cause. Many of the skills and perspectives regarding therapeutic choices that are developed here are as relevant to those who are sick as to those who are well. But I am writing this book mainly for all who consider themselves well despite occasional or even persistent nagging doubts. Your sense of well-being requires conviction to withstand the badgering assaults of health-promotion programs. Some of you are overcoming encounters with illness; others are still trying to put such encounters into perspective. Some of you are burdened with forebodings; others are fatalistic. If you feel you are well despite all this, you have an unshakable inherent sense of invincibility. This book is written to provide the wherewithal to bolster that conviction. It is not designed to obviate the need for seeking help when your conviction seems shaky. If you feel such a need, *Worried Sick* is designed to make you an active participant in the choosing of treatments among the many that various professional purveyors promulgate and even aggressively market. It is written so that you will have the courage to take responsibility for rationally considering these options.

We all need to become the most sophisticated of "health-care" consumers. We have all experienced heartburn and heartache, backache and neck pain, unfamiliar bowel function, peculiar sensations, days in the doldrums, realizations of physical limits, insomnia, and myriad other predicaments — and we will again. These are unpleasant, disconcerting, personal, even noxious experiences; these are morbid events that test the limits of our sense of invincibility. *Worried Sick* is written to bolster the personal resources that facilitate coping, whether we attempt such on our own or we negotiate professional guidance. And our coping is in dreadful need of bolstering. The wealth of health information disseminated by all sorts of health-care vendors, including those in the medical profession, may be intended as helpful but often is not. Much of this information does violence to our sense of invincibility without doing equivalent good for our health or longevity. This book levels the playing field.

My approach is imbued with the teachings of Karl Popper. Popper moved the philosophy of science into the modern era. He placed on us all the responsibility to doubt, to question, and always to try to refute each successive putative "truth." Truth, he taught, is only the hypothesis that is yet to be disproved. I have spent my career as a medical educator under this banner, teaching at the bedsides of a vast array of very sick patients at my home institution and as visiting professor at over a hundred others. *Worried Sick* is crafted to inform the well reader how to feel well. Rest assured I understand the plight and circumstance of those who are not so fortunate as to be well. Otherwise, I could not appreciate the challenges to the sense of wellness faced by those who are well. When I'm done with you, you will not be as vulnerable to pronouncements that are presumptuous if not self-serving.

In crafting *Worried Sick*, I have relied on an experience that is typically uncommon for mainline academic physicians. Thirty years ago I realized that nearly all my patients were faced with a plight that was barely mentioned during the years I spent learning to be a physician; patients leave the office or hospital and then contend with the impact of their illness on daily life and on their expectations. Thirty years ago I commenced a study of one aspect of that plight: the need to maintain substantial gainful employment. My interest in the "illness of work incapacity" has taken me far afield, forcing me to explore workplaces, analyze work and work contexts, and probe the sociopolitical constraints imposed on the interface between the medical community and the permanently and transiently disabled. This book is imbued with my understanding of the social consequences of illness.

Likewise, an understanding of medicalization permeates the book. The study of the interplay between illness and work demanded a more intimate knowledge of the perceptions of illness and of its consequence for people who had not sought medical attention. From the perspective of the physician, these people who were not yet patients were well. However, my work, some work by predecessors, and a vast current literature has dissected the construct "well" as it pertains to life in the community. To be well is not to be free of symptoms — of morbidity — continuously or for long periods of time. It is abnormal to escape heartburn and heartache, backache and headache, sad days and days when we're aware of our bowels. Sometimes we tell others of our predicaments, describing our plight as we perceive it in our own idioms of distress. But whether we tell someone or not, we are challenged to cope with these predicaments of life and of living. To be well is to be able to cope with morbid episodes. And coping may not be easy. It can be thwarted by the intensity of the morbidity, or by complicating and confounding factors.

Medicalization is one such confounding factor. Medicalization is the process by which the morbidity is framed by the person as a medical illness for which medical treatment could or should be sought. To do so, it must seem reasonable to ascribe the symptoms to a medical disease. The Victorians could medicalize the female orgasm, whereas we can medicalize its absence. Medicalization superimposes a scientific idiom of distress on the common sense. Common sense is not common, temporally or geographically, and if it is sense, it is sense that is highly susceptible to presuppositions, magical thinking, and market pressures.

Most importantly, *Worried Sick* is imbued with critical, rigorous science. I've already admitted to being a committed refutationist, a follower of the teachings of Popper. I started my investigative career as a geneticist, moved on to study immunochemistry, and spent my first decade on faculty as a physical biochemist. I only closed my laboratory when I found that contending with the other three passions of my academic career was more than a plateful. However, I have a keen appreciation for the scientific method at its most rigorous. I have applied that razor to my own epidemiological studies and to the relevant epidemiological studies of others. The result is a definition of uncertainty, even a quantification of uncertainty. The result is not — not now and maybe not ever — a definition of certainty. The best I can tell you is how uncertain I am about any assertion of fact I make, and how certain I am about any tenet I declare to be rubbish. This is an elegant philosophy of science but a demanding philosophy of life. How much uncertainty we tolerate about any fact relates to our own personal value system. Suppose I tell you that if 1,000 well people take a particular drug every day, all will be living in five years' time, whereas only 500 will survive without the drug. Most of us would value the drug greatly, even if its longer-term toxicities were unknown. Would you value the drug if I told you that after five years, there were only 510 survivors? Do you think it is possible to reliably measure the difference between 510 surviving on the drug and 500 surviving without the drug? If so, do you think it is meaningful? Is it worth the bother of swallowing the pills, the risk of short-term toxicities, and the uncertainties in the long run? Would 550 survivors on the drug seem more compelling? We will revisit this scenario in chapter 2 and the notion of medical uncertainty from the patient's perspective repeatedly throughout the book.

Worried Sick is a treatise on medicalization that is informed by science, clinical reality, and an analysis of life's morbid experiences. I intend to suggest ways of coping with some of the morbidities that are unavoidable in the course of living as a well person. I intend to demonstrate how to discern instances when medicine can offer you insights in that regard. And I intend to teach you how to avoid iatrogenicity, medical interventions that cause harm. Armed with skepticism and a critical intellect, it is possible to safely and effectively benefit from modern medicine without being harmed in the process. Armed with informed skepticism, it is possible to design a rational health-care delivery system. It is not my intent to speak ill of your doctor, or even of doctors generally. I am examining the institution of medicine that molds the behavior of physicians and that waits upon your complaint. I have no compunctions about sharing the bad with the good that results from that examination. I have no compunctions about suggesting a system of health insurance that underwrites only the good, only those items among all that have been studied that have been shown to have a meaningfully advantageous benefit-to-risk ratio.

This book has fourteen chapters. Several confront the inevitability of death. Yes, we will all die. The issue for me is not so much how or why we die, but when and how we lived. In the academy and in the lay mind, the proximate cause of death is foremost, so that great energy and great wealth is expended trying to spare you death from a particular cause without considering whether you will die at the same time from some other cause. This medicalization of dying hides under the Orwellian banner of "Health Promotion, Disease Prevention," affectionately termed "hippie-dippie" for the acronym HPDP by the self-important insiders. The idea is that all of us are time bombs. We harbor bundles of risk factors and face potential hazards that someday will rise up, smite us ill, and carry us off. Hippie-dippie promises to modify and mollify our mortal risks. Who can resist? Anyone who has read *Worried Sick.*

Other chapters step back from the myth of immortality to examine the medicalization of the morbid predicaments of life. This theme will make you uncomfortable at first blush. Once I educate you, you will be able to go before your physician with such complaints as "Doc, I feel awful. Could it be in my mind?" or "Doc, my back is killing me. I can't figure out why I can't cope with this episode." I daresay most of you would find the first complaint off-putting if not infuriating, and the second counterintuitive. I will undertake this exercise in semiotics to change your idioms of distress so that they reflect your predicament rather than personal and medical presuppositions. You will learn how psychosocial challenges to our sense of invincibility can cause us to focus on physical and emotional symptoms so that the symptoms seem more the issue than the challenges that caused us to focus in the first place. Don't read something abnormal, weak, or weak-minded into this assertion; it is describing a normal dynamic. Until this concept is grasped, myriad approaches offered by others to help with the symptoms will seem seductive. Pursuing help for the surrogate complaint seldom provides relief, often exacerbates the symptoms, and always and forever changes your sense of well-being.

Teaching the well how to critically approach the medical treatment act is something of a heresy. After all, I am teaching that neither naïveté nor trust can be counted on to serve you well. Most of the lessons, the object lessons I will teach, are heretical as well. Without criticism and controversy, the weaknesses of our beliefs never surface. My goal is to provide readers with the skills to assume responsibility for assessing their health status in the face of the barrage of information that they will confront in the days and years to come. Each of the fourteen chapters is an object lesson; each tackles a topic of immediate relevance and teaches a particular skill set. I have ordered the topics so that the skills complement and build on one another. It is certainly reasonable to skip to the chapter you find most relevant to you. I have made some allowances in the design of the chapters for picking and choosing. However, I urge you to read the book in sequence. I am not setting out to turn you into biostatisticians and epidemiologists. I am setting out to mold your critical skills so that you can recognize and contend with the unfounded assertions, tortured and massaged data, and egregious marketing that has always been present but is now industrialized. There is no other way to avoid sacrificing the sense that you are well to medicalization, or worse yet, losing your actual wellness to iatrogenicity, the illnesses that are caused by medical treatments. And there is no other way to recruit you to my "hidden" agenda: fomenting a debate that demystifies "modern" medicine so that we can promulgate a rational health-care delivery system and underwrite its cost.

chapter one

The Methuselah Complex

Man has no dominion over the breath of life,
neither to retain that flicker of life nor the
power to determine the day of death.
— Ecclesiastes 8:8

Do you know when you want to die?

If you could, would you choose the date?

"Never" is not an option; the death rate is one per person. "When?" is the profound and bedeviling enigma. Ending one's own life raises great issues in moral relativism, as great as does ending the life of another. Prolonging life also raises issues in moral relativism. Should we go to lengths to prolong all life, or just life we deem sufficiently high in quality? Hence, "When?" is pregnant with, "How goes the journey?"

These are questions for the ages. The authors of the Old Testament weighed in: foreknowledge of the time of one's death would be a heavy burden, not a blessing. Furthermore, if a world without death becomes a world without birth, the specter is bleak and joyless. Rather, death is viewed as inevitable and the imponderability of its imperative assuaged with notions of afterlife. Longevity is treated as a sign of purposefulness if not holiness. The Old Testament offers up Abraham, Moses, and that statistical outlier for the ages, Methuselah, the grandfather of Noah, whose age at death is usually translated as 969 years. Some scholars choose a different Sumerian dialect for translation or convert to lunar years and come up closer to eighty-five — exceptional, not too shabby for the time of the Great Flood, and not fatuous as is 969. Are we, the residents of the modern resource-advantaged world, likely to live to be eighty-five? Can we aspire to be purposeful for eighty-five years? Are highly functioning octogenarians still statistical outliers?

Daily, we are offered the image of the baby-boom generation going on forever, making impossible demands on successive generations to provide pensions, health care, and community. That, too, is fatuous. However, more of us are living longer than did our parents. Clearly, the likelihood that we will enjoy life as an octogenarian has increased over the course of the twentieth century. Far less clear is whether the likelihood of becoming a nonagenarian has increased similarly. It has certainly not done so at anything like the same rate as the likelihood of being an octogenarian. The effect is so striking that it has caused many of us to wonder if there is not a fixed longevity for our species, set around eighty-five years of age. Some have likened this to a warranty: you are off warranty at eighty-five, beyond is a bonus, and well beyond is a statistical oddity. This projected demographic is consistent with current population trends. With one caveat, these hard facts seem unlikely to change. It is possible that molecular biology can alter the fixed longevity of our species. But don't hold your breath. None of us will live to see that — and maybe no one ever will.

Eighty-five (± a little bit) appears to be the programmed life expectancy for our species. I grant that the science is imperfect. But eighty-five is a linchpin of my personal philosophy of life. I, for one, do not care how many diseases I harbor on my eighty-fifth birthday, though I prefer not to know that they are creeping up on me. I, for one, do not care which of these diseases carries me off as long as the leaving is gentle and the legacy meaningful. Perhaps the best we can reasonably hope for is eighty-five years of life free of morbidities that overwhelm our wherewithal to cope, then to die in our sleep on our eighty-fifth birthday.

Unfortunately, not all of us will arrive at our eighty-fifth birthday with tranquility or, having done so, have a peaceful passing. Fortunate, indeed, are the octogenarians of today who have the wits and faculties to contend with life's demands. But time soon whittles away even their higher level of functional capacity. Month by month they face days when they do not perform as usual and even feel the need to take to bed. Inexorably, activities of daily living, activities they always took for granted, become an insurmountable challenge. They will come to take their place among the frail elderly. They will lean on canes by the graveside of their friends. They do not merit a disease label, such as "Alzheimer's"; they merit awe, compassion, and community.

The hope is faint that contemporary medical science will shepherd more of the high-functioning octogenarians into the very meager ranks of the high-functioning nonagenarians. It is, however, possible to provide comfort and support for these octogenarians through the transition toward decrepitude and in their final passage. Friendship, community, and love are defensible as prescriptions, clinical interventions, and targets for public policy and expenditure. To advocate otherwise, including measures purporting to increase the lifespan beyond eighty-five, is to harbor delusions of immortality. Heroic efforts on behalf of the highly functioning octogenarians will accomplish little of substance. We can, perhaps, alter the proximate cause of death — that is, the diagnosis on the death certificate — but I am aware of no data to support the premise that we can alter the date of death. This is not to advocate therapeutic nihilism. It is the invoking of the age-old ethic of medicine to contend with the reality of our aging and our mortality. When the high-functioning octogenarian declines, it is because her or his time is nearing. When death supervenes, it is because it is her or his time. That is the real proximate cause of death. It does not matter how many diseases are vying for coupe de grâce. It only matters that the journey was as gratifying as possible.

One might be tempted to ascribe the increasing longevity in North America to past medical programs that promote health and to ongoing medical care. Science tempers any such hubris (we return to this realization in chapter 14). Health-adverse behaviors and cardiovascular risk factors may relate to the proximate cause of death, but they account for less than 25 percent of the hazard to longevity. This might explain why multiple assaults on health-adverse behaviors and cardiovascular risk factors have uncertain effects on all-cause mortality. They might change the proximate cause of death, but they do not alter its timing.

While the best clinical management of frailty in octogenarians may be only support, comfort, and community, I welcome aggressive efforts to increase the likelihood that more members of future birth cohorts will close the story of their lives as highly functional octogenarians. Many people in the resource-advantaged world still lag behind. Who die before their time? Who live to a ripe old age?

Understanding the good fortune of vibrant octogenarians requires understanding the hazards to well-being that lurk in the course of living. These life-course hazards are aspects of our interactive and integrative worlds, our ecosystems, that can powerfully influence our biology and, thereby, our fate. Much of this is captured by measures of socioeconomic status (SES). There is an incontrovertible relationship between SES and longevity. But do not be misled into assuming SES is simply a measure of income status. Longevity is more dependent on how poor you are relative to those who are advantaged in your ecosystem. For example, the greater the gap in income between the rich and the poor (the

"Robin Hood effect") across states in the United States, the sooner the poor die. This relationship between income gap and longevity holds across the advanced world. Also, do not be misled into assuming SES is a measure of health-care expenditures; it isn't, not in North America or elsewhere. SES is a measure of the salutary nature of the neighborhood in which you live and the context in which you pursue gainful employment.

A handmaiden of SES is educational status. For example, people born between the world wars who managed to average twelve years of education are likely to live some seven years longer than the low-SES strata of their birth cohort. For the advantaged octogenarians, the transitions to doldrums, decrepitude, and demise are telescoped into the last year or so of life. The disadvantaged in their birth cohort commence these transitions earlier in life and suffer through their painstaking unfolding. They labor in jobs that are less rewarding, satisfying, or secure (see chapter 12). They live under clouds of persistent pain and pervasive work incapacity. Their life is shorter and less sweet.

The octogenarian and great German pathologist Rudolf Virchow (1821–1902) developed a notion of "natural" as opposed to "artificial" diseases and epidemics. He considered typhus, scurvy, tuberculosis, and mental disease to be "artificial" because they were primarily due to social conditions: "The artificial epidemics are attributes of society, products of a false culture that is not distributed to all classes. They point toward deficiencies produced by the structure of the state or society, and strike therefore primarily those classes which do not enjoy the advantages of the culture."

The stratum of society that dies before its time falls victim to an "artificial epidemic." "Artificial epidemics" account for 75 percent of mortal hazard. They will not respond to pharmaceuticals nor can they be surgically excised. They play out well beyond the walls of the clinic and the hospital. They are not considered the proper target of the "Health Promotion, Disease Prevention" initiatives of contemporary medicine. Rather, contemporary medicine nibbles at the frays of the other 25 percent of mortal hazard. These are the health-adverse behaviors and other biological "risk factors" that we hear so much about. Any agenda that ignores the other 75 percent does little to serve the "Public Health." For most people who are enjoying an SES they perceive as adequate, even advantaged, there is little to do to increase their longevity since they are already likely to approach the magical eighty-five when their time is near. For the disadvantaged, those who perceive their SES as lacking, adjusting cholesterol and screening for cancer is little match for the mortal hazard of their situation in life.

Evidence-Based Medicine

These and other topics have occupied the careers of thousands of clinical investigators. The literature they have produced is enormous and varied. The quality of the science ranges from the overtly flawed through the anecdotal to the elegant. The intent of the science is less heterogeneous. Throughout history, clinical investigators have sought the evidence that would ground their treatments. In times past, astute observation of reproducible health effects was the only scientific method. It served well to identify such breakthroughs as colchicine for gout 2,000 years ago, vitamin B12 for pernicious anemia eighty years ago, and streptomycin for tuberculosis sixty years ago.

The observational method also left a paper trail and legacy of false starts, false inferences, and adverse effects of medical treatment (iatrogenicity). Tonsillectomy, for the prevention of childhood pharyngitis, is an example many older readers will recall. We learned the hard way that most children outgrow recurrent pharyngitis with or without tonsillectomy. Recently, we have learned the same lesson for "ear infections" in childhood. The triumph of the last fifty years is the development of methodologies to test whether clinical inferences are valid before they are unleashed on the ill. These methodologies try to ensure that an association drawn between a stated health effect and any drug, surgical procedure, dietary change, or other intervention is genuine. Their success derives from the design of the clinical trials and the statistical methods to handle the data. Some academic disciplines are devoted to pushing back the frontier of this methodological triumph, and certain licensing agencies, beginning with the Food and Drug Administration (FDA) in the 1960s, now demand evidence of safety and efficacy before pharmaceuticals can be marketed (see chapter 9).

The ethic, the methodology, and the regulations have converged to create the modern clinical trials enterprise. It is an enormous enterprise, spewing forth trials in the thousands and data points in the millions each year. Its output threatened to overwhelm comprehensibility and effectiveness. The result is the spawning of yet another discipline devoted to making sense of all this output — "evidence-based medicine," or EBM. Around the world, groups of investigators are sifting through all the evidence to sort the wheat from the chaff. Yes, there is chaff. Some trials were designed less well than others because nuances that improve design were unappreciated or ignored, or because of execution or even faults in data analysis. Yet it's not rational, or feasible, simply to rely on the most adequate trials for diagnosis and treatment. Having contended with debates as to which trial is best, one is often faced with results that pertain to particular patient groups and still are likely to be inconsistent. So the investigators revisit the "more acceptable" trials and attempt to decide, or even mathematically model, which are the least flawed and, therefore, which conclusions are least likely to be spurious. I am not belittling this effort. It is spearheaded by the Cochrane Collaboration, a ten-year-old multinational undertaking supported by various federal coffers. (No pharmaceutical industry monies are involved — yet. There are pressures in that regard.) The collaboration has 10,000 participants divided into work groups according to clinical topics. It has a registry of some 500,000 studies and has already produced some 4,000 evidentiary reviews, with nearly as many in the pipeline and plans for 7,000 beyond that.

Reviews from the Cochrane Collaboration pertain to nearly every topic covered in this book, and I have taken advantage of all of them. I also discuss their limitations in many chapters and in the relevant section of the annotated readings. The collaboration, like other EBM investigators, is committed to methodological excellence. The working groups try to discern whether there *is* evidence. For the clinician and the well person faced with a decision, however, that is only the first issue. If there is evidence for some health effect, the next point is whether the evidence is likely to be reliable or whether the next clinical trial will discount it. If it is likely to be reliable, is the effect meaningful and, therefore, worthwhile? Or is the effect too trivial to bother with or not worth the tradeoff in risk? This was the point of the hypothetical trial I put forward in the introduction. Without this frame of reference, our values will be uninformed and our decisions naïve. I intend to provide a frame of reference for decisions that relate to mortality and to symptoms (morbidity) and other aspects of the quality of life. As we will see, it is more difficult to make rational decisions about quality of life, given the vagaries of health effects in this area.

The supplementary readings for the introduction and this chapter include an expanded discussion on life-course epidemiology, the construct that underlies all of my longevity arguments. No one should be as concerned about the proximate cause of their demise as they are about the likelihood their course in life will be satisfying. It matters little what carries one off, as long as it was her or his time and the journey was gratifying.

chapter two

The Heart of
the Matter

Interventional cardiology and cardiovascular surgery are the cash cows of, if not the engines driving, all that is indefensible about the American health-care delivery system. I'm not accusing interventional cardiologists and cardiovascular surgeons of malfeasance. Some may be deserving of such condemnation, but I assume that most are caught up in the folly of peer review. They are so convinced that what they do advantages patients, they are hell-bent to do it better. Furthermore, they are so handsomely rewarded, in acclaim if not monetarily, that it would seem counterintuitive if not absurd to question what they do. Not only would they get their backs up, but many also would rally to their support with a vengeance: grateful patients who assume they'd be dead were it not for their stent or bypass, hospital administrators who live off the overhead of their endeavors, profiteering suppliers and manufacturers of all the necessary widgets and putatively necessary drugs, and "health" insurers who skim off the top of the enormous cash flow.

Fortunately, interventional cardiologists are so cocksure in their work that they have long been willing to accept federal and industry monies to study their effectiveness. We are swimming in such data. The best of science does not presuppose the outcome; the worst tries to support rather than disprove presuppositions. The best of science stands on its own; the worst hides behind the approval of colleagues of like mind. Interventional cardiology suffers the latter, much to the encouragement of the industry it spawns and the media coverage that industry underwrites. It falls upon us, the patient or potential patient and the physicians committed to the well-being of their patient, to sift through the mountains of data. All one needs is a razor: Is the study methodologically sound enough to believe? Is the result reproducible? And, most importantly, was anything meaningful accomplished?

The Folly of Peer Review

From time to time, every one of us gets a "bee in our bonnet." We have an idea that is so appealing, we can't let it go. It doesn't matter if others are less certain, or even call us superstitious. The belief is so comfortable, so plausible, we defend it vigorously. That's human nature. Physicians are human. Sometimes our beliefs turn out to be correct, to be prescient. Sometimes they don't. Not long ago, tonsils were removed because they were swollen and uteruses because they were lumpy. We got it wrong with stents, too. Let me tell you how.

Fifty years ago, heart attacks were a scourge. Everyone knew a working-age man who'd dropped dead from one. Medicine seemed stymied. That's when it became clear that the large arteries that feed the heart muscle, the coronary arteries, were clogged by atherosclerotic plaque in nearly every man who had a heart attack. Cardiac surgery had made great strides in fixing leaky heart valves, so why not fix clogged arteries? Removing the clog was too difficult, so pioneering surgeons developed methods for creating blood vessels that bypassed the obstructing plaques. Thus was born "coronary artery bypass graft" surgery, the CABG. It was firmly believed that if the blockage was bypassed, the patient was saved.

There were skeptics. Skeptics foment controversy, and controversy is the fuel for progress. Otherwise, we remain stubbornly complacent about our beliefs. Thanks to the skeptics, thousands of men with heart pain were enrolled in trials in the United States and Europe comparing CABG surgery with medical treatment. These studies went on for over a decade, until around 1980. The results were not encouraging: with the exception of a small group, the patients who had CABG did not live any longer than those treated medically. Besides, a significant percentage of CABG patients died before they could leave the hospital, about half had a stormy recovery, nearly that many had memory loss at a year, and half suffered cognitive decline at five years that was beyond that observed in their birth cohort. But it's not easy to give up a belief. Besides, there is a small subset, about 3 percent of all patients, with a particular blockage that is helped. Treated medically, only 65 percent of this subset survived for five years; 85 percent if they survived CABG. See, said the believers, there is some truth to our belief that plaques were *the* evil. With improved skills and techniques, more than 3 percent should be helped. Progress was slow and uncertain. Rather than question the basic belief, the problem was thought to be that the grafts did not function for long.

That's when another idea came along from Switzerland: rather than bypass the blockage, put a balloon into its center, blow the balloon up, and smash the plaque, thereby opening up the vessel. That's called angioplasty. It is less of an ordeal than CABG, but no more effective. Again, it was noted that the vessel rapidly clogged again. Maybe that's why the procedure was not as helpful as was believed it should be.

Enter stents. These are wire tubes that are inserted into the artery after the plaque is smashed. Then the artery can't clog again, it was believed. Wrong. These plain stents clogged at least as quickly as arteries without them. The patients did no better than if the stent was not inserted, which is no better than if the plaque was not smashed, which is no better than if the patient had a CABG, which is no better than medical treatment (and medical treatment has advanced).

Undaunted and unbowed, the believers leaped at the next idea: coat the stent with drugs that interfere with clotting and thereby keep the vessel open. Finally they made a difference. Patients were worse off for this idea.

Cardiologists and cardiac surgeons still have this bee in their bonnet. They talk about new procedures, new widgets and gizmos, the particular timing of the procedures, and anything else rather than wonder if their basic belief is wrong. They manage to sting over a million American hearts each year with the bee in their bonnet.

You have two options: you can avoid this sting or survive it. I prefer the former, and not just because CABG and angioplasty and stents cannot be shown to offer any important advantage. Remember when heart attacks were a scourge, some fifty years ago? They no longer are: in one generation, the chance of having a heart attack dropped 40 percent. And the chance of living five years after your first heart attack increased from 50 percent to 96 percent. You can increase it further, to 98 percent, with a touch of aspirin, but little else makes much of a difference. We don't know why heart attacks are no longer so common or so evil. Medicine deserves little if any credit. But heart attacks are no longer your father's heart attacks. I'll take my chances with the baby aspirin, thank you.

The Devil Is in the Details

Will you? Can all these strutting cardiologists and heart surgeons be fooling themselves, and nearly all the rest of us? Myocardial infarction and heart attack, cerebral vascular accident and stroke, atherosclerosis and hardening of the arteries, and myriad related terms are darlings of the lay medical press. Pharmaceutical and hospital marketing budgets conspire to hang coronary artery disease like an imprecation over North America. Pills, diets, and all manner of "health-promoting" regimens are purveyed. Failing all else, there's a technological solution. We should rejoice at the marvels of modern cardiovascular surgery and interventional cardiology. The practitioners of these crafts are heroes who bypass concretions in our hardened coronary arteries or pummel them with angioplasties. These are technological poultices for our stricken hearts touted to ward off the grim reaper. They are saving us from the scourge of our time. We should all be poised to avail ourselves of these wonders. Interventional cardiology and cardiovascular surgery are lifesaving. They are priceless, we are told.

If I can't convince you otherwise, at least let me arm you with the data that demands you ask pointed questions whenever cardiovascular interventions are offered to you or your loved ones.

All diseases have their own histories. Bubonic plague changed the course of the Middle Ages in Europe and then disappeared — inexplicably, since all elements that supported the pandemic were unchanged: rats, squalor, lice, the bacillus, etc. Rheumatoid arthritis is a twentieth-century disease, peaking in incidence and severity in midcentury. Despite the fact that the pharmaceuticals in use at the time did little if anything to modify its course, rheumatoid arthritis has been on the wane ever since. Even tuberculosis was on the wane in the early twentieth century, long before streptomycin, the first effective antibiotic for its treatment, was discovered.

Heart attacks and strokes are twentieth-century diseases. Since peaking near midcentury, their incidence has been diminishing in all age groups. This trend started before "prevention" was purported to be effective and continues despite the minimal-to-marginal effectiveness of public-health agendas to modify "risk factors." Of course, the diminished incidence of strokes and even heart attacks is less striking in octogenarians, but that's an issue in proximate-cause epidemiology. Proximate-cause epidemiology is the exercise that attempts to deduce which of the mortal hazards operating at the time of death is most likely to be causal. In our culture, everybody has to die from something, some proximate cause. All octogenarians are going to die. There is no proximate-cause epidemiological survey (or death certificate) that countenances "it was her time." That's why the decrease in the incidence of strokes, for example, is much more striking in sixty-year-old people than in octogenarians.

There is no scientific reason for "Heart Attack and Stroke" to hang as an imprecation over the American people. Yes, we all will know people who died before their time from heart attacks and strokes. I certainly do not belittle the tragedy. But we know far, far fewer people who died before their time than did our parents. Aside from the socioeconomically disadvantaged and those few whose families are riddled with premature cardiovascular tragedies, death before our time by myocardial infarction or stroke, although it bedeviled earlier generations, need not much concern ours.

This does not seem to make sense. We are taught that some behaviors must be avoided since they predispose to coronary artery disease. We are taught that biochemical markers of risk must be identified and modified. And we are taught to be vigilant for symptoms suggestive of pending ischemic damage so that we can expeditiously avail ourselves of the wonders of modern invasive cardiology and cardiovascular surgery. Women are instructed that fatigue is alarming, as it may be a symptom of heart disease. I will address the "risk factors" and "health-adverse behaviors" sophistry in the next chapter. Here, invasive cardiology and cardiovascular surgery for coronary artery disease are my targets.

Angina for Sure

Let's assume that our next chest pain is angina. (I will dissect that assumption below.) Angina is a form of exercise-induced chest pain caused by inadequate blood flow to a portion of the heart muscle (myocardium). Myocardial blood flow (perfusion) normally increases to support the nutritional demands of exercising. Angina results when more is demanded than the blood supply to that portion can support, usually because flow through one or more coronary arteries is compromised in the setting of atherosclerosis. The underperfused portion of heart muscle is near death because of inadequate oxygenation. This ischemic myocardium spews out chemicals that communicate its plight to local nociceptive (pain) nerve endings. The pain typically precludes further exercise. Without the added demand, blood supply is adequate and the pain resolves, leaving behind a portion of the heart muscle at risk for further ischemia, and even death (myocardial infarction, or "heart attack").

What can be done? There are medical options that are not often touted in the lay press. Unfortunately, they are not touted in the American clinical setting either. Rather, if they are mentioned at all, it is often as a trial with the tacit, if not explicit, understanding that these medical options are merely temporizing. A real American would want to be fixed. A real American would want the abnormality in perfusion repaired. Isn't that the triumph of modern invasive cardiology? I venture to say that nearly every medical student, medical resident, and practicing physician would stand and applaud. I venture to say that this is the common sense. I will show you the science that demonstrates this belief system to be wrong.

Granted, there has been a technological triumph. Interventional cardiologists and cardiovascular surgeons are able to alter the blood supply of the heart with a remarkably low, though far from negligible, incidence of catastrophe. These practitioners find this low incidence acceptable. But let me again introduce the concept of Type II Medical Malpractice. Type I Medical Malpractice is familiar; medical or surgical performance is unacceptable. Type II Medical Malpractice is doing something to patients very well that was not needed in the first place. Type II Medical Malpractice is a scourge. Doing violence to the ischemic myocardium or its vasculature is a prime example. Furthermore, if any procedure doesn't work, there is no acceptable risk. Interventional cardiology and cardiovascular surgery for atherosclerosis-associated ischemic disease is dripping Type II Malpractice. I base this heresy on a compelling and robust science.

Atherosclerosis is a process that leads to the formation of plaques that cause focal narrowing of coronary arteries and arteries elsewhere. It has a complex pathogenesis that involves lipid deposition in the vessel lining, a proliferative response of some cells in the vessel wall, and finally calcification. We all are developing, if not harboring, the resultant atherosclerotic plaques. They are found in the coronary arteries of many young men and are ubiquitous in octogenarians. They tend to form near the origin of the main coronary vessels that supply the more muscular left ventricle. The narrowing can be impressive, even occlusive. Plaques are present in nearly everyone who has suffered a myocardial infarction. They are present in nearly everyone who has angina. But they are not present in everyone with myocardial infarction and angina. And they are present in many an adult who has never experienced either. In fact, they can occlude a coronary artery of a person who has never had either angina or myocardial infarction but who is fortunate to "grow" collaterals, compensatory blood vessels branching off of other coronary arteries. There is more to angina and myocardial infarction than just the presence of plaques. That much has been clear for decades. However, until recently the villain was said to be the plaque itself, which directly or indirectly blocks blood flow to the heart muscle, thereby causing angina if not a myocardial infarction. Today's revision of this theory is that the younger, smaller plaque is prone to developing abnormalities that allow for blood clots to form. The blood clots break off and do their evil downstream, blocking blood flow to the heart muscle and causing infarction.

The large, mature occluding plaques develop slowly enough to allow for collaterals to compensate. This revisionist theory is responsible for a new wave of experimental pharmacology. However, the occluding-plaque theory drives current practice.

There are ingenious ways to diminish the effects of the occluding plaque on blood flow, either by removing the plaque or circumventing it. The hope was that such maneuvers would do more than change blood flow in the patient's heart — they would advantage the patient. Early on, several of these theories were put to the test. By put to the test, I mean a randomized controlled trial of the intervention. In other words, patients with angina were randomized to receive either the intervention designed to address the plaque directly or an intervention not so designed. One of the earliest "good ideas" involved pericardial poudrage — the sprinkling of a powder around the heart. The wrapping of the heart, the pericardium, is a smooth-surfaced sack. It normally supplements the coronary arteries as a source of nutrition and oxygenation for the myocardium. This contribution is quite small but not trivial. Putting a powder into the pericardial sac causes highly vascular granulation tissue to form, which, theory held, would more effectively supplement the diminished contribution of the atherosclerotic coronary arteries. In a randomized controlled trial, all patients were anaesthetized and underwent a skin incision; only half had pericardial poudrage. Half of both groups woke to discover that their severe anginal condition was gone. The control patients had to have this sham surgery because there was no other way to test if the procedure was effective in alleviating the symptom of angina. It turned out that the particular surgery added no benefit to the surgical event. I will discuss the "placebo effect" and ethics of sham surgery in chapters 9 and 13.

Pericardial poudrage was relegated to the archives, but not the idea of circumventing the occluding plaques. In 1959 another randomized sham-controlled surgical trial for the treatment of angina was published. This time an artery near the heart but not supplying the heart was ligated (tied) in the hope of shunting more blood to the coronary circulation. Let me emphasize that again the control group underwent a sham procedure, a surgical procedure designed to be futile and not too dangerous but a surgical procedure nonetheless. A sugar pill might be an adequate control if the experiment is to test the effectiveness of another pill. And no surgery might be a reasonable control if the experiment is testing whether surgery alters the probability of a "hard," unequivocal, and unambiguous outcome such as death. However, there is no other way to test whether any elective surgical procedure is effective in palliating a symptom such as angina than to have a sham surgical control. A trial that compared surgery with nonsurgical treatment will not suffice. I find no ethical dilemma in subjecting patients to sham surgery for this purpose. To unleash any unproven elective procedures on a trusting public based on inductive reasoning and hubris is unethical, in my view. The result of the 1959 sham-controlled surgical trial also was disappointing, and surgery for coronary artery disease fell on hard times. Not for long; cardiac surgeons are resilient. Theory prevailed: something had to be done about circumventing plaques.

Cardiac surgery was making great strides in the repair of congenital and acquired diseases of the heart valves. The same technical competence was brought to bear on plaques in the form of bypass surgery, the fashioning of CABGs to physically circumvent occluding plaques. An industry was born, but not without its critics. In response to these critics, three large, randomized controlled multicenter trials of CABG surgery were undertaken in the late 1970s. Hundreds of patients with stable anginal syndromes were recruited and randomly divided into two groups. One group had CABG bypass surgery. However, sham surgery was not considered appropriate or ethical, so the other group received the optimal medical therapy of the day. Patients in one of these trials were followed for five years and those in the other two for over a decade. The results were reported in the mid-1980s. The primary outcome studied was death.

For 97 percent of the CABG patients in all three trials, there was no survival benefit from the surgery. There was a subset in all three trials with a particularly noxious distribution of plaques prominently involving the Left Main Coronary Artery (so-called Left Main Disease) that enjoyed a survival advantage consequent to CABG. On medical therapy, the five-year survival for patients with stable angina and Left Main Disease was 65 percent; it was 85 percent if they underwent CABG. So CABG can provide a survival advantage, save a life if you will, for a small subset at high risk of death. For nearly everyone else, 97 percent of patients with angina, *there is no discernible survival advantage*! And there are prices to pay for CABGs, many of which have come to light in the past decade. I am not referring to the transfer of wealth, although it's unconscionable for a largely bogus procedure. I am not even referring to the anguish of the cardiac catheterizations required before surgery, or the 2 to 8 percent perioperative mortality (depending on the experience of the surgical team and the frailty of the surgical victim), or the challenges of recovery and healing. I am referring to the fact that nearly 50 percent of CABG patients have to cope with significant emotional distress, mainly depression, in the first six months following surgery, and nearly as many acquire easily measured cognitive deficits persisting one year after surgery. For some, dementia is the only clinically important result of having their coronary artery anatomy successfully rearranged. Medical therapy has advanced significantly in the past fifteen years, so that the "control" group would do even better today. There is no data to suggest that CABG is more effective today than it was fifteen years ago.

If you still are not convinced that there is no reason for anyone with angina to submit to a CABG for survival's sake, maybe the U.S. Veterans Administration multicenter, randomized controlled trial of CABG for "crescendo angina" will carry the day. Crescendo angina is one of several labels that denote angina so severe it occurs even without exertion. Classically, it was thought to bode evil both in terms of impending myocardial infarction and death. The VA trial disabused us fifteen years ago; the two-month incidence of death was 2 percent and five-year less than 10 percent, and that was true whether or not the patient was subjected to a CABG.

CABGs should have been relegated to the archives twenty years ago. They have not been. In fact, over 500,000 are still done annually in the United States. This is an incidence that far outstrips all other countries, including the majority of resource-advantaged countries whose life expectancy exceeds that in the United States. The cardiovascular surgery community trumpets the demonstrated survival benefit, but it seldom mentions the fact that the vaunted benefit pertains only to the 3 percent of all comers with the special Left Main blockages. Oh, the cardiovascular surgery community speaks of benefit to patients who have multiple blockages in multiple vessels, but the basis for that claim is marginal. It derives from a reanalysis of the data from the trials I mentioned, a "secondary" or "subset" analysis that is an indefensible statistical maneuver. Even so, the effectiveness is minimal. And the surgical community has not overwhelmed us with forewarnings of the demonstrated downside; in addition to the adverse outcomes discussed above, an alarming number of people (depending on their level of activity prior to the CABG) never return to the workforce or describe themselves as well and enjoying life. Needless to say, the cardiovascular surgical community does not warm to such a condemnation. The retort, in public, is that the CABG technique has been refined since the old trials. However, the data I just mentioned regarding in-hospital mortality and cognitive deficits pertain to recent experience, not just to the early days. Still the cardiovascular surgical community is convinced it is doing better, technically better in terms of how the bypasses are created. The consensus among these surgeons is that the patients are doing so well there is no need to attempt to scientifically "show me" they wouldn't do even better without the surgery. The consensus is that the three classic trials are dated; experience and consensus bears out the theory that by-passing plaques with the latest techniques supersedes the science. A colleague of mine, a prominent, respected, senior cardiovascular surgeon renowned for technical prowess, put it to me this way: "Nortin, if you were to hold a diseased gray heart in your hand and watch it turn pink when you established full flow through a graft, you wouldn't question the benefit of CABG." My response was that he clearly felt triumphant, but did this luminous event translate into any meaningful outcome for the patient? Not likely.

As discussed in the supplementary readings for this chapter, outcomes must be defined before the study commences in order to minimize the risk of being fooled. In the three classic studies, the primary outcome is unequivocal; death is death. Nearly all studies since these three have used a combined outcome termed a "composite end point," usually death or myocardial infarction or "need" for CABG as defined by the judgment of the treating cardiologists and cardiovascular surgeons. In all these subsequent studies, whether studies of surgery or interventional cardiology, the interventions do not alter the likelihood of death. They may alter the likelihood of nonfatal myocardial infarction, but that is an inconsistent result. They often alter the decision that the patient should undergo CABG, or undergo CABG again. However, defining the surgical indications is always a subjective exercise that samples the prejudice of the investigator and the gullibility of the subject. Beware of "composite end point" studies; they demand scrutiny. This caveat will color our subsequent discussions.

The cardiovascular surgery community has two powerful allies: it is supported by an enormously profitable, codependent, interventional cardiology industry, and it is such a darling of the lay press that seems wedded to applauding technology for technology's sake. As a result, an untenable clinical hypothesis has become a social construction. It is commonly believed, by physicians and the laity alike, that if a patient has angina, any putatively offending plaques must be circumvented.

The need to find occluding plaques has been elevated to an unalienable right of Americans who are suffering, or might be suffering, angina. For three decades, American cardiology had no higher calling. Could so many cardiologists have been fooling themselves and, pari passu, their patients, whom they shepherd before cardiovascular surgeons? To be kind, cardiology took the lead in trying to spare its patients the rigors of cardiovascular surgery, but not by questioning its premise. Rather, gaining momentum since the 1990s, cardiology has touted another approach to increasing the perfusion of partially occluded coronary arteries, an approach that was in their purview as a modification of the cardiac catheterization procedure. Interventional cardiologists have perfected the skill of threading all kinds of tubes through our arteries or veins into all sorts of cardiac nooks and crannies. Furthermore, the biotechnology industry is leaping to create profitable widgets to put at the end of the catheters that do violence to putatively offending, occluding plaques. First, special catheters were invented with balloon tips so that the tip can be inserted into the narrows of the vessel and inflated, thereby literally breaking asunder the plaque (so-called angioplasty). Not surprisingly, many a vessel so pummeled would reocclude, usually starting with a blood clot. Also not surprisingly, the outcome for the patient was little different if the pummeled vessel remained patent or not.

However, the Holy Grail for these interventional cardiologists was to maintain the patency of vessels whose plaques they pummeled. Recently, they have come to leaving behind a stent designed to keep the vessel patent. And they have recruited all sorts of pharmaceutical inventiveness to that end, most designed to inhibit blood clots forming at the site of the stent. The number of angioplasties in the United States each year doubles the number of CABGs. That's right: angioplasty has not supplanted CABG, yet. Many an unsuspecting soul has been afforded both. After all, the explicit understanding between cardiologist and patient is that angioplasty and stenting are "less invasive" (they are not less expensive), but should the outcome be unfavorable, CABG is the fallback. And if the CABG "fails," another CABG is the fallback. The resulting transfer of wealth keeps escalating, with cardiologists and cardiovascular surgeons and their respective minions enjoying the fruits of their labors and providing fodder for an enormous supporting industry. I have too long heard terms such as "throughput" and "units of care" bandied about to describe the management of patients with coronary artery disease in the less-than-hallowed halls of American academic health centers, terms that have come to color all aspects of hospital care in America.

These are my interpretations of the systematic trials that found CABG to be no more effective than medical therapy in improving the likelihood that a patient will live to eighty-five. I believe that the morbidity of and mortality from CABGs suffered by the 97 percent who gain no survival advantage overwhelms the 20 percent improvement in survival that benefits the vaunted 3 percent with Left Main Disease. As for angioplasties, interventional cardiology is so convinced it is on the right track that there is no need for similar trials using "medical treatment" as the control. There is an occasional trial with medical controls, as discussed in the supplemental readings, that long left little reason to allow any-one to violate your coronary arteries. Quite recently, two trials were published that should assuage whatever doubt remains.

In the first, over 2,000 patients who had persistent occlusion of the vessel that caused their heart attack were all treated with optimal medical therapy and randomized so that half also received angioplasty and stenting with a drug-eluting stent. There was no reduction in death, or recurrent heart attacks, or heart failure for four years after stenting. After that, the patients who had stents were worse off.

The U.S. Department of Veterans Affairs Office of Research and Development had the resolve to perform a similar multicenter trial, the "COURAGE Trial," in their hospitals and in many outside the VA's system. They provided optimal med-ical care to over 2,000 patients with objective evidence of myocardial ischemia. Half were randomized to also have angioplasty, usually with stent placement. The angioplasty/stent therapy did not save a life; it didn't even spare anyone a heart attack over the next five years. Their conclusion was that angioplasty "did not reduce the risk of death, myocardial infarction, or other major cardiovascu-lar events" when added to medical therapy for "stable coronary artery disease." CABG and angioplasty and stenting should be consigned to the annals of good ideas that proved bad.

However, interventional cardiology and its fellow travelers have too much at stake to yield easily. The argument is offered that angioplasty and stenting must be done at a particular point in the disease history, and only with a particular kind of plaque. After all, there have been many, many trials comparing one form of angioplasty with another, and others probing whether the timing of angioplasty, close to a clinical event or not, matters. There are small differences, usually apparent in the "need" to go on to CABG or the incidence of myocardial infarction but never in patient survival. There also have been many, many trials testing whether a particular form of angioplasty offers an advantage over an-other form or over CABG. No doubt more will be forthcoming. No doubt there will continue to be papers that compare CABG with angioplasty and discern no important clinical difference, which is interpreted that angioplasty is as good as CABG and gentler. My interpretation is that angioplasty is as bad as CABG and at least as costly, but gentler.

Furthermore, the argument that there is a "golden hour" soon after the heart attack when angioplasty works would be laughable were it not so dangerous. This argument can render all of us worried whenever we have chest discomfort, worried enough to seek reassurance. The diabolical nature of the argument escalates when we hear that symptoms can be atypical, particularly in women who are forewarned regarding fatigue or menopausal symptoms. We are urged never to hesitate; take thee to the nearest emergency department posthaste — no leisurely taxi ride for you any more, it's EMS or nothing. Reassurance may prove Sisyphean; we are likely to hear a "maybe." Cardiology and radiology are hell-bent to develop noninvasive imaging techniques capable of seeing the plaques in all too many of us, including the many who are concerned enough to seek re-assurance for chest discomfort. The "golden hour" might serve a public-health agenda if the interventions could be shown to be helpful. As it is, the "golden hour" is naught but an unconscionable marketing scheme.

I submit that interventional cardiology and cardiovascular surgery have written one of the bleakest chapters in the history of Western medicine. If there was never another CABG or angioplasty performed or stent placed, patients with heart disease would be better off. Clearly, all this is missing the forest for the trees. There is something basically wrong with the theory that calls for violence to the offending, occluding plaque. To abandon the theory would shut down in-terventional cardiology, nearly all of cardiovascular surgery, and many surgical supply houses and biotechnology firms. It would dramatically downsize most hospitals in the United States and free up over $100 billion annually. And that's just the direct costs: the price of evaluations leading to cardiac catheterization and the process of surgery with all the costs of hospitalization, surgeons, anes-thetists, drugs, and intensive-care units. There are "indirect" costs that relate to income substitution and lost productivity. There's also the personal indirect cost of becoming a "cardiac patient" or even a "cardiac cripple." The former is the fate of all, the latter the fate of too many who are hidden from the popular view. We are regaled by the legends of public figures, politicians, and football coaches that rebound from CABGs or angioplasties as if nothing had transpired. They are the exception. As I will explain in chapter 12, if you had no job au-tonomy before sliding down this cardiovascular algorithm, you will likely end up on someone's disability role. Sadness will be your fate.

I would suggest that readers who live in "advanced" countries other than the United States thank their lucky stars, or their politicians, or their physicians. The national health-insurance schemes of other resource-advantaged coun-tries cost a quarter of what we spend on those who are insured, have a third of our "overhead" or less, and eschew much of the Type II Medical Malpractice that I decry in this chapter and many others. Survival statistics in all advanced countries exceed ours; their citizenry enjoys more years of high-quality life. Physicians in these other countries can be heard bemoaning the fact that they are less wealthy than the American interventionalists (though not less wealthy than so-called "cognitive" physicians). The bureaucrats in these other advanced countries can be heard bemoaning their relative lack of power, their lesser numbers, and the fact that their compensation pales in comparison to American hospital administrators, who view themselves as grandiose corporate leaders commanding more compensation than a U.S. president, senator, governor, or even most successful college football coaches.

Stop the tirade, you say. Maybe CABG and angioplasty don't save lives. Maybe their value is in improving symptoms, such as reducing angina. There is precious little scientific data addressing this issue. There is an enormous trial under way, still unpublished, comparing modern medical therapy with angioplasty. One wonders if such a trial can be carried out in the United States, where the medically treated "control" group is likely to feel slighted if not underserved. Trials of invasive procedures with symptoms as end points require sham controls. I favor such for many an unproved invasive procedure. However, the literature relating to CABGs, angioplasties, and stents is so extensive that one can infer the results of a sham-controlled trial. First, remember the sham surgery trials where half the subjects experienced symptomatic relief whether in the sham or the putatively effective groups? That is generally the result of thousands of placebo-controlled, randomized trials of pharmaceuticals for angina. For the agents that pass regulatory muster, the effectiveness was a bit more than the 50 percent response rate found in the placebo group. Does this mean that angina is "in your mind"? Some of the explanation relates to the natural history of angina; it is an intermittent and remittent symptom complex, meaning it can go away even though the plaques don't. Maybe that relates to collateral vessel formation. But maybe, just maybe, some of the explanation is "in your mind." Maybe participating in a trial where you might be afforded benefit helps you deal with the anticipation of the pain more effectively or allows you to circumvent precipitating angina by subtle alterations in behavior. Those are plausible forms of "in your mind." For me, "in your mind" is reasonable enough as an explanation for the time being.

However, in the clinical setting, rather than the clinical trial setting, the relevant "mind" is not just the patient's but the treating physician's as well. Medical therapy of a symptom such as angina is not simply the prescription of a pharmaceutical. It is a treatment act of far greater dimension. The attitude of the physician will color the attitude of the patient and prejudice the effectiveness of the treatment act. We have compelling data to that effect in rheumatology, in the treatment of painful joints. If the attitude the physician projects emphasizes concerns about toxicities or ineffectiveness, the patient is less likely to be on the prescribed agent for long. In cardiology circles, the prejudice is so strong toward invasive procedures that few patients can suffer angina without receiving some form of violent beneficence, or receiving it again. Both the patient's and the doctor's prejudice favors the invasive procedures, so that few patients can countenance the likelihood that all was in vain. For the patient, interventional cardiology and cardiovascular surgery for coronary artery disease become truth.

Stroke

While we're on this tack, note that the most cerebral of subspecialties, neurology, has countenanced interventionalist inroads. The parallels with interventional cardiology and cardiovascular surgery are obvious; in this case the invasive neuroradiologists are manning the catheters and the neurosurgeons are bypassing the plaques. The parallel with angina is called a "transient ischemic attack," or TIA. This is the development of highly disconcerting neurological deficits that totally reverse within twenty-four hours. How does one know they will disappear? If they don't, you have suffered a stroke (some refer to this as a "brain attack" to emphasize the parallels with heart attacks). People with TIAs all have plaques in the four major vessels that course through the neck to feed the brain. Unlike the heart, these main vessels join up as a circle before entering the brain, so that diminished flow in one can be compensated for by the flow in the others. Of the four vessels, the internal carotid arteries are amenable to plaque intervention — either removal or a delicate stenting procedure that, in very experienced hands, can be accomplished without too many catastrophes.

Debate raged as to whether the patient was better off for the effort. A large, randomized controlled trial offered the answer, though the public is generally offered just part of the answer. If you have TIAs *and* a very tightly occluded internal carotid artery feeding the side of the brain that is transiently ischemic, surgical removal of the plaque (carotid endarterectomy) will afford you a meaningful reduction in your risk of suffering a stroke on that side — meaningful enough to justify the surgical risks, which are substantial. *But . . .* that surgery will not improve your longevity: you are likely to die at the same time, often of a stroke on the other side or of cardiac disease. Maybe the quality of your life will be benefited if you are spared the stroke on the same side as the surgery, but that's no more than a maybe.

You will not be surprised to learn, given the open season on coronary arteries, that stenting of a tightly occluded carotid artery has been sanctioned by the FDA in patients who are too sick to undergo the more invasive surgical removal of the plaques, or endarterectomy. You will also not be surprised to learn that the stentorian doctors and the stent purveyors think they are on to something. They had a major setback when a large trial comparing stenting with carotid endarterectomy had to be stopped because there were fewer deaths and strokes with endarterectomy than with stenting. Trust me, there are several other trials under way using different stents and different techniques, all trying to match endarterectomy — which is damn near useless.

While we're on the TIA topic, there was another trial that excites the interventional neuroradiologists and is causing hospitals across the United States to staff "Stroke Units," likened to "Coronary Care Units." If one develops a focal neurological deficit (a stroke), and undergoes a cerebral angiogram (like a cardiac catheterization but of the brain's vessels) within three hours, and has a blockage from a blood clot, then infusing drugs directly into the occluded cerebral artery to dissolve the clot improves the likelihood of a more complete recovery. That assumes that you are not among the 6 percent in whom the infusion causes far more catastrophic bleeding into the brain than nearly all strokes. I'll take my chances with the natural history. Hopefully, the deficit will turn out to be a TIA, in which case taking aspirin will decrease the likelihood of recurrence of a TIA, and maybe the occurrence of a stroke. And if a stroke is my fate, it is more likely to be mild and to occur near my eighty-fifth birthday than was true of prior generations.

Angina

So, coronary artery disease is no longer a scourge. And interventional cardiology and cardiovascular surgery are no solution. However, angina is an awful experience. And, yes, you can die from a myocardial infarction with or without first suffering angina. Given the state of the science and the unconscionable state of American cardiology and cardiovascular surgery, what is a well person to do?

First, we must find a primary-care physician who feels compelled to keep our welfare at the center of the treatment act. It is easy to find physicians with that ethic. It is nearly impossible to find physicians who can serve the ethic well any more. All the perspective and wisdom one would hope for is squelched by a "health-care delivery system" that denigrates the spending of time with a patient. The U.S. "health-care delivery system" will pay our primary-care physician the same if we present with angina whether we are expeditiously referred on to a cardiologist or treated to/with a discourse designed to overcome our preconception that we need to have our heart fixed. The U.S. "health-care delivery system" does not support a lengthy discussion between a well person and a physician aimed at defining contingencies prior to the experiencing of angina or a myocardial infarction. If such a physician is identified, we should seek to discuss these contingencies when we are well. This is not an "annual physical examination," which is entirely useless, as we'll discuss in the next chapters. This treatment act is to discuss codicils to our living will that pertain to events that fall far short of a catastrophe. For one, we might explain that should we end up in an emergency room with chest pain from myocardial ischemia, with or without a completed infarction, we want nothing done to the heart unless it is supported by compelling scientific data as to meaningful beneficial outcomes. If this physician is not comfortable with the relevant literature, ask for a referral to some physician who is. This is the only way to know our own mind in this regard, to consider options when we are well and able to consider why someone's "best" advice is "best" for us. Today, for me, that means no angioplasties, stents, or CABGs. Since I have no interest in such, there is never a reason to "define my coronary anatomy" with a cardiac catheterization study.

Once we have an expanded living will, we can safely approach the medical establishment with a complaint of chest pain knowing our sage physician will stand between Type II Medical Malpractice and us. If the pain is awful, meet this sage physician in the emergency room. The standard management of an acute myocardial infarction in the United States is dripping as much Type II Medical Practice as the approach to angina. Most hospitals have algorithms, or cookbook roadmaps that are designed to find reasons to usher you into the cardiac catheterization suite en route to doing violence to your coronary arteries. No one will ask you if you know how beneficial all these bells and whistles are for you. You need someone else, someone who is not in pain and not fearful, to advocate for you. Or you need to consider your options long before you are in such a fearful, painful state.

So, let's take the case of less severe chest pain. We should not fear to approach our wise physician with such a complaint. Describe the pain. Explain that it is too severe, or atypical, or pervasive for us to cope with on our own. We are seeking insight free of the pressure to find a putatively offending occlusive plaque. If it's angina, we want the best of modern medical therapy. That includes pharmaceuticals with some small but important effect on the frequency and intensity of episodes. That includes pharmaceuticals that decrease the likelihood of suffering an infarction before you have the time to form collaterals, baby aspirin for one. That may include other agents that interfere with the pathogenesis of coronary artery disease, including agents that work on lipids if you like the long shot. We'll have more to say about that in the next chapter. How do we know if the chest pain is angina?

Classically, angina is a severe squeezing pain in the center of your chest precipitated by exercise, relieved by rest. It is described as so pervasive that few can do anything but stop all exertion. The pain has a tendency to radiate into the left arm, even as far as the base of the thumb. And if you place nitroglycerine under your tongue during an attack, you will promptly substitute a headache for the chest pain. If you have symptoms of this nature, it is nearly certain you have angina.

Variations in this story may still be angina. Cardiology and its industry are committed to developing a test that makes the diagnosis of angina when the symptoms are atypical. This effort is driven by the belief that the diagnosis of angina is critical since it leads to all the wonders I decry above. I, obviously, see no pressing need to "make" the diagnosis of angina. Furthermore, all the tests — from exercising while monitoring your electrocardiogram (EKG) to exercise tests that more directly monitor the perfusion of your heart muscle — are not up to making the diagnosis of angina, or excluding it either, with compelling validity. They are all bedeviled with false negatives and false positives. They are all expensive and all anxiety provoking.

So, what is one to do if the chest pain may be angina — or not? We must negotiate with our physician a clinically meaningful approach to the differential diagnosis of chest pain. There are entities that can be defined, some of which you want to know about because something can be done that advantages you in an important way. Some are tumors, some lung diseases, some are other vascular diseases, some afflict your esophagus or stomach, etc. As long as the diagnostic exercise is defined and delineated up front and holds a meaningful promise for a meaningful outcome, we should go along with it. Otherwise, why bother? Let's take our chances on natural history, get on with our lives, and trust our physician to do the worrying.

In the supplementary reading for this chapter, I expand on several of the insights that require an understanding of experimental design and data analysis. I also illustrate the fashion in which the latter can be abused.

chapter three

Risky Business
Cholesterol, Blood Sugar, and Blood Pressure

Cognitive dissonance is the confusion we experience when we attempt to meld two contradictory ideas. Americans who are concerned with their health are reeling from cognitive dissonance: obesity, high blood pressure, diabetes, and high blood cholesterol are epidemic threats to our lives, yet America is graying so rapidly that nothing can save the Social Security and Medicare funds from collapse.

This chapter and many that follow will teach you how to filter the pronouncements of authorities that relate to your health. With a few skills and rules, the exercise is far less tenuous than that which we undertake every day in every other arena. After all, most health pronouncements are offered as "science," and science is quantifiable. The challenge is not that the terminology is unfamiliar; the terminology the media has learned to spew is now parlance. The challenge is in knowing how to discern the "science" in the cacophony so that you can ask if the pronouncement is meaningful to you. I will teach this with some of the most familiar "scares of the week."

Getting Comfortable in Your Cholesterol

There is no question that blood "cholesterol" is a "risk factor." But it's not much of a risk factor. If you have no extraordinary family history, yet you have extraordinarily high low-density lipoprotein (LDL) cholesterol and low high-density lipoprotein (HDL) cholesterol, it will cost you a year or two of life expectancy. Nearly all who are labeled "high cholesterol" are far from the extreme and have minimal risk. Nearly all labeled "high cholesterol" are contending with a reduction in life expectancy of months. Do you think a reduction of months of life expectancy is meaningful, or even measurable?

There is no question that the "statin" family of drugs can lower cholesterol. There is no question that these drugs advantage members of families with a particular genetic disease that causes heart attacks (myocardial infarctions) when very young. There is no question that lowering cholesterol in patients who have already suffered a myocardial infarction will result in a very small though measurable decrease in the likelihood that they will suffer another myocardial infarction and a smaller, barely measurable increase in their survival. This is termed "secondary prevention," or preventing recurrent disease. However, there is a serious question as to whether statin treatment affords any meaningful advantage to all the rest of us who have not suffered a myocardial infarction. Can we recruit science to answer that most relevant question, or even assuage the doubt? Are statins useful for the primary prevention of heart disease?

Consider the following scientific protocol. A program was set up to screen the blood cholesterol of healthy men age forty-five to sixty-four. Of those with high cholesterol, 6,595 agreed to participate in a five-year, randomized placebo-controlled trial of pravastatin, the "statin" marketed under the brand name Pravachol by the Bristol-Myers Squibb Pharmaceutical Company, which funded the trial. That means that every morning for the five years, these men took a pill. For 3,302 men, that pill contained 40 mg of pravastatin, and for the remainder the morning pill contained a pharmacologically inert substance, a placebo. The main results are presented in Table 1. This pivotal study was published in the *New England Journal of Medicine* in 1995. It is called the West of Scotland Study because it was a multicenter study conducted by a consortium of investigators, the West of Scotland Coronary Prevention Study Group. It remains the most compelling study for all who argue that statins are important for the "primary prevention" of cardiac disease. The result elevated statins to the forefront in public-health policy considerations. It has driven statins to the forefront in recommendations by advisory panels of such organizations at the American Heart Association. Thanks to the fallout from this study, Americans know that cholesterol is bad and statins are good. Questioning the credo is heresy. There are parallels to the fashion in which the results of the trials of CABG surgery (see chapter 2) have gained such influence that the efficacy of CABG is an American "truth." Just as we debunked the CABG "truth," we must decide if science compels us, the well people, toward cholesterol screening and treatment if our cholesterol level is said to be "high."

Let's examine the table from the bottom up. Pravachol (in high dose) saved

TABLE 1. The West of Scotland Pravastatin Study

Outcomes over the Five Years	For 3,293 on Placebo: Number (percentage)	For 3,302 on Pravastatin: Number (percentage)
Nonfatal heart attacks	204 (6.5)	143 (4.6)
Deaths by heart attack	52 (1.7)	38 (1.2)
Deaths by cancer	49 (1.5)	44 (1.3)
Noncardiovascular death	62 (1.9)	56 (1.7)
Deaths by any cause	135 (4.1)	106 (3.2)

Source: Adapted from Shepherd et al. (1995).

no lives; the difference between the numbers who died from any cause is neither statistically nor clinically meaningful. There was also no difference in the
likelihood of death from noncardiovascular causes. That's important for two
reasons: deaths from stroke were not avoided, and violent deaths did not increase. The latter was a finding in several earlier studies of the effect of other
cholesterol-lowering drugs. Pravachol did not increase cancer deaths, either.
And . . . Pravachol did not protect one from suffering a definite fatal myocardial
infarction! The difference between the percent who suffered a fatal myocardial
infarction on placebo and on Pravachol is 1.7 percent–1.2 percent = 0.5 percent.
That difference is not statistically significant, nor is it clinically meaningful.
When the investigators shifted ten deaths out of the "Noncardiovascular death"
category into the "Deaths by heart attack" category because these ten might
have died from a heart attack, the difference is 1.9–1.3 = 0.6 percent. That difference is barely statistically significant; it would happen by chance 4.2 times in a
100, slightly less than the consensus cutoff for statistical significance of 5 times
in 100.[1]

 So the authors of the paper concluded that pravastatin saved lives. To my eye
they are massaging the data beyond the reasonable, a tendency that is all too
common and that has been derided as "data torturing." Even granting them
their secondary analysis, a difference of 0.6 percent is not clinically meaningful. There is simply too much "noise" in any clinical trial to ever be confident
of such a small difference. There are many sources of such "noise." Some represent flaws in design, execution, or analysis of the trial, sometimes reflecting
prejudice on the part of the investigators, or even malfeasance. We will exam-

 1. These cutoffs are arbitrary; it depends on how much you are willing to gamble that an
infrequent event is too infrequent to occur by chance alone. I muse that winning a state
lottery is such an event; there must be some unknown force.

ine examples of such in subsequent chapters. However, even the most elegant of trials can fall victim to "randomization errors." Bear with me through this explanation. It is a crucial concept and necessary if you are to be a match for all the seductive marketing schemes based on trials yielding small differences in outcomes.

The principle of a randomized controlled drug trial is that the comparison groups are comparable in every way except for the exposure to the drug being studied. Some of the comparability can be assured by design: gender, age, even socioeconomic status and the like can be matched as subjects are assigned to study groups. If an even distribution of measured attributes is not assured in the process of assignment to groups, any detected discordance can be compensated for in the design of the statistical analysis of the data. However, some crucial attributes cannot be measured. Some remain hidden because they are not yet defined (for example, genetic factors that determine collateral vessel growth and therefore the likelihood of healing a myocardial infarction). Some remain hidden because measurement is not feasible. For example, one might like to match the groups for coronary artery anatomy so that as many individuals with severe, but asymptomatic, atherosclerosis end up in the pravastatin as in the placebo groups. However, that would entail exposing over 6,000 well men to the hazards of a cardiac catheterization. (Yes, there are hazards to cardiac catheterization — important complications in a few percent and the death of a few men — that are hard to justify for the sake of randomization.) So one assumes/hopes the random assignment of the men to Pravachol or placebo will equalize these unmeasured confounders. But what if it doesn't? What if instead of 50 – 50, those with severe subclinical atherosclerosis distribute 49 – 51, or 48 – 52? That's not too improbable a skew. And maybe the distribution of those with pristine coronary arteries was similarly skewed, but in the opposite direction. Such randomization error can well account for the 0.6 percent difference in outcome and, since it is not measured, remain hidden. For that reason, I discount as unbelievable any statistically significant result that represents a tiny outcome. My cutoff for credibility is at least a 2 percent difference in a clinically meaningful outcome. There are others who are even more stringent. This issue in uncertainty does not seem to trouble many who design and analyze drug trials, and certainly not many who trumpet the results. That is your first health-related caveat emptor.

Is 2 percent a solution? Is it clinically meaningful? Is it meaningful to you? Two percent reduction in nonfatal heart attacks over five years is what we're being offered in the top line of the table as the highly statistically significant finding, likely to occur by chance less than one time in 1,000. If a well man with high cholesterol takes 40 mg of Pravachol every day, his risk of a nonfatal myocardial infarction over the course of five years is reduced nearly 2 percent: 6.5 percent – 4.6 percent = 1.9 percent. Again, I ask, is this important to you? Consider the following before you answer.

In the paper and in subsequent marketing, the purveyors of Pravachol and their fellow travelers seldom describe the result as a 1.9 percent reduction in likelihood of suffering a nonfatal heart attack in five years, which is the reduction in *absolute* risk. They are wont to talk about reduction as *relative*-risk reduction, which is the percentage that the risk on placebo would be reduced if one were to swallow Pravachol — 1.9/6.5 = .29, or 29 percent; that is, you're 29 percent less likely to suffer a nonfatal heart attack if you take Pravachol. That's true, too, and it certainly seems impressive. But the absolute reduction in likelihood is what is meaningful to you — and that's 2 percent. NEVER LET ANYONE TALK OF RELATIVE-RISK REDUCTION WITHOUT DEMANDING A STATEMENT OF ABSOLUTE-RISK REDUCTION. Is this 2 percent reduction in absolute risk of not suffering a fatal heart attack in five years worth your taking Pravachol every morning?

In the previous chapter, I point out that my likelihood of surviving for five years after my first heart attack was about 95 percent. If I take a daily baby aspirin, the likelihood rises to about 97.5 percent. That's a 2.5 percent absolute-risk reduction. (It's half of my total risk of 5 percent, so it's a 50 percent relative-risk reduction.) There have been many studies of the hazards of long-term low-dose aspirin therapy. There may be a very small increase in the likelihood of intestinal bleeding, but that hazard is overwhelmed by the 2.5 percent reduction in the absolute risk of death before my time once I've suffered my first heart attack. If you have a heart attack, it makes sense to take a baby aspirin daily for the rest of your life. But should you, as a well person who has never had a heart attack or a gastrointestinal bleeding episode, decide to take a baby aspirin every day as a precaution against having your first attack? The absolute-risk reduction for the primary prevention of a heart attack, if there's any risk reduction at all, is miniscule. The absolute risk of intestinal bleeding from taking a baby aspirin every day is also miniscule. It's your call.

What about statins? How do you come to a similar personal benefit/risk assessment for a statin? Does the 1.9 percent reduction in risk of nonfatal heart attack advantage a well person with high blood cholesterol enough to justify taking Pravachol forever? Many elements enter into such a personal benefit/risk assessment. Cost may be an issue for you. It certainly is for the "health-care delivery system." The costs of a screening program and the treatment of 7 percent or more (the lower limit of "normal" is forever sinking by consensus of various "experts") of males between the ages of forty-five and sixty-four are substantial. The pharmacoeconomists leap to that challenge. They typically focus on the 0.6 percent absolute reduction in the risk for death from definite/possible heart attacks, or the 0.6 percent I dismissed as unreliable. If you accept the 0.6 percent as valid, you can calculate the number of people you need to treat (the "Number Needed to Treat" has been given the acronym NNT) for five years to save one life. The result of such NNT calculations based on the West of Scotland Study is generally in the 200 range.[2] You can also calculate the number of lives you will save in five years for the cost of having all the well men swallow Pravachol. Generally, if the calculation comes out less than $50,000 (U.S.) per year of life saved, the drug is deemed worthy and the purveyor gains an edge with the FDA, with managed care and other insurers, Medicare and Medicaid, prescribing physicians and you. A cost per life-year gained for primary prevention with pravastatin in the United Kingdom was calculated to be $34,640 in 1997. If, as I suspect, Pravachol saves no lives, then we are all paying a great deal of money for nothing.

If cost is not your issue — probably because you don't have to think about paying out of pocket — are there other personal risks to taking Pravachol that might mollify the 1.9 percent reduction in the risk of a nonfatal heart attack? You may get a rash, or a headache, or some nausea, but if you do, you can stop the therapy. But statins can cause a severe, even deadly destruction of muscles. That's rare, but the benefits are too slight to tolerate much risk of catastrophe. One statin, Baycol, was pulled from the market because of fifty or more cases of fatal muscle damage. Fewer such catastrophes have been reported for the other statins, but there are catastrophes reported with exposure to each along with a number of cases with milder and reversible muscle toxicity.[3] There's the rub. I can't tell you the long-term risk of statins; they are a unique class of agents, and our long-term experience is limited. We can gain a modicum of re-

2. Of course, this depends on which outcome you choose to treat for. If you assume you can effectively treat to prevent both fatal and nonfatal heart attacks, the NNT per year with Pravachol has been calculated at 217. This is similar to the calculation for another study treating well people with a different statin. The calculations for treating ill people with established coronary heart disease vary between 63 and 167.

3. Post-marketing monitoring for drug toxicity (i.e., after regulatory approval) is neither systematic nor comprehensive in the short or long term. Systematic post-marketing surveillance is called Phase IV drug trials. They are not required. In fact, systematic Phase IV data is seldom pursued unless driven by a product-liability lawsuit. The FDA relies on Phase III

assurance from the West of Scotland cohort. Over the course of a decade after the study ended, nothing unusual emerged from an analysis of administrative data (mainly hospital records). For all I know, subtle muscle disease, or liver disease, or cognitive impairment is the fate of some. For all I know, the recent suggestion that statins increase the incidence of osteoarthritis of the hip will prove prescient. For all I know, a few will come to regret that the "standard of care" practiced by their physician and the direct-to-consumer marketing on television, by a former football coach, was allowed to color the sense that they were well.

Ten percent of all drugs approved for marketing by the FDA between 1975 and 1999 were subsequently either withdrawn from the market because of adverse reactions or labeled with a "black box" indicating special hazards. There is much to be said for avoiding the use of any new drug unless there is compelling data that it offers an important benefit that does not derive from older agents. I do not allow "samples" in my clinic and do not allow pharmaceutical "detail" people to try to convince me that the agent they market is indispensable. I do not want to be swayed by the convenience of samples nor delegate benefit/risk assessments. I assume responsibility for assessing the available clinical trials as to efficacy of the touted drug. And I wait several years to prescribe any "me too" agent or novel agent with equivocal benefit. I want the empirical, practice-based, inefficient, post-marketing surveillance system to offer up some reassurance that prescribing any putatively more-effective or as-effective (but more convenient) agent has no dire consequences.

Even if my uneasiness about long-term toxicity of statins turns out to be unfounded, there remains the risk of "negative labeling." We have known for twenty years that many people feel stigmatized by the knowledge that they have "high" cholesterol. Once labeled, they feel vulnerable. Their coping skills are challenged. They can rapidly disappear from the ranks of the well forever. The same consequence of labeling has been shown for the "hypertension," "sickle trait," and several other diagnoses.

Other statins have been tested for effectiveness in primary prevention, in-

---

randomized controlled trials. These often recruit thousands of subjects, seek the statistical power to detect the small difference in effectiveness I decry, and last a year or a few years. Post-marketing, the agent can be prescribed to tens of thousands for many years. As with Baychol, it only takes the appearance of fifty tragedies from unique complications to spot the toxicity and assign its cause. An important increase in the incidence of a disease with a significant background incidence — dementia, for example — would be missed if we rely solely on a haphazard reporting mechanism.

cluding a trial of lovostatin in well U.S. Air Force personnel with normal blood cholesterol. However, no study offers more compelling support for a "public health" agenda to pharmacologically lower the blood cholesterol of well people than the West of Scotland Study. Most other studies are negative; a few suggest harm. The Air Force prophylactic statin study has results consonant with, but no more compelling than, the West of Scotland Study in demonstrating the slight efficacy of lovostatin. To further muddy the waters, the West of Scotland result did not reproduce in a randomized controlled trial in the United States called the Antihypertensive and Lipid-lowering Treatment to Prevent Heart Attack Trial — Lipid-Lowering Treatment (ALLHAT-LLT). Over 10,000 men and women, age fifty-five or older, were randomized to receive pravastatin or "usual care" in a trial conducted in some 500 different clinics around the country. Pravastatin did not reduce either all-cause mortality (absolute-risk reduction = 0.4 percent) or coronary heart disease events (absolute-risk reduction = 1.1 percent) compared to "usual care."

The statins were developed because spectacular Nobel Prize – winning basic science (by Konrad Block, Michael Brown, Joe Goldstein, and others) pointed the way. The development of the statins is a triumph of applied biochemistry. However, the "translational" science, which seeks clinical effectiveness, is nearly as disappointing as the basic science is illuminating. Statins have a crucial role to play in the treatment of some rare genetic disorders of cholesterol metabolism and a defensible role in secondary prevention, preventing a second heart attack. As for primary prevention, with its potentially huge market of well people, statins should be viewed as a false start and an object lesson. But there are billions of dollars of profit at stake for most of the major pharmaceutical firms. Marketing dollars flow into the coffers of advertising firms, of professional organizations, of "thought leaders" among cardiologists, endocrinologists, and prescribing physicians, and of political war chests and political action committees. Several voices have decried this marketing campaign. In September 2005 a class-action lawsuit was brought against Pfizer, alleging that the company engaged in a massive campaign to convince doctors and patients that its statin, Lipitor, is beneficial treatment for nearly everyone with high cholesterol — despite the lack of evidence in major segments of the population and the puny evidence discussed above in middle-aged men. Several organizations have tried to dampen the enthusiasm. For example, the American College of Physicians weighed in on the debate on cholesterol screening and treatment in 1996 with conservative guidelines. Today in the United States, cholesterol screening is considered good medicine. Today, one is more likely to hear of cardiologists bemoaning the fact that it is difficult to get patients to take their prescribed statins consistently over long periods. Even the Centers for Disease Control and Prevention (CDC) is bemoaning the fact that Massachusetts was the only state to reach the 80 percent screening goal by 2003.

I don't applaud all the chest beating. Rather, the fact that cardiologists like statins more than their patients is one of my illustrations of how noncompliance can be "homeostatic." Homeostasis is a term coined by Walter Bradford Cannon, a professor of physiology at Harvard Medical School, to capture one of the great insights of biology developed in his 1932 treatise, *The Wisdom of the Body*. Cannon's theory was that biological systems are invested in mechanisms to maintain stability when disturbed. The theory proposes a kind of force/counterforce leading to stability. Cannon was prepared to generalize the concept of homeostasis to social structures. The term has evolved to include elements of equilibrium, balance, even harmony. So, by suggesting that "noncompliance can be homeostatic," I am acknowledging those circumstances where the advice is unfounded or the prescription unhelpful.

Now you know why I won't let any well-meaning colleague check my blood cholesterol or any other lipid level. Now you know why I want to endow those of you who are still well with the sophistication to be the keepers of your own wellness. It's a minefield out there.

The Metabolic Syndrome

The hypothesis that cholesterol and various lipids are atherogenic — predisposing to plaques in our arteries and thereby to heart attacks and stroke — has been around for over fifty years. Lipid metabolism has challenged generations of investigators. This challenge won't go away, nor should it; lipid metabolism harbors secrets relevant to coronary artery disease and to atherosclerosis elsewhere. That even holds for cholesterol metabolism. After all, if you already have had one heart attack, lowering blood cholesterol is of slight but measurable effectiveness in preventing another. That is to say that if you are in the subset of patients already ill from atherosclerotic coronary artery disease, the benefit/risk ratio of pharmacologically manipulating your cholesterol metabolism can be argued to justify the intervention. If you are not in that subset, if you are not even a patient and thus still well in spite of whatever atherosclerosis you harbor, the effects of manipulating your cholesterol metabolism are too puny to discern reliably and therefore not clearly worth your while. There are lipids and lipoproteins, many involved in cholesterol metabolism, that are also playing a part in the pathogenesis of atherosclerosis and are small, though independent, markers of the likelihood that you will suffer a heart attack (i.e., risk factors). However, the data that we currently have about pharmaceutical agents that manipulate these to our benefit is even less impressive than that which we have just dissected for cholesterol.

There are several reasons all this "translational" effort seems to be going nowhere quickly. First, as discussed in chapter 1, in an advanced, industrialized country, at least 75 percent of the hazard to longevity can be captured with measures of socioeconomic status and job satisfaction. These are life-course sociopolitical realities that operate whether or not you behave in a manner adverse to your health and whether or not you have biological risk factors for earlier death. Health-adverse behaviors and the known biological risk factors are vying to take their toll on the other 25 percent of your likelihood of living to a ripe old age, and they do so in an interactive fashion. It is challenging to isolate these elements of proximate-cause epidemiology, one from the other. It has proven daunting to manipulate them in isolation to your benefit. Perhaps that's because the elements of proximate-cause epidemiology are not so independent.

The possibility that the biological factors were integrative was recognized some years ago. It was postulated that a particular clinical presentation was so likely to eventuate in cardiovascular disaster that it deserved denoting as a syndrome; "Syndrome X" was coined over a decade ago. Today, Syndrome X is generally called the "Metabolic Syndrome." The hallmarks are the abnormal accumulation of body fat resulting in central obesity, decreased insulin sensitivity leading to adult-onset diabetes, and abnormalities in blood lipids associated with high blood cholesterol. The full-blown extremes of the Metabolic Syndrome is the kiss of death in terms of the 25 percent of the hazard to your longevity that can be ascribed to biological proximate causes; it is atherogenic and diabetogenic, thereby predisposing to hypertension, heart attacks, renal failure, strokes, and other portals for leaving this life. The Metabolic Syndrome is often helped along by tobacco abuse and is far more likely to afflict people who are already marked by chronic stress at work or their lower socioeconomic status in advanced societies.

In 2001 an "expert panel," convened by the National Institutes of Health (NIH), took a stab at criteria for the Metabolic Syndrome. To qualify, they said, one must have three or more of the following:

1. A waist circumference > 102 cm (40 inches) in men and > 88 cm (35 inches) in women.
2. Hypertriglyceridemia defined as > 150 mg/dl.
3. Low HDL cholesterol defined as < 40 mg/dl in men and < 50 mg/dl in women.
4. High blood pressure defined as > 130/85 mg/dl.
5. High fasting glucose defined as > 110 mg/dl.

If you use these criteria, the age-adjusted prevalence of the Metabolic Syndrome in the United States is 23.7 percent. For those age sixty to sixty-nine, the prevalence is 43.5 percent! Furthermore, the prevalence is comparable in white men, white women, and African American women but lower in African American men. That's very peculiar epidemiology. Nearly all other studies probing associations of race/ethnicity with risk to longevity favor the white population over the African American (although these putative associations with race/ethnicity are really associations with SES and probably have little to do with race/ethnicity itself[4] — with the possible exception of birth weight). Not only are the associations with ethnicity peculiar, the prevalence also is striking. Do you really think that 43 percent of Americans age sixty to sixty-nine should be medicalized as having the Metabolic Syndrome? Could it be that this definition is nonsense? After all, it is certain that more Americans are living longer despite their putative Metabolic Syndrome. Maybe robustness in body configuration and in metabolism is responsible for improving longevity, and not a curse. In fact, the less robust among the elderly live less long. There is a recent analysis of the risks to hearts and lives from the Metabolic Syndrome in Finnish men that suggests that the term should be reserved for individuals at the top quartile of the population the NIH "expert panel" defined as having the syndrome, since little risk was established for the remainder.

Full-blown, the Metabolic Syndrome is easy to spot, and its victims are not well people — not for long. It's spotting the incomplete syndrome and the early

4. After a century of presumption and assumption, modern science is finally deconstructing the construct of "race." There are genetic differences between populations with differing ancestral continents of origin. However, the genomic similarities are far more striking than the differences. Furthermore, in an outbred population such as the citizenry of the United States, the genomic differences are further blurred. Ethnic and racial labeling is on the shakiest of genetic grounds. The labels should be used with caution so as not to reinforce untenable stereotypes or to mask the sociocultural variables that are far more influential in terms of longevity and other health outcomes (Kaplan and Bennett 2003; R. S. Cooper et al. 2003) Geographic ancestry and explicit genetic information will supersede notions of race with further progress in human genetics (Bamshad 2005).

stages in the well population that is our next contentious topic. If you exhibit a little bit of the elements of the Metabolic Syndrome, should you be marked, marketed to, and segregated as a ticking time bomb? Do the data on Finnish men generalize to other populations and to women? Even the spokespersons for the American Diabetes Association and European Association for the Study of Diabetes are arguing that the construct, the "Metabolic Syndrome," is premature, not prescient. It leads to the notion that there might be a common pathophysiology to these cardiovascular risk factors; insulin resistance has long been a contender in this regard, and some are touting an inflammatory disorder affecting blood vessels. The debate about the existence of the Metabolic Syndrome is getting heated. It is fueled by vested interests, not all of which are pure and intellectual. Those who want us to treat each element with drugs argue that the Metabolic Syndrome is a statistical artifact and not a real entity. This argument is voiced most notably by those who bear the American Diabetes Association's imprimatur. Those who favor the existence of the syndrome advocate "lifestyle" modifications, including diet, as essential. Of course, when diet fails there's always a statin to fall back on. These proponents tend to unfurl the banner of the American Heart Association. Since no common denominator has been established, we will examine the epidemiology of three principal attributes in the criteria: obesity, diabetes, and hypertension.

Body mass index (designated by the acronym BMI and also called the Quatelet index) describes the heft of a person, taking into account both weight and height. The calculation is simple: it's your weight in kilograms divided by the square of your height in meters. So if you weigh 200 pounds and you're 6 feet tall, your BMI = 27.1. BMI is a risk factor for dying before your time. But, like all the risk factors that are elements of the Metabolic Syndrome, the relationship between BMI and longevity is not linear — it's U-shaped. Some of the plots of proximate-cause versus mortal hazard are more J-shaped than U-shaped, but none is linear. Here's a prototype curve for people in the community, plotting increasing likelihood of death before your time against increasing BMI.

U

BMI →

That means that at a very high BMI and at a very low BMI, your likelihood of dying too soon increases dramatically. If your BMI much exceeds 30, you have the disease "morbid obesity" and you are no longer a well person. If your BMI is very low, you either have anorexia nervosa or some yet-to-be-diagnosed inflammatory, neoplastic, or infectious disease. Regardless, you're in trouble. Between very high and very low, increasing BMI is a very gentle risk factor. It is somewhat less gentle if you carry discordant weight in your belly. Divide the circumference of your waist by the circumference at your hips. The greater your gut-butt ratio is over 1.0 for a man and 0.9 for a woman, the greater your risk of dying before your time. But you are still on the gentle upward slope of the base of the U-shaped curve until you are approaching a BMI of 30. If SES is taken into account, the slope is gentle indeed.

The image of the U-shaped curve and the shallowness of its upward slopes engender cognitive dissonance. Daily we are bombarded with warnings about the dire consequences of chunkiness. Losing weight is a public-health imperative. Aren't love handles stigmata and a jelly belly a harbinger of doom? Imagine the consternation in public-health circles, let alone all the stakeholders in the weight-reduction industry, when two papers appeared in 2005, both from divisions of the CDC, that supported the notion of the flat-based, U-shaped curve. Cardiovascular risk factors have declined considerably over the past forty years in all BMI groups, to the extent that being overweight (BMI between 25 and 30) was no longer a risk for death before your time. The backlash to this epidemiology was swift and loud, so that the director of the CDC urged the public to ignore the finding. However, the readers of this book know better. We also know better than to accept all the portending (and the prescribing that will follow) about the U.S. epidemic of "obesity."

Perhaps the small risk, and therefore the limited potential yield, explains the disappointing results of all those trials of weight loss rather than the usual explanation — recidivism. Most trials of weight loss are plagued by noncompliance. In fact, there is a hint that recurrent recidivism, so-called "yo-yo" weight loss or weight cycling, is more likely to cost you time on the earth than if you left well enough alone. This brings me to the hype that obesity is a new American epidemic, a plague upon our houses. True, the average weight of Americans is increasing. True, also, the average life expectancy is increasing. That should engender cognitive dissonance for all those in public health policy who want the masses to get themselves to the valley of the U-shaped curve even if that means finding the purveyors of various diets and putative weight-reducing drugs seductive. "Normal body weight" is a social construction. As long as we stay away from the sides of the U-shaped curve, we are not faced with escalating mortal hazard. To argue otherwise is to pervert science; defining obesity short of the steep slope is a social construction that creates a vast marketplace for unnecessary and unproven remedies. Furthermore, I wonder if we won't learn that the entire U-shaped curve is slowly shifting to the right, so that "morbid obesity" in my generation will be less weighty than that in the generations to come. There is precedent with almost all such measures — as long as societies don't stratify, don't increase their income gap, and don't force more into the ranks of the disavowed.

Blood sugar also has a U-shaped curve, though an asymmetric one. Very few well people suffer very low blood sugar (hypoglycemia). Nearly all who feel weak or feel faint at times need to be disabused if someone told them they have "low blood sugar." They almost certainly do not, and there is no yield in medicalizing them in this fashion. If we exclude people on insulin therapy, or people who have had gastric surgery, hypoglycemia is very, very rare. It is a presenting feature of a pancreatic tumor that secretes insulin. It can occur four to five hours after a meal, but that is an extraordinarily rare event usually presaging full-blown diabetes. An enormous amount of our endocrine system is committed to making sure we don't suffer hypoglycemia, even if we nearly starve to death. So the U-shaped curve rises sharply at the low end, but the risk for death before your time rises very gradually toward the high end of the distribution. Furthermore, aging broadens the curve, so that the valley sets at a higher blood sugar; that is, "normal" blood sugar is age dependent.

So, who has diabetes?

If you don't make insulin, you are not a well person. You have type 1 diabetes, and without insulin therapy, you will soon die. Type I diabetes usually starts in childhood or young adulthood. Your blood sugar (glucose) will escalate, but the glucose will not be able to enter the cells of most of your organs without insulin. Those cells will go to extremes in the attempt to utilize alternative energy sources, and you will be worse off as a result. If you are to survive with type 1 diabetes, you must inject yourself with insulin from the onset of your illness. The more meticulously you administer insulin therapy, attempting to keep your blood sugar normal all the time, the more risk you run of hypoglycemia, which can damage the brain and even kill. But the trade-off makes sense if the vascular complications of type 1 diabetes are postponed.

The landmark study suggesting this benefit used "surrogate" measures of outcome, measures that may not be directly important to you but which are sensitive to change, readily detectable, and likely to presage events that are important. Meticulous control of the blood sugar of patients with type 1 diabetes will delay the development of changes in the eyes, delay the tendency of the kidneys to leak more trace amounts of protein into the urine than normal, and protect the peripheral nerves from damage (neuropathy). These are changes that reflect damage to small vessels, called microcirculatory disease. These are the data suggesting that bathing tissues in fluids high in glucose causes microcirculatory damage. The data that meticulous control of blood glucose postpones damage to large vessels is suggestive, but only became so after the patients in the trial were followed for seventeen years. It is the larger vessel (macrovascular) atherosclerotic disease that associates with heart attacks, strokes, and peripheral vascular disease that often ravage patients with type 1 diabetes decades before others in their birth cohort. Certainly the surrogate microcirculatory measures have much more face value than if we were told only that meticulous insulin dosing can normalize the blood sugar. The seventeen-year follow-up validates them.

There has been a debate since the discovery of insulin as to whether tight control in type 1 diabetes was worth the fiddle and the risk of hypoglycemia. With the surrogate measures in hand and the follow-up data as to postponing coronary artery disease, that debate is largely stilled. I am offering up this précis on type 1 diabetes because it colors all thinking about high blood sugar (hyperglycemia) in people who do make insulin, people labeled as having type 2 diabetes (also called adult onset diabetes mellitus [AODM] or non–insulin dependent diabetes mellitus [NIDDM]). In fact, such people make more insulin than normal, but the insulin appears less effective; this is known as insulin resistance. People with type 2 diabetes are usually identified in midlife or later and are at increased risk for the same vascular complications as the type 1 patients, but the risk plays out much later in life. These people can be found on the upward slope of the asymmetric U-shaped curve for blood sugar. Where is the cutoff to abnormal, to type 2 diabetes? Shouldn't the cutoff be adjusted for age? After all, the older you are, the more likely your blood sugar is elevated, but the less likely hyperglycemia will have time to wreak havoc or deprive you of your longevity. Furthermore, those in the upper range of normal are more likely to be farther up the slope as they age. Should we label the upper limits of normal "pre-abnormal," or should we shift the definition of normal further and further toward lower blood glucose levels? Do we know that if we declare a cutoff and treat the hyperglycemia so defined, we will advantage these people? Very few hyperglycemic well people know they are hyperglycemic. Some urinate more frequently, but that's a fact of life for many aging men and women, hyperglycemic or not. The issue is, can we protect the hyperglycemic well people from severe vascular disease or death before their time?

Several august panels, speaking for equally august professional bodies, are convinced that we can, and therefore we should be more liberal with the cutoff. The result is that the cutoff is progressively lowered by consensus. It follows that the prevalence of type 2 diabetes is escalating. If we keep lowering the cutoff, pretty soon all of us will age into type 2 diabetes, and even more will be labeled as having the Metabolic Syndrome. The public-health world is alarming us about yet another epidemic that the public-health world itself is creating by virtue of changing the rules for labeling. Screening programs are now advised. And, in parallel with the reasoning for treating type 1 diabetes, meticulous management of blood sugar is called for, in this case resorting to pills designed to increase the efficiency of the patients' endogenous insulin responsiveness before resorting to insulin therapy.

These pills, so-called oral hypoglycemic agents, were first introduced some fifty years ago. This is another of the hot spots of pharmaceutical development: second-, third-, and fourth-generation oral hypoglycemic agents are marketed along with novel agents, and there is much more "in the pipeline." This is another enormous marketplace, ranking with the statins we discussed above, and the antihypertensive agents we're about to examine. With the oral hypoglycemics, too, the advisors to the august bodies and the members of the panels often have financial ties to the marketplace, one way or another. Nonetheless, they are convinced they are doing right to pharmacologically stem the tide of type 2 diabetes, and they have convinced most payers, most providers, the lay press, and most patients, who are told their blood sugar is too high.

I have doubts.

My reflexive cynicism was planted some thirty-five years ago by the first major randomized controlled trial of an oral hypoglycemic, obviously a first-generation agent. That agent was compared to diet therapy and insulin therapy in a multicenter trial. The subjects taking the first-generation oral hypoglycemic agent were likely to die *sooner* than the other two groups. These were the early days of multicenter randomized controlled trials. This famous trial has been used ever since to teach about errors in design and data analysis. It had serious flaws and may have led to an incorrect conclusion or . . . maybe not. Besides, very few trials of oral hypoglycemic agents since have been powered to consider such dramatic, definitive outcomes as death. Most are looking at surrogate outcomes to generate the data upon which the FDA bases the decision to license the product for sale as a prescription pharmaceutical. There were nagging doubts even in the diabetes research and treatment community until 1998, when those doubts were largely laid to rest.

I still have doubts.

In 1998 the results of the UK Prospective Diabetes Study (UKPDS) were published in *Lancet*. The stated intent of the study was to determine whether improved blood glucose control did more than manage surrogate measures. Did it advantage, or disadvantage, the patient with type 2 diabetes in terms of macrovascular disease and its ravages, including heart attacks and death? This study bears scrutiny. The fact that the investigators, the United Kingdom Diabetes Study Group, had the temerity to undertake such a study is remarkable in and of itself. The investigators couldn't recruit subjects with long-standing hyperglycemia who are at greatest risk of vascular catastrophe and expect a fair test of the hypothesis that treatment was beneficial; if there were no benefit, it would be argued that they had closed the door when the cows were already out of the barn. To stand even a remote chance of an interpretable result requires enrolling and following a very large, relatively young population for a very long time. Otherwise there is too little likelihood of untoward outcomes in the control group to expect to be able to discern an effect in the experimental groups. This multicenter, practice-based study started enrolling the almost 4,000 newly diagnosed patients with type 2 diabetes in the 1970s. To qualify for enrollment, patients had to be forty-eight to sixty years old, with fasting blood glucose levels of 110–270 after three months of dieting. The patients were nearly all white, a third were male, and they had an average BMI of 28. About a third smoked, and 20 percent were sedentary. On average they had normal blood pressures, though a third were considered hypertensive and enrolled in an embedded second study of controlling both blood sugar and blood pressure. We know nothing of their SES, a critical confounder (see chapter 1). They were randomized so that a third received "conventional" therapy and the remainder "intensive" therapy. The "conventional" group attended clinics every three months to receive advice and encouragement from a dietician. The intensive group was further randomized to receive insulin therapy, a first-generation hypoglycemic agent, or a second-generation hypoglycemic agent. Patients were followed an average of ten years. The study closed in September 1997.

These were not naïve investigators. To the contrary, they were prepared to apply all that biostatistics could offer to challenges such as crossover, dropout, missing data, noncompliance, and treatment failure. Some of the findings are strikingly disconcerting: it is clear that the intensive therapies caused weight gain. It is clear that the intensive hypoglycemic therapies reduced blood glucose, sometimes too much, so that there was an impressive increase in episodes of symptomatic hypoglycemia. Some of the findings are disconcertingly marginal: there is a suggestion that intensive therapies decreased the likelihood of some microvascular complications, notably the surrogate measures of leakage of protein from blood vessels in the retina or in the kidney. However, this effect did not translate into fewer patients suffering from kidney or eye damage. Intensive therapy did not alter the likelihood of peripheral neuropathy. It is also abundantly clear that there was no advantage from intensive therapies in terms of macrovascular complications, that is, no decrease in heart attacks, strokes, or important peripheral vascular disease, including amputations. And there was no decrease in all-cause or in diabetes-specific mortality!

Ten years of intensive therapy offered no real advantage for 1,000 middle-aged, hyperglycemic people. So why in the name of science would anyone declare the UKPDS supportive of intensive therapy, including intensive therapy with oral hypoglycemics? Is it because the surrogate measures moved in the right direction? Wasn't the rationale of undertaking the UKPDS in the first place to demonstrate benefit beyond surrogate measures? How about the weight gain, a surrogate measure that does not bode well? From my perspective, the UKPDS is an argument for "conventional" therapy and not pharmaceutical interventions. Furthermore, there is good reason to be wary of the next generation of hypoglycemic agents, even if they are more effective in terms of surrogate outcomes. One such agent, triglitazone, which offers a novel way to enhance endogenous insulin efficiency, has already been withdrawn from the market because of liver toxicity. Should physicians leap to prescribe similar drugs as soon as they are released? Hardly.

The UKPDS group published a secondary analysis in 2000, torturing the same data to derive an association that is more consistent with their preconceived notion that treating the high blood glucose in type 2 diabetes treats the patient in some meaningful way. The secondary analysis was based on the fact that some of the patients responded more readily and completely than others to their brand of treatment and therefore were less hyperglycemic over time. The secondary analysis demonstrates that the greater the exposure to hyperglycemia over time, the higher the incidence of microvascular and macrovascular events, including all cause- and diabetes-related death. The relationship between control of blood sugar and the reduction in the relative risk of untoward outcomes is linear and with a low slope, meaning that you're increasingly a bit more likely to be spared adverse events than if you were not treated to lower your blood sugar. It's not a particularly impressive result from all the massaging of data. That's why we are told about the absolute-risk reduction, which is not linear but log-linear, meaning if you have an extraordinarily high blood sugar, you may actually benefit, although the benefit is more in the way of the surrogate than the clinically overt outcomes. Sorry to have to take you through this argument, but someone must. Read the last few sentences again; you'll see how this log-linear relationship can lead to importunate claims of benefit that capture your doctor's attention as well as yours and warm the hearts of all who hold stakes, in industry and in medicine, in the purveyance of oral hypoglycemic agents. Nonetheless, this enthusiasm is based on a secondary analysis. The vaunted relationship might not pertain to the blood sugar at all. The relationship might reflect some other unmeasured risk factor (SES, for example). Furthermore, the authors' assertion that reducing exposure to hyperglycemia might reduce risk is admittedly hypothetical. This seems a tenuous hypothesis upon which to base the present massive investment in treatment.

Tenuous or not, it is an inference that is gaining steadily on ground that is increasingly fertile for the spate of pharmaceuticals approaching the market-place. There is a blood test (hemoglobin A1c level) that measures the amount of glucose attached to hemoglobin (glycosylated hemoglobin), which indicates the degree to which the body is exposed to elevated blood sugar. Not surprisingly, this is a value that associates with the risk for cardiovascular disease in diabetics. Doctors like to have a simple blood test to "monitor" therapy, and patients are comfortable thinking they're better off because the hemoglobin A1c (or blood pressure or cholesterol) is lower. The surrogate blood test becomes the "disease." That has happened for type 2 diabetes in practice. It is even applauded in print by the likes of H. C. Gerstein of McMaster University, the North American epicenter of evidence-based medicine. In an editorial in the august *Annals of Internal Medicine*, Gerstein declares "Potential Financial Conflicts of Interest" in his business relationships with Aventis, Lilly, and Novo Nordisk — all pharmaceutical firms heavily committed to purveying agents for the treatment of type 2 diabetes.

Monitoring blood sugar and/or hemoglobin A1c and treating when "abnormal" became the mantra of the American Diabetes Association in 2006. It was declared one of the criteria of the Ambulatory Care Quality Alliance form measuring health-care quality. And it is promulgated as one of the educational mainstays of internal medicine by the American College of Physicians. All this and more to treat surrogate measures despite the clear message of the UKPDS trial that clinically important benefits are elusive. All this and more has caused another 1.5 million Americans to be labeled "diabetic" each year, and to be treated as aggressively as necessary to normalize their blood sugar. Caveat emptor.

Hypertension is the last component of the "Metabolic Syndrome" on our plate. Hypertension has a J-shaped curve. As with cholesterol and blood sugar, defining the point of abnormality on the curve short of the steep sides has been delegated to experts in committees, experts who nearly always declare "potential conflicts of interest" with the patients' betterment. In defining the cutoff of normal, these committees try to weigh elements of benefit/risk and cost/benefit when neither the risk imputed by the surrogate measurement (here, blood pressure) nor the benefit of the potential interventions (here, antihypertensive drugs) can be precisely defined. The exercise degenerates rapidly to prejudices that play out in small-group psychology. For hypertension this exercise recently produced the "Seventh Report of the Joint National Committee on Prevention, Detection, Evaluation, and Treatment of High Blood Pressure." As the reader has become painfully aware, the worlds of cardiology and cardiovascular epidemiology swim in acronyms. Every trial, committee, most classes of drugs, and many surgical procedures are referred to by their acronym, often an acronym that can be pronounced (CABG, GUSTO, CASS, SHEP, RITA-2, and many others have passed before you but I've spared you many, many more). The recent pronouncement about hypertension was by JNC 7. The committee classified levels that earlier committees called normal and high-normal as "prehypertension." Over 90 percent of us will qualify for hypertension by the time we're octogenarians. So what does it mean to be normal if no one is?

No doubt the treatment of severe hypertension is to the advantage of my patient. Aggressively treating severe hypertension improves life expectancy, though it does not fully normalize it. There have been dozens of enormous, costly, randomized controlled trials of treating mild hypertension with various pharmaceuticals seeking evidence for effectiveness beyond just lowering the blood pressure. It is a daunting literature, and quite telling. The likelihood of important benefit from antihypertensive therapy across these trials is highly varied. It is never dramatic. In fact, the vast majority demonstrates no change in mortality consequent to treatment. There is a decrease in the likelihood of stroke in a few, and myocardial infarction in fewer. Two of these trials are object lessons.

1. It's not all good! MR FIT is an acronym for the Multiple Risk Factor Intervention Trial, a famous multicenter U.S. trial initiated in 1973 with the screening of 361,662 men age thirty-three to forty-seven years. Most were followed as late as 1990. Much was measured and many papers published. Embedded in this experience early on were trials of antihypertensive agents, obviously older agents used in a "step" fashion that commences with the milder drugs. The surprise finding was that hypertensive patients who were treated with gentle diuretics fared poorly, an observation that led to creative explanations. It is likely that the excess mortality reflected dose-dependent drug toxicity (elec-

trolyte disturbances), although personally I would not discount randomization errors. Regardless, it is worth emphasizing that treating well people with mild hypertension with drugs has a disconcertingly tight benefit/risk ratio. No well person should be persuaded otherwise. By the way, a recent analysis of the MR FIT cohort, sixteen years after inception, documents that SES overwhelms and subsumes all of the measured biological risk factors for all-cause mortality as well as most other mortal and morbid end points.

2. It's not all bad! Speaking of gentle antihypertensive therapy, it has become clear that such will advantage the elderly with systolic hypertension, and that's the majority of the elderly. In fact, this is the only group of well patients with mild hypertension that I have reason to feel confident that I am helping them by treating their mild hypertension. The elderly are likely to enjoy a meaningful benefit in cardiovascular morbidity, a meaningful decrease in the incidence of stroke, and perhaps a touch of extra longevity. However, I can only justify a gentle and inexpensive single drug regimen. Furthermore, another randomized controlled trial, the TONE study, demonstrated that gentle weight reduction in the more robust and gentle reduction of salt intake in the less robust spares the elderly as much grief as gentle diuretic therapy. That gives the elderly a choice. The same pertains to the less elderly. That was the implication of the "PREMIER" trial, in which 800 mildly hypertensive adults, mean age fifty, were randomized to various behavior modifications. Behavior modification in the PREMIER trial is as effective in lowering blood pressure as low-dose combination pharmaceuticals, if the recent meta-analysis of 354 randomized, double-blind, placebo-controlled trials captured the latter.

This is not to say that the medical literature does not strongly advocate the use of drugs in the treatment of well younger people with mild hypertension. This is one of the literatures that is scarred by vested interest. The brouhaha over the effectiveness of a class of antihypertensive drugs, the calcium channel antagonists, is instructive. The controversy commenced with the publication of a trial in the *Journal of the American Medical Association* (*JAMA*) purporting to demonstrate increased likelihood of myocardial infarction in patients treated with a particular calcium channel blocker. In the next year, the medical literature was peppered with nearly seventy commentaries, some with multiple authors, taking a stand on this issue. It turns out that the authors who supported the use of calcium channel blockers as antihypertensive agents were far more likely to admit a financial arrangement with pharmaceutical companies that purvey these agents. Likewise, authors who took a stand against using the calcium channel blockers were far more likely to have a vested interest in pharmaceutical firms that purvey competing classes of antihypertensive drugs. Alas.

By the way, the association with increased mortality that initiated the brouhaha proved irreproducible in subsequent trials. However, it is sensible to be wary of all claims of pharmaceutical benefit for well people who have mild hypertension, particularly for benefit from newer, more expensive agents. The same ALLHAT trial that I mentioned earlier in this chapter because no benefit from treatment with pravastatin was discerned also sought differential benefit across classes of antihypertensive agents. Over 33,000 participants age fifty-five or older with mild hypertension were randomized to treatment with a standard, inexpensive diuretic, or a drug of the calcium channel blocker class, or a drug of the angiotensin-converting enzyme (ACE) inhibitor class. Those treated with the old-fashioned, inexpensive diuretic were less likely to suffer a major cardiovascular event during five years of follow-up. Maybe, as MR FIT suggests, they would have been even better off not treated.

But that is not a conclusion shared by the antihypertension community. For this community, if an exceedingly high blood pressure is exceedingly bad for you, then "normal" blood pressure is the goal. It's an argument reminiscent of the hemoglobin A1c argument, and it has strong advocacy in the academy intertwined with a powerful investment by the pharmaceutical industry. Fortunately, this sophism is running amuck, skewered by the debate over the TROPHY trial. This was a randomized controlled four-year trial comparing the effectiveness of an expensive new drug, candesartan, compared to placebo in preventing people with "prehypertension" from rising to the criteria for hypertension. The trial was underwritten by AstraZeneca LP, the manufacturer. The analysis of the data was said to show an important benefit at two years that became trivial at four years, leading the authors to conclude that "treatment of prehypertension appears to be feasible." The study design and data analysis were to be tellingly criticized in subsequent editorials. The profit motives driving these studies have been decried yet again. However, I have no doubt that we will be bombarded with more assaults on "prehypertension," although there will need to be great inventiveness with the criteria as the international trend in blood pressure has been drifting downward in recent decades.

We've now examined the elements of the "Metabolic Syndrome" and dissected the degree to which they are noxious. In each instance, a well person needs to be out on a limb (figuratively, of the U-shaped curve) before the hazard is clinically meaningful enough to warrant being labeled obese, or diabetic, or hypertensive. In each instance, the data that suggests we can intervene effectively, short of the extremes, is tenuous at best.

What about people at the extremes? The data is suggestive and is bolstered by a series of papers that examines the benefit to the patient of treating the hypertension of a patient with both type 2 diabetes and hypertension. It is clear that hypertension and diabetes are synergistic evils. Much of this information derives from secondary analyses of many of the hypertension drug trials to which we have already referred. Investigators went back to the data to extract the subjects who had coincident type 2 diabetes and hypertension. In fact, most of the effectiveness demonstrated in these trials is restricted to the stratum of hypertensive patients who were also diabetic. That includes the SHEP trial; the annual cardiovascular event rate among 4,149 nondiabetic elderly patients decreased from about 3.5 percent to 2.5 percent consequent to treating their systolic hypertension, but for the 583 with type 2 diabetes it decreased from just over 6 percent to about 4 percent, a slightly more credible benefit.

The analysis of the UKPDS trial is even more illuminating, particularly since embedded in that trial were some 4,000 patients with hypertension and type 2 diabetes; after a complex allocation scheme, 1,000 were randomized to either tight or less tight blood-pressure control. The incidence of almost all end points was less in the patients whose blood pressure was tightly controlled. For example, if the systolic blood pressure was maintained below 120 mm of mercury, there were 7 deaths per 1,000 people per year. If the systolic blood pressure could not be maintained below 160, there were 20 deaths per 1,000 persons per year. Seems like an impressive reduction? About 13 people in 1,000 (1.3 percent) with diabetes and hypertension who would have died that year will live to die another year. Suppose I grant, begrudgingly, that we can measure this difference. This is the order of magnitude of benefit in four other trials similar to UKPDS. They, too, have acronyms: ABCD, MDRD, HOT, and AASK. The result is consistent. However, to achieve the blood pressure reduction goal in all these trials, the patient was not on a simple, gentle regimen. To the contrary, these patients were taking on average three antihypertensive agents, each agent with its set of problems.

For patients with type 2 diabetes and hypertension, given the trade-offs and uncertainties, the decision to treat or not to treat with hypoglycemic agents is easier. The decision to treat with multiple antihypertensive drugs is challenging; it requires a dialogue. Most patients who have had the opportunity to build a relationship of trust with their physician will resort to, "What would you do,

Doc?" Thanks to the ALLHAT data, prescribing an inexpensive, gentle diuretic is an appealing option. I might even be tempted to advise changing lifestyle, although to do so is a cop-out since the science supporting that advice is as tenuous as the science that documents compliance — as will become clear in the next chapter.

The supplementary reading for this chapter is comprehensive. Many of the points on data analysis are revisited for further emphasis and clarification.

chapter four

You Are Not
What You Eat

In 2005 it was considered reprehensible to feed your child butter; today, it's reprehensible to feed your child margarine. You must be thin, but not too thin. Bran is fast fading as a salutary "must" that lowers your cholesterol and burnishes your colon. Now eating some fish will save your life thanks to omega-3 content, unless the mercury content does you in first. A diet low in carbohydrate is good for you, or not. A diet low in fat is good for you, or not. Red meats are bad, except maybe a little is okay; white meats are good unless toxic substances lurk in the juices.

The print and broadcast media are committed to dishing up the scare of the week and the cure of the weekend. The public is insatiable. Nearly all of this has an authoritative source: some governmental agency, a disease-specific, not-for-profit association or foundation, the public relations department of some medical school, or an earnest and smiling scientist. Major medical journals (*JAMA*, *New England Journal of Medicine*, and others) have public relations departments that forewarn the press of an upcoming newsworthy article, many of which are displayed online before they are in print. Nearly all of this advantages some producer or purveyor and spells harder times for some other. And we, the gullible, swallow any drivel or babble that we are told relates to health. We are far less gullible when it comes to the pronouncements by our politicians, or by those hawking other wares. We listen, with a prepared mind, for nuanced duplicity when it comes to our pocketbook or our sense of community. We accept only the pronouncements that pass this filter, and we do so tentatively. Caveat emptor is our way of life. We are all too aware that the pronouncements of politicians are qualitative and value laden, if not as corrupted as the doublespeak of "used-car salesmen." Mention our health and we are patsies.

Literature such as we reviewed in the previous chapter provides fodder for my cynicism. Epidemiology often seems to have lost its way. In fact, epidemiology may lose its credibility given its tendency to declare last month's "good" this month's "evil." Epidemiology has evolved from a science of the epidemic to its contemporary mission of probing for associations between less-dramatic exposures and less-cataclysmic health effects. To wit, modern epidemiology has enlightened us as to the association between smoking and lung cancer, inhalation of certain types of asbestos fibers and mesathelioma, alcohol consumption and motor vehicle accidents. Giddy with such successes, modern epidemiology is probing for associations between exposures that are difficult to define and health effects that clearly have multiple causal associations.

Epidemiology has acquired near religious beliefs that statistical modeling is a match for any degree of variability and uncertainty in the definition of exposure, and probability theory and its imperious p-values are a match for discerning tiny health effects. In chapter 3 we examined the UKPDS and West of Scotland pravastatin trials as examples of the pitfalls in defining exposure (Who has type 2 diabetes? Who's cholesterol is high?) and both for issues in whether the outcome was meaningful. These were randomized controlled trials in which the investigators had some control over the exposure (the drugs), and still the results are equivocal and the authors' interpretations unconvincing.

Nonetheless, these randomized controlled trials stand head and shoulders above observational studies. Epidemiology falls flat on its face when it tries to tease minor exposures and minor health effects by observing all the glorious variability that is humanity. Biases and confounders lie in wait for any epidemiologist trying to tease minor events and influences out of the complexity of life. Condemnation lies in waiting for any epidemiologist who is willing to analyze data with the goal of supporting a preconceived notion ("data dredging") rather than testing a hypothesis. Most disconcerting is the fact that much of this epidemiology is generated in trials that are supported by companies that are purveying, or wish to purvey, the pharmaceutical under study. Recent analyses of the published results of such industry-sponsored trials document systematic biases that favor the drug or the foodstuff when compared to trials of the same drug sponsored by other sources. The reader of *Worried Sick* will take little for granted in the future.

Something Is Fishy

Let's take the example of the hype over the salutary nature of a diet rich in fish harboring omega-3 fatty acids. As is true for many of the putatively lifesaving diets that are hyped, someone first noted that people elsewhere are living longer and have diets that seem distinctive. The dearth of atherosclerotic disease among the Eskimos of Greenland and the longevity of rural native Japanese, and the fact that their diets are rich in seafood, was held up as more than coincidence. No one seems concerned that these are genetically distinctive populations living in countries with distinctive socioeconomic structures. The notions that eating fish — or a Mediterranean diet, or green vegetables, or less meat, or more carbohydrate, or less saturated fats, or whatever promises the fountain of youth — easily gain credibility. To test the inference with a randomized controlled trial seeking differential effects on clinically important outcomes in a well population is prohibitive. It's daunting to test a pharmaceutical where you can administer pills that contain either the active agents or a placebo. Can you imagine controlling the diets of half the sample for decades, waiting to see how many die? Even modern epidemiology has no such hubris. But modern epidemiology comes close with its belief that it can test inferences as to subtle risk just by observing large populations at work and play.

The pitfall of the unmeasured confounder may explain the tiny survival benefit observed for those among 22,000 Greek adults who adhered more tightly to a "Mediterranean diet" over the course of forty-four months of observation. Multiple confounders were taken into account, but not SES. This is not to say there's no biological effect from adding olive oil and nuts to your diet, even a low-fat diet. Your lipid profile will look better, more pleasing to those who define risks and hazards. But the reduction in hazard is very small. Don't feel remiss if you don't like nuts or olives. This, too, is much ado about the miniscule.

I feel the same about the craze to eat fish, or at least consume the particular omega-3 fatty acids found in finfish or shellfish. There is a suggestion that modest consumption of fish will reduce the relative risk of coronary death by about 30 percent, but it will decrease the absolute risk of death before your time very little and all-cause mortality not at all (see chapter 1). It will not protect you from any manifestation of coronary artery disease other than death. There is no hint of a benefit in terms of cancer. So, there's a whiff of white smoke. Then there's the fear factor, fear of the contaminants in our waters contaminating seafood and threatening our very survival. There's something counterintuitive about this fear, since the Japanese are thriving despite their diet. Nonetheless, it is the sort of trivial epidemiology that promulgates fear. The compromise is that fish is good, but not too much fish. If you are beginning to wonder why we are swimming in such pronouncements, realize they are "peer reviewed" and federally supported.

Take the example of the famous "Nurses' Health Study" based at Harvard. In 1976, 121,700 registered nurses, all women between the ages of thirty and fifty-five and nearly all white, were enrolled into the study, with an extensive questionnaire probing all kinds of details about their lifestyle and medical history. Every two years since, follow-up questionnaires were sent to update information and identify new major illnesses. In 1980, 1984, 1986, 1990, and 1994, the women were asked how often they consumed particular foods, on average, in the prior year, with a scale ranging from "almost never" to "six or more times per day." During sixteen years of follow-up, amounting to 1,307,157 years of life that 100,000 responding nurses lived, there were almost 500 deaths ascribed to coronary heart disease and 1,000 nonfatal heart attacks. Think of it: after sixteen years, only 0.5 percent of the cohort was dead, and another 1 percent had suffered a nonfatal heart attack. Even if every one of these 1,500 women avoided fish all their lives, and the remaining 98,500 women ate fish often, I would still be skeptical. I would wonder what else was going on that we weren't measuring.

Of course, the exposure was not so binary, nor was it uniform year by year, nor can it be measured that reliably (short of a food diary, the recall of dietary habits for a year is problematic). In fact, forty-one of the women who suffered a fatal heart attack recalled eating fish less than once per month and twenty-five more than once a month; the remaining 400 fatalities were spread out between these extremes of fish consumption. By inspection, the raw data looks pretty unpromising if your belief is that eating fish is good for you.

The investigators were undaunted, however, statistically modeling the data to account for differences in age, BMI, cigarette smoking, hypertension, blood cholesterol, type 2 diabetes, and the like to come up with relative risks that suggested a statistically significant protective effect of eating fish. Of course, the absolute reduction in risk was miniscule and not apparent until the data was massaged statistically. Such modeling of small effects is susceptible to confounding. For example, "job satisfaction" has been an issue for the nursing profession, and the lack of it is a mortal risk (see chapter 12) that was not considered in the statistical modeling. But the investigators are enamored of their methodology. They even estimated the content of omega-3 fatty acids that was being consumed and advised we all partake. Perhaps you'd prefer I say, Where's the beef?

I don't want to leave you with the impression that all observational studies are doomed to wallow in the trivial or the irrelevant, or that the Nurses' Health Study has no redeeming features. The study has been the source of a number of important insights. For example, it was shown that nurses who chose to have silicon breast implants were no more likely than their peers to suffer rheumatoid arthritis or any other major systemic rheumatic disease. The observational design is a match for that insight because both the exposure (breast implants) and the health effect (systemic rheumatic diseases) are well defined. The design is even a match for probing for biological risk factors for death or myocardial infarction, although there are challenges to defining the exposure (for example, blood sugar, cholesterol, or blood pressure) when the measure can vary considerably over the course of observation. However, trying to define dietary exposures, or stressful exposures, or level of physical activity, or other aspects of the fabric of daily life over decades of observation requires multiple suppositions and approximations. Any investigator or funding agency with the temerity to try is begging to be wrong. The investigators involved in the Nurses' Health Study have no such qualms. They analyzed this enormous data ready to see if habitual intake of caffeinated beverages increased the risk of hypertension; no such relationship was discerned. And it doesn't matter in terms of coronary heart disease if the nurses tended to choose a diet lower in sugar and higher in protein and fat over the course of twenty years. Both observations are consonant with my prejudices. But I take the "science" with a grain of salt.

Others don't. For example, recent analysis of the Nurses' Health Study coupled with an analysis of its companion study in men, the Health Professionals Follow-up Study, is the engine behind the national fear of trans-fatty acids (margarines and many commercial cooking oils). Trans-fatty acids are manufactured by a chemical process that converts vegetable oils into semisolid fats, which the wisdom of the past held to be better for you in terms of cardiovascular risk factors. Cardiovascular risk factors were trumped by the Nurses' Health Study. Of the nearly 80,000 nurses followed for nearly two decades, 1,200 suffered nonfatal heart attacks and 500 fatal ones. Remember, the nurses had been asked annually "how often, on average, she had consumed" a particular quantity of sixty-one foods. Over the course of twenty years, the nurses consumed progressively less of all kinds of fats. Furthermore, the very small hazard from fat intake was not dependent on the type of fat. However, if the data was further massaged to consider the degree to which fat as an energy source was substituted for carbohydrate, trans-fat seemed to be uniquely hazardous, particularly in thin nurses younger than sixty-five for whom trans-fat accounted for more than 2 percent of their energy intake. The investigators never bothered to publish the number of nurses with and without heart attacks in the highest and lowest quintiles of trans-fat consumption, or even the absolute risks. All we have is the relative risk reduction based on comparing the quintiles. The multivariate relative risk is 1.33. That 33 percent increase is based on a tiny number of nurses whose dietary intake over two decades is at best approximated. This data analysis, coupled with the influence of the Harvard Schools of Medicine and Public Health, has had an enormous impact on margarine sales. Cities and states are banning margarine from restaurants and fast-food chains are removing it from their fryers. And no doubt the plaintiff's bar is lurking to provide a legal remedy for all who were supposedly poisoned by margarine. And all because of a tiny association that was dredged out of an enormous data set that is "soft" in the center. Do you really think any of us can recall our dietary intake last year with the exactitude prerequisite to the analysis?

The Battle of the Food Pyramid

Most readers are aware that there are zealots for low-fat diets, zealots for low-carbohydrate diets, and all other combinations. These zealots have vast followings and often mind-boggling profit margins from their books, health spas, and the like. All the hype has forced some systematic studies. We will have much to say about the Women's Health Initiative in chapter 11. This was a federal initiative, funded with great sums, investigating a number of issues relevant to the health of American women. It included a randomized controlled trial of dietary modification for the primary prevention of invasive breast cancer, colorectal cancer, and cardiovascular disease. Almost 49,000 postmenopausal women were enrolled and followed from 1993 to 2005. A low-fat diet made no difference in any important outcome. The true believers were not to be convinced; they remain true believers in the benefit of diet despite these studies because the women were "healthier than anticipated." I am delighted that they were. I am convinced that a low-fat diet is a silly way to seek a longer, healthier life.

The Euphemism of the Good Lifestyle

Other cohort studies have examined the relationship between leisure-time physical activity and all-cause mortality and cardiac outcomes. These studies find an inverse relationship between activity and mortality. All of these studies factor in biological risk factors and health-adverse behaviors, such as tobacco abuse. But these studies do not consider SES. Who is likely to spend an hour or two each week exercising for fun? Who is likely to choose to walk the stairs rather than take an elevator? Is it the advantaged person whose work is not physically demanding? How many blue-collar production workers or materials handlers or field hands want to ride an exercise bicycle after work?

However, there are studies that are designed to ask some lifestyle questions in a fashion that might provide meaningful insights. Most examine population at high risk for the particular health effect and are experimental in design. They are usually randomized controlled trials and demanding of resources. But they are less susceptible to confounding and bias. More often than not, these studies trump the notions based on observational data. That's why a voluminous observational literature suggests antioxidant vitamins protect you from cardiac disease, but the experimental literature finds no such benefit.

Let me mention four randomized controlled trials that tested the effectiveness of lifestyle alterations that the investigators thought should advantage the subjects. All relied on surrogate measures of outcome. All inform our common sense and influence the thinking of the members of committees convened to advise the common good.

1. In 1997 the DASH collaborative research group published a trial on the effects of dietary patterns on blood pressure. Nearly 500 normal adults were enrolled. For three weeks they were fed an average American diet, low in fruits and vegetables. For the next eight weeks they were randomized to continue the control diet, eat a diet rich in fruits and vegetables, or eat a diet rich in fruits and vegetables but reduced in saturated and total fats. Sodium intake and body weight were maintained at constant levels. The experimental diets were associated with a lowering of blood pressure, particularly in the subjects whose blood pressures were in the upper tertile at inception of the cohort. Subsequent studies suggest that reducing the carbohydrate results in further improvement in surrogate measures and therefore might result in improved clinical outcomes.

2. In 2001 the Finnish Diabetes Prevention Study Group published a multicenter randomized controlled study of the effectiveness of lifestyle alteration in preventing type 2 diabetes. They enrolled some 500 middle-aged people who were clearly overweight (average BMI = 31). All had impaired glucose tolerance as well. The intervention group each had seven sessions with dieticians the first year and quarterly thereafter to instruct, urge, and monitor compliance with an exercise regimen and a diet tailored to be high in fiber, lower in calories, and low in saturated fats. The control group received educational material and instruction at entry and annually for the three years of the study. The interven-

tion group lost more weight than the control group and had less progression in the degree of glucose intolerance.

3. The Diabetes Prevention Program Research Group published the results of its three-year trial in 2002. They had recruited over 3,000 overweight people (average BMI = 34) with mild glucose intolerance. These were randomly assigned to receive routine care plus a placebo, routine care plus metformin, or an intensive program aimed at lifestyle modification. Metformin is an interesting hypoglycemic agent that is unique in not having weight gain as a common side effect. The study originally included a fourth limb on triglitazone but, as I mentioned in chapter 3, the FDA withdrew that drug in 1998 because of liver toxicity. The intensive program started with a sixteen-session curriculum taught one-to-one covering diet, exercise, and behavior modification. Monthly individual and group sessions for reinforcement followed this. After three years, more impressive progression in glucose intolerance was demonstrated in the placebo group compared to the other two, with the lowest incidence in the lifestyle group. Both intervention groups lost weight in the first year; the metformin group was nearly back to baseline by the end of the study and the lifestyle group well on its way toward baseline.

4. A recent randomized trial, the "PREMIER" trial, of comprehensive lifestyle modification demonstrates that persons with early hypertension can lose weight and improve control of blood pressure at eighteen months. The trial had three arms: advice, a group that targeted established guidelines, and a group like the second that also followed the DASH regimen referenced in number 1 above.

There you have it: a wealth of research data at our disposal. We are most confident that surrogate outcomes can be altered to a small degree by guesses at the best diet. It is this sort of information that an expert panel, convened by the National Institute of Medicine in Washington, D.C., brought to the table. Their proclamation of "New Dietary Guidelines" poured forth on September 4, 2002, expanding the recommended daily intake of carbohydrate and fat and doubling the amount of exercise recommended daily from thirty minutes to one hour.

If I am teaching as intended, the reader will smirk.

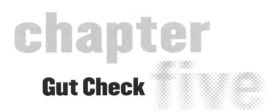

chapter five

Gut Check

About 1 percent of the U.S. population dies each year; let's say that's 3 million people. The proximate cause of death for 1 million is designated as cardiovascular disease. The proximate cause of death for another 0.6 million is malignant neoplasms (i.e., cancer). The great majority of cancer deaths occur after age sixty-five, well after age sixty-five.

One-quarter of the 600,000 cancer deaths are from lung cancer. About 10 percent are from colorectal cancer, followed closely by death from prostate and breast cancer. This chapter considers whether a well person is well advised to go to lengths to be spared the fate of death by colorectal cancer. There are options that will decrease the likelihood of acquiring colorectal cancer in the first place. There are options that will decrease the likelihood of dying from colon cancer. However, the very existence of these options does not mandate their choosing. One needs assurance that choosing these options will prolong pleasant time on this earth.

If choosing the options does nothing more than alter the proximate cause of dying at the same time, the choosing is far less compelling. It is certain that most older people whose death is ascribed to cardiovascular disease harbored undetected breast, prostate, and/or colon cancer. It is certain that a significant number of the older people whose proximate cause of death was breast or prostate or colon cancer had comorbidities — coincident diseases, including cardiovascular disease — vying to be their grim reaper. One wants reassurance that avoiding colon cancer is more than an exercise in futility in terms of longevity and quality of life. Options for avoiding death from breast cancer and prostate cancer are subjected to scrutiny in the next two chapters. Here we are concerned with defining the basis for contending with the specter of becoming one of the 60,000 Americans that will have colorectal cancer certified on their death certificates as the cause of death.

Colorectal cancer is a relatively indolent disease. From the time of diagnosis, the five-year survival (including those whose cancer was completely resected) is around 50 percent. Compare that with 3 percent for pancreatic cancer, 10 percent for lung cancer, and 70 percent for breast cancer. It follows that it is hard to justify any colon cancer screening in an octogenarian. By eighty-five, many diseases are vying to be fatal before you are ninety. The other extreme of the age spectrum is more problematic. The death of a young person is a tragedy regardless the cause. If a disease-specific tragedy such as death from colon cancer can be avoided, what would stay our hand? The disease is so rare in young people that to save a life you will be forced to screen the haystack looking for the needle. That means all those well young people will be exposed to procedures and risks for precious little yield. You will soon learn that the risks to the well population, albeit rare, overwhelm the gain to the even more rare young person with colorectal cancer. For the young well population, screening is reserved for those with a family history of diseases that predispose to colorectal cancer (genetic diseases that cause the growth of polyps) and for those whose parent or sibling died young from colon cancer.

When is a well person not too young or too old to justify screening? The answer is much debated. One would think it would be relatively straightforward. After all, the answer could be based on an analysis of the age-dependent efficiency of the various screening options. There is no doubt that screening is too inefficient to undertake in octogenarians or people much under fifty. However, there is daunting variability in the statistics that define efficiency between fifty and eighty, variability that derives from individual differences in the biology of patients and in the efficiency or proficiency of screeners. Some critical data is simply missing, forcing guesses and approximations. As a result, the definition of age-dependent efficiency depends on the suppositions underlying the statistical modeling.

That is just the start of the complexity. There is the issue of values. How many colorectal cancers are you willing to miss? How many young well people are you willing to expose to the risks of screening to spare one young person death from colorectal cancer? Expert panels, one after another, have studied this issue. Some of the scholars leading this effort are colleagues of mine at the University of North Carolina, notably David Ransohoff and Robert Sandler and their protégé Michael Pignone, who authored the most recent proclamation by the U.S. Preventive Services Task Force on this topic. In spite of my entreaties, even my colleagues are unwilling to depart from the standard for statistical modeling in this field. That modeling considers death by colorectal cancer to be the important outcome. I want a more meaningful outcome. I want to know how many years of good life would be lost to colon cancer were it not for screening. If screening spares you death by colorectal cancer, but you die at the same time from something else, was the screening valuable?

Perhaps screening would be valuable if the death experience was altered from torment to sudden death. However, there is no way to predict that likelihood. I take comfort in the arguments set forth in chapter 1. Will screening for colorectal cancer make it more likely that you will live out your eighty-five years on earth? I am not seduced by interventions that do no more than change the proximate cause of death. With that as my philosophy, I will attempt to display the fashion on which one might base a choice to undergo screening for colorectal cancer.

Notice that I am avoiding the issue of expense. This is the era of "managed wealth" in medicine, that is, managing to foster the transfer of wealth to whatever provider is in control at the moment (see chapter 14). To serve this transfer of wealth, many analyses are designed to assess cost/benefit ratios rather than risk/benefit ratios. However, "cost" is a will-o'-the-wisp. Recent analyses take $1,000 or so as the "cost" of colonoscopy, for example. As one friend, colleague, and finely honed wag from Britain likes to say, "There's a thousand-dollar bill in every American cecum; you just have to get up there and get it." But it need not be $1,000. The procedure is tedious and demands compulsivity, some dexterity, and patience. But it does not require more than procedure-specific training. In two controlled studies, nurse practitioners have been trained to perform colonoscopy with proficiency indistinguishable from that of the gastroenterologists who trained them, at a fraction of the "cost." I'll focus on risk/benefit considerations and not belabor cost/benefit issues further.

Let's start with the absurd. If you lack a colon, you won't have colon cancer. Why not remove all colons at age fifty? Imagine that laparoscopists have honed their techniques so that colectomies can be done on outpatients and the terminal small bowel can be fashioned into a pouch that is attached to the rectal sphincters. Most of you would have normal bowel function, or a tendency toward diarrhea easily managed with medications. Some 20 percent would have more of a challenge with bowel habits. However, colorectal cancer would be expunged from your mortal fears. The expense would be reasonable, perhaps five to ten screening colonoscopy equivalents. Serious complications, either requiring major surgery or leading to death, could be reduced to 1 in 1,000. Would you do it? Would you do it if gastroenterologists, or GI surgeons, recommended it? Would you be persuaded if it were an option promulgated by august professional bodies and indemnified by your "health" insurer? When I get done with you, I would hope you would consider such a scenario to be a parody. However, remember this scenario when you read chapter 7 on prostate cancer. Today, laparoscopic surgery is nearly refined enough to offer out-patient colectomies, but the likelihood of diarrhea is so high and the likelihood of even rare operative complications so intolerable that such a recommendation would be absurd.

Short of colectomy, there are screening options that promise to detect your colon cancer before it is a problem for you. To understand the limitations of these options, one must first understand the enemy.

The Natural History of Colorectal Cancer: An Overview

With a few exceptions, all the tissues and organs of our bodies turn over and renew, each controlled by an internal rhythm that causes older cells to die at the same rate that younger cells take their place. The process is elegantly orchestrated so that our tissues and organs maintain their architecture and function throughout our lives for most organs in most of us. Minor aberrancies in turnover are common, often recognized as an extra tissue structure or new growth, which is called a neoplasm. Sometimes we refer to the neoplasm as a tumor. If it maintains the biology of the organ from which it arose, it is a benign tumor. There are many benign tumors, incidental findings in many of us — lipomas (fatty tumors under the skin) and uterine leiomyomas (fibroids), to name two. There are also common benign neoplasms that we are not wont to label tumors, such as Heberden's nodes (the bumps that grow as we age at the joints near the tips of the fingers), skin tags, and nasal polyps. All of these are examples of benign tumors that will always constrain their biology to that of their tissue of origin, rest assured.

There are benign tumors that have potential to undergo a transformation in their biology, casting off some critical features of the biology of their tissues of origin. Some acquire architectural characteristics that are distinctive. The cells of some lose the need to associate with like cells to turn over normally. Some cells acquire a biology that is far less discriminatory as to their nurturing neighborhood. If they acquire these last two features, they can take up residence elsewhere in the body, commandeering the host tissue to serve their needs. These distant explants are metastases, and their tumor of origin is a "malignant" tumor — a cancer.

Soft-tissue cancers — cancers arising from solid organs other than the brain

— come in two general types: bad and evil. No cancer is "good." The bad soft-tissue cancer develops in a relatively predictable fashion, over time and through the stages I just alluded to. Cervical cancer and prostate cancer (see chapter 7) are examples, as is colorectal cancer. The time that malignant neoplasms spend in a prelethal state is referred to as the "dwell time." There is always variability in the dwell time, between tumor types and from person to person. If the dwell time of a particular tumor type is not too short, screening is feasible and "staging" can be useful. Hence, screening with cervical "Pap" smears leads to a defensible algorithm for interventions for the stages of cervical cancer. Our brief in this chapter is to decide whether there is an analogous algorithm for colorectal cancer that is also defensible. Various authors estimate the dwell time for a polyp to transform into colorectal cancer to be at least a decade, if not two.

By definition, "evil" cancers have brief dwell times. They undergo the transformation to the biology of metastasis too quickly to permit staging or even screening. Some may arise already endowed with the biology of metastasis. We will learn in the next chapter that "breast cancer" is so heterogeneous that some tumors manifest "bad" biology and others "evil" biology, confounding all attempts to design and interpret screening programs. Colorectal cancer is just "bad."

Benign tumors are common in the colon and rectum as we age. Most are polyps on a stalk, like a grape, comprised of cells representative of the normal lining cells of the colon. Some grow sizeable on the end of the stalk. Other benign tumors arise from the lining on a broader base and are termed adenomas. Half the adenomas have distorted architecture. These also have the potential to grow in place, in situ, even to the extent of blocking the lumen of the colon and thereby obstructing the bowel.

Colorectal cancer always starts in these benign tumors, we think. The adenomas, particularly those with distorted architecture, are most likely to transform further, so that cells that normally are restricted to the lining of the colon are observed in the deeper layers. These cells are on their way toward metastatic biology. However, their metastatic biology is relatively specific; they prefer to take up residence in the local lymph nodes and the liver, the sites to which blood and lymph from the colon drain. Their metastatic biology is not such that these cells use the bloodstream to widely metastasize to lungs, brain, and elsewhere. Metastatic colorectal cancer is a chronic debilitating disease. One aspect, colonic obstruction, is surgically remedial. In fact, there are studies from the Mayo Clinic that should call a halt to performing radical surgery for obstruction in the frail elderly in the quest for "cure." A simple bypass procedure with a colostomy is palliative; it can allow for a tolerable and comfortable end of life without the trauma and risks of aggressive therapy.

The Natural History of Colorectal Cancer: The Devil Is in the Details

From autopsy studies, we have a reasonable idea of the age-dependent prevalence of the early stages in the evolution of colorectal cancer. About 1 percent of people at age fifty have at least one polyp, and the population acquires polyps at a rate of about 1 percent per year after age fifty. We also know that at age fifty, a person has about a 2 percent chance of dying from colorectal cancer over the next thirty years. And we know that at age fifty, a person has about a 60 percent chance of dying from all causes over the next thirty years! There's the rub.

Suppose there was a screening technique that could reduce a person's chance of dying after age fifty from colorectal cancer by 60 percent. Caveat emptor. You know, from our earlier discussions, to be wary of any assertion based on relative risk or relative risk reduction; that 60 percent reduction means your 2 percent chance of dying from colorectal cancer in the next thirty years is reduced to 0.8 percent, but your chance of dying for all causes is not meaningfully reduced.

This is the forest. Some of the trees are interesting enough for us to examine them. But don't let these considerations cause you to lose your way in the forest, or forget that's where you are. Most epidemiologists in this field, most policy makers, most gastroenterologists and all who do colonoscopy for a living are wandering among the trees. Is the 1.2 percent reduction in absolute risk of dying from colorectal cancer a reliable figure? If so, is it meaningful to you? Let's tackle the reliability issue first. Then we can examine your values.

Screening for Colorectal Cancer by FOBT

FOBT is the acronym for "Fecal Occult Blood Testing," a method of testing a small sample of stool for trace amounts of blood. It's indelicate, but at least it's safe. It's also inexpensive, until you start designing FOBT screening programs that involve lots of samplings from lots of people. FOBT has been around for generations, in spite of well-documented inherent limitations: some polyps, particularly adenomatous polyps and most colorectal cancers, bleed, but not all and not all of the time. That latter fact limits the sensitivity of FOBT — that is, the false-negative rate — and is the reason most FOBT screening programs call for multiple samples. There are even more factors that limit the specificity of FOBT, or its false-positive rate. Firstly, it is normal to lose a few milliliters of blood into the bowel daily, so that if the FOBT test is too sensitive, all of us will be positive. Secondly, there are noncancerous lesions with a propensity to bleed. For example, tiny arteriovenous malformations are common in the elderly. Bleeding from the oropharynx, particularly the gums, and from gastritis and peptic ulcer disease also occurs. Finally, the FOBT is not specific for human blood; ingesting a rare steak can cause a false positive.

It is only in the past decade that screening for colorectal cancer by FOBT has been subjected to careful scientific scrutiny. There are now several randomized controlled trials. They are all similar to the first, the Minnesota Colon Cancer Control Study, published in 1993. The cohort was comprised of some 47,000 adults between the ages of fifty and eighty at inception. They were randomized to a group that had FOBT annually, a group that had FOBT biennially, and a control group, and they were followed for thirteen years. About 90 percent in the tested groups had at least one FOBT, and about half were fully compliant with the protocol. Over the course of the study, there were some eighty deaths from colorectal cancer in the group screened annually but about 120 in the biennial and control groups. This is a tiny difference given that 47,000 were enrolled in the study. Nonetheless, the statistical modeling of the data managed to endow this tiny reduction in disease-specific mortality with statistical significance. There was absolutely no difference in all-cause mortality across the groups, about 3,300 in each group. To spare forty people over the age of fifty death by colon cancer required identifying these "true positives" among the 75 percent of the 47,000 tested who had false positives. That means over 20,000 people underwent a diagnostic study to determine if the positive FOBT was a false positive or one of forty true positives. This testing included 12,246 colonoscopies. Of these, four resulted in perforation of the colon (all requiring surgery) and eleven resulted in serious bleeding (three requiring surgery).

So, if you rely on FOBT as a screening modality, you would have to screen about 1,000 people over the age of fifty for a decade to spare one death by colorectal cancer. You would not decrease all-cause mortality. And if you rely on colonoscopy as your gold standard to determine if a positive FOBT was a true or a false positive, for every person spared death by colon cancer, a person with a normal bowel would suffer a serious, nonfatal complication of the diagnostic algorithm — damage to the colon caused by colonoscopy.

Annual FOBT survived the scientific scrutiny of expert panels for most of the past decade. Until recently, colonoscopy was not advised as the preferred method of sorting out the positive test. There was concern about the hazards and costs of colonoscopy. There was also concern about its accuracy. One study recruited 183 patients with positive FOBT to undergo two colonoscopies by two different experienced colonoscopists on the same day. The first colonoscopist removed all the polyps and adenomas that were discovered, 289 in all. The second found another eighty-nine that the first missed. Some of this false negativity is a reflection of how rushed the colonoscopist is inclined to be; the slower the colonoscope is withdrawn, the more likely polyps are found.

Shying away from colonoscopy, the expert panels prior to 2000 tended to advise flexible sigmoidoscopy to follow up on a positive FOBT. The flexible sigmoidoscope is inserted into the colon a distance of 60 cm; the colonoscope is inserted twice as far, all the way to the small intestine. The majority of colorectal cancers arise within 60 cm of the anus, but many hide further up. Flexible sigmoidoscopy takes less time, requires less dexterity and fewer support personnel, and is performed without sedation (although only a gastroenterologist could imagine it is not seriously unpleasant). The general feeling a decade ago was that annual FOBT on three samples was advisable, relying on flexible sigmoidoscopy to verify positives.

Then came the year 2000. Two papers appeared in the *New England Journal of Medicine*, cross-sectional studies that essentially reiterated the obvious. If you do flexible sigmoidoscopy you will miss all cancers beyond the reach of that scope, a substantial minority. An accompanying editorial questioned why we don't just "go the distance." The lay medical press was already intimately involved with colorectal cancer screening. Katie Couric, then the host of NBC's *Today Show*, was the bereaved widow of a young man who had recently died of colorectal cancer. March 2000 was designated as "Colon Cancer Awareness Month" and a five-part documentary was aired on the *Today Show*, including Ms. Couric's own colonoscopy. Before the end of 2000, Medicare decided to support colorectal cancer screening, including colonoscopy, and this — no surprise — was followed by a major increase in colonoscopies in Medicare recipients. The American Cancer Society was at the heels of health insurers to the same end. The general consensus has evolved to cut to the chase, to forego FOBT and flexible sigmoidoscopy and go directly to colonoscopy with a periodicity based on some guess at the dwell time. The zeal is such that the medical community is downplaying the iatrogenic downsides. Fortunately, a paper has appeared that makes the case for sparing all average-risk people under age fifty this right of passage. Fortunately, as well, the 2002 recommendations of the

U.S. Preventive Services Task Force mentioned previously waffles on the issue of colonoscopy.

The result is that all of us who have yet to submit to colonoscopy have to contend with the trumpeting of others who have undergone screening colonoscopy, with the common wisdom that it makes sense, with the likely recommendation of a primary-care physician, and the complicity of the gastroenterology community with this sophistry. As for me, I'll pass on FOBT and forgo screening colonoscopy. I will admit that I submitted to a flexible sigmoidoscopy at about age fifty-five. There were no abnormalities. So I know I am very, very unlikely to die before my time from colorectal cancer and exceedingly unlikely to die from colorectal cancer arising in the distal colon and rectum. Acquiescing to the procedure was not a lapse in logic; it was performed because of complications when I was recovering from a ruptured appendix. I would not have cared if a polyp or two were found (although such would play with my sense of invincibility). If there was a broad-based adenoma, I would want it biopsied as it might be a so-called high-risk lesion that could cost me time on earth. But if a polyp was found, an adenoma on a stalk, I would want it left alone. It is too unlikely to cause me grief to warrant the potential complications of its removal. Yes, most of the complications of sigmoidoscopy and colonoscopy result from snaring and cutting the stalk of these polyps. Leave them alone. I realize that reimbursement for the procedure escalates with every polyp that is snared. I'd suggest they find another source of income. However, I know no colonoscopist, even some who are trained in epidemiology, who can restrain from the snaring. They will justify their zeal with, "We are not sure of the dwell time." Give me a break. Let my polyps go.

One negative flexible sigmoidoscopy at age fifty-five is more than good enough for me. I may still develop colon cancer. I may even die from, rather than with, colon cancer. But I don't care if I die of colorectal cancer, as long as it's my time to die anyway, hopefully at a ripe old age.

You will have to make up your own mind.

Colorectal Cancer Prevention

Two recent randomized placebo-controlled trials of aspirin have demonstrated a decrease in the incidence of recurrent adenomas in patients who had an adenoma removed. There was a statistically significant reduction in incidence in patients who took low doses of aspirin compared to those taking higher doses

TABLE 2. The Efficacy of Aspirin Prophylaxis

Outcome	Number Needed to Treat (NNT) to Prevent/Cause One Outcome	Duration of Treatment (years)
1. Secondary Prevention		
Recurrence of adenoma	10	2.5
Recurrence of advanced cancer	19	2.8
2. Primary Prevention		
Heart attack (fatal or not)	50 – 250	5
Colorectal cancer	471–962	>5
Death from colorectal cancer	1,250	10–20+
3. Adverse Events		
Gastrointestinal bleeding	100	1.5
Major GI hemorrhage	300–800	4–6
Hemorrhagic stroke	800	4–6

Source: Adapted from Imperiale (2003).

or placebo. This is a population at higher risk for colorectal cancer since they already demonstrated that proclivity. An intervention that is designed to prevent recurrence is termed "secondary"; primary prevention is the attempt to prevent the first episode. When the data is closely examined, it is clear that the magnitude of benefit is quite small, so that the benefit/risk ratio for primary prevention is prohibitive and for secondary prevention, marginal. Thomas Imperiale ran the numbers with the result presented in Table 2. Several people would pay the price of the primary prevention of one death from colorectal cancer by trying to survive major gastrointestinal hemorrhaging. The trade-off for the primary prevention of a heart attack death is not so lopsided, but it is not compelling either. Secondary prevention of a heart attack is readily justified. Secondary prevention of colorectal cancer is a close choice.

As an aside, the observations regarding aspirin and secondary prevention of colorectal cancer caused Merck and Pfizer to see if Vioxx and Celebrex might provide such benefit with less risk. That led to the realization of the cardiotoxicity of Vioxx and the brouhaha I will discuss in chapter 9. However, aside from the cardiotoxicity, the Vioxx trial suggests some decrease in the likelihood of polyp formation. However, when the U.S. Preventive Services Task Force examined all published evidence, they were not convinced that taking aspirin or any of the other nonsteroidal anti-inflammatory drugs, including Celebrex and Vioxx, protects you from colon cancer and recommends against taking these drugs for that purpose.

A published detailed analysis prevents me from offering the same suggestion regarding dietary fiber. If you're eating a lot of bran, it's because you like bran or what it does for your bowel regularity. It will not save your life.

A Path through the Woods

Most people, most physicians, and many endoscopists have not picked their way through the state of the art as we have just done. We know the current approach to colorectal cancer screening is a sitting duck as soon as anyone has an alternative that makes more sense. Clinical science is not static, and screening for colorectal cancer is a topic ripe with fame and fortune. New approaches to screening are on the way. I urge you to be very, very wary.

There even are new approaches begging to cross the line to the bedside that are scientifically seductive. However, they have inherent limitations that demand close inspection by you, even if they pass muster with the FDA.

One tries to define more subsets of people at high enough risk to make the risk/benefit ratio of screening colonoscopy defensible. I have already mentioned two subsets of well people. The first have a family history of the genetic diseases that cause multiple polyps. For them, genetic screening is possible and colonoscopy, if not colectomy, reasonable. The second subset has a history of colon cancer in a young, first-degree relative. However, there is feverish activity trying to define genes that infer susceptibility to colorectal cancer on those of us who are in the vast majority. If you can define those at greatest risk, the risk/benefit of screening colonoscopy might favor the procedure. However, genotypes that infer slight increases in risk do not alter the risk/benefit ratio sufficiently to change our argument. To do so would require genotypes that infer considerable risk and therefore define the vast majority of people at risk. Then tens of thousands would be subjected to screening colonoscopy annually, not millions. I doubt there is such a genetic influence. For the vast majority of us, the risk for colorectal cancer may be stochastic — that is, risk operates by the luck of the draw.

Another approach in the pipeline is to discover a better alternative to FOBT. For example, reagents that only recognize human blood eliminate the false positive consequent to eating a rare steak; but that hardly improves FOBT. It turns out that the more malignant lesions not only bleed, they shed abnormal cells and cell fragments bearing tumor-specific DNA, RNA, and protein traces. Finding these tumor-specific traces, in theory, would eliminate all false positives. It would not eliminate false negatives (tumors that didn't shed when you sample), so sensitivity will have to be defined. The limitation to fecal molecular screening is in the technology. All the techniques depend on chemical reagents that are persnickety. They can be rendered magnificently specific and sensitive in pure systems where there are few unknown chemicals. Much effort will be required to define how they perform when their target has to be isolated from feces sampled from millions of people. Then there's the cost . . .

Finally, the radiologists are weighing in with "virtual colonoscopy." One swallows a capsule that contains a miniaturized camera that transmits images of the inside of the bowel while in transit. Many images are generated, requiring much time in analysis. Those committed to examining the images are pretty good at spotting lesions. The advantage is the patient avoids the risks and unpleasantness of colonoscopy.

I suspect that a defensible approach to screening that spares us the risk of dying from colorectal cancer before our time will remain a will-o'-the-wisp for some time to come. In the supplementary readings, I expand on all of these arguments.

chapter

Breast Cancer
Prevention
Screening the Evidence

This chapter is particularly challenging to write. Breast cancer is a topic that seldom countenances dispassionate, let alone objective, treatment. There is good reason for that. The topic roils with gender issues and object lessons in medical heuristics. Even today, when they are widely recognized, the existence of gender biases cannot be overemphasized. No one should be deprived of care of the highest quality for any reason, including gender, ethnicity, and ancestral continent of origin. However, the outcry to redress the gender issues by providing empathic and effective remedies carries an inherent hazard. We need to address past wrongs, but attempts to do so that are ill conceived may not benefit those who justly feel poorly served. Iatrogenicity is the term for any medical action that causes harm. There is no question that the saga of breast cancer is more notable for iatrogenicity than for benefit. I am writing so that no such reproach will pertain in the future. Unfortunately, that future has yet to arrive. It is my intent in this chapter to examine many of the false starts of the past century in detail so that the reader understands the fallacies that drove them. Before undertaking this exercise, let me demonstrate the challenge of protecting women from death from breast cancer.

The Women of Malmö

In 1976 some 42,000 of the women of Malmö, Sweden, had birth years falling between 1908 and 1932. Half were randomly selected to be invited by letter to participate in mammographic screening every 18 to 24 months for a decade. Both the screened and unscreened women were followed from 1976 to 2001, fifteen years after the study ended. Since Sweden has a national health-insurance scheme, survival and detection of breast cancer for each women could be determined. A total of 2,525 cases of breast cancer were registered. In the invited group, 1,320 women developed breast cancer (91 percent invasive). Of these, 584 women died, but only 212 (36.3 percent) died from their breast cancer; the others died with their breast cancer. In the control group, 1,205 women developed breast cancer (93 percent invasive), of whom 588 died, 274 (46.6 percent) from their breast cancer. There were 9,279 total deaths in the invited group and 9,514 in the control group. These observations, themselves, tell us very little about risk from breast cancer and whether screening mammography altered the risks. That requires an analysis that considers the age-dependence of cancer-related outcomes, and the difference between the decade of the trial and the following fifteen years. Table 3 presents the age relationship to cases of breast cancer stratified by whether the cases occurred during the decade of the randomized trial or the fifteen years after. Incidence is the number of new cases in a given period of observation. The unit of observation here, as for most epidemiological studies, is "1,000 person years." So an incidence of 3.43 means that 3.43 out of 1,000 women developed breast cancer each year. Table 3 illustrates one of the principal messages of the Malmö experience. Screening mammography did not detect any more cases in any age group during or after randomization.

But we don't screen to find cancer. We screen to find the cancers that kill women before their time. With or without mammography, some three to four breast cancers were detected in every 1,000 women each year. That means three to four women out of every 1,000 underwent some form of biopsy each year that yielded a positive result. How many more women underwent a biopsy that was negative? How many women with the positive biopsy had invasive cancer? How many women with invasive cancer died of something else or would have died of something else sooner than they would have died from breast cancer? For the women who were found to have noninvasive cancer, and for the women who were found to have cancer that would not have caused them grief in their lifetime, and for the women who are treated for invasive cancer when some other disease is more likely their reaper, mammographic screening is an exercise in overdiagnosis and overtreatment.

The Malmö experience offers answers relevant to the women of Malmö. We will explore the fashion in which this experience might not generalize to the United States. For example, if U.S. radiologists were more inclined to call mammograms "suspicious," the false-positive rate would escalate. If U.S. patholo-

TABLE 3. The Malmö Trial of Mammographic Screening

Interval Observed	Age at Randomization	Invited Group		Control Group	
		Cases	Incidence	Cases	Incidence
Randomized	55–69	438	3.43	324	2.53
	45–54	303	2.77	257	2.41
Follow-up	55–69	342	2.89	374	3.14
	45–54	237	3.66	240	3.64

Source: Adapted from Zackrisson et al. (2006).

gists were more inclined to call lesions "invasive," that too would skew the data (see below).

The women of Malmö who were age fifty-five to sixty-nine at randomization are highly informative. This is an aged cohort twenty-five years later; 60 percent had already died. More cancers had been detected in this cohort than in the control during the screening decade. Let's assume that the lifetime risk of breast cancer is 8 percent, and the lifetime risk of dying from breast cancer is 2.5 percent. The number of women one needs to screen from age fifty-five on in order to prevent one breast cancer death is 250 (assuming surgery or medical treatment really works). However, this screening of 250 will detect two other women with treatable breast cancer that would not have been their proximate cause of death. In other words, screening will lead to the treatment of three women, for two of whom the treatment is unnecessary. That's the best-case scenario for screening postmenopausal women. There is no best-case scenario for younger women without family histories of early death from breast cancer.

We will return to screening, the thesis of this chapter. These considerations are relevant to all women, and to those of us interested in "health care" reform (chapter 14). First, I need the reader to understand something about the consequences of detecting breast cancer.

Mastectomy

For much of the twentieth century, heuristics drove surgeons to "heroics" that both boggle the mind and curdle the blood, culminating in the "super-radical" mastectomy. The surgical cure for breast cancer demanded extirpating the primary tumor and every site to which the tumor was likely to have spread (metastasized). Surgeons vied for the distinction of invading neck, chest wall, and chest cavity in pursuit of any lymph node that might harbor a metastasis. No matter how extensive and morbid, surgery was considered a noble enterprise; the scalpel was the instrument of cure, not of mutilation. There was, however, at least one doubter in the hallowed halls of the academy. Oliver Cope, professor of surgery at the Massachusetts General Hospital, was a cultured, genteel man and a renowned innovative surgeon specializing in surgery of the neck. In the 1960s, at the sunset of his career, he realized that the radical mastectomy had not discernibly improved the five-year survival of patients compared to historical controls. The five-year survival of women in earlier generations who had not been afforded the cutting-edge of modern medicine was no worse (about 50 percent). I cherish the memory of a mentoring session with him when I was a medical student; he calmly and convincingly put forth this revolutionary notion. No medical journal would publish Cope's observation; it failed "peer" review. Cope had no peer. He settled for an article in a women's magazine. Regardless, Oliver Cope ignited the controversy that led to the work of Bernard Fisher and his collaborators in the United States and Umberto Veronesi and his collaborators in Italy.

In the 1970s, Fisher and his colleagues commenced randomized controlled trials of the various surgical approaches to the treatment of a woman with a palpable, cancerous, small (2 cm or so) breast lump but no palpable lymph nodes in her axilla or evidence of metastatic disease elsewhere. One trial dealt with the aggressiveness of mastectomy. Another probed the relative effectiveness of breast-conserving surgery. In the former trial, one-third of the women received radical mastectomy (the breast was removed along with the underlying musculature and the regional lymph nodes), one-third underwent simple mastectomy (just the breast is removed) followed by radiation therapy of the axilla, and one-third underwent simple mastectomy alone with a biopsy of the adjacent nodes. If that biopsy was positive for metastatic cancer, half underwent radical mastectomy and the other half had irradiation. These women were followed for twenty-five years. Women with negative nodes had a 50 percent likelihood of surviving for ten years without evidence of recurrent disease, while those with positive nodes had a 50 percent likelihood of surviving only for five years without recurrence. Neither radiation therapy nor more extensive surgery made a difference after twenty-five years of follow-up. These results at twenty-five years are commensurate with the results published in 1985 after ten years of follow-up. The 1985 paper turned medical heuristics upside down regarding the cure of breast cancer. It also inflamed the women's movement. After all, rather than being heroic, radical mastectomy turns out to be mutilating. There must be a gentler way to treat breast cancer, gentler even than simple mastectomy followed by irradiation. Furthermore, given the survival differential favoring node-negative, and therefore putatively early, disease, can't we find these tumors earlier, before they are palpable lumps? Both points remain well taken, to say the least.

The first led to the demonstration that breast-conserving therapy served as well as simple mastectomy. In fact, in the U.S. trial, lumpectomy was as effective as mastectomy whether or not it was followed by irradiation. True, radiation therapy after lumpectomy reduces the local recurrence rate to that of simple mastectomy, but it does nothing for disease-free survival, the likelihood of distant metastases, or overall survival. It took twenty-five years for science to incontrovertibly refute the "the more you cut, the more you cure" heuristic touted by two generations of surgeons. No longer should any woman with a small breast cancer be offered mastectomy without due consideration of breast-conserving alternatives.

The second point — the more advanced the disease, the more likely it is lethal — is the rallying cry for early detection. It led to the flowering of mammography and continues to be its driving force today. Early detection followed by a breast-conserving surgical cure is the Holy Grail. Certainly, such an approach holds more promise of cancer-free longevity than medical therapy of early or established disease. The evidence that we can "cure" metastatic breast cancer with nonsurgical therapy, even today, is anything but compelling. In fact, the evidence that we can even prolong life demands scrutiny.

Medical oncology wields therapeutic zeal that harkens to the "to cut is to cure" zeal of the midcentury cancer surgeons that now elicits disdain. The oncology community touts its advancements. However, the improvements are likely to be more apparent than real. Much of the so-called advance can be ascribed to "lead time bias." Our ability to detect metastases has steadily increased. Therefore, the breast cancer that might have been deemed nonmetastatic a decade ago can be shown to be metastatic today and be labeled as such. However, it is more likely to have a natural history approaching its "nonmetastatic" than "metastatic" forebear. We are fooled to think the "improved" survival reflects effective treatment of metastatic disease rather than this difference in staging.

The late Alvan Feinstein, the pioneering epidemiologist from Yale, called this the "Will Rogers Phenomenon," alluding to Rogers' Depression-era sarcasm that when the "Okies" left Oklahoma for California, they raised the mean IQ of both states. The Will Rogers Phenomenon aside, the literature regarding the effectiveness of variations in radiation therapy and chemotherapy following lumpectomy is as disappointing as it is extensive. There is some benefit to chemotherapy for operable lesions in premenopausal women. But by and large the topic of adjuvant chemotherapy, chemotherapy given to supplement the benefits of the surgery, begs the refutationist treatment I am applying to all the topics in this book. Such a treatment would uncover a push to "cure" that takes advantage of a science as marginal as demonstrated in chapter 2 for CABGs, that promotes hubris, and that is far more efficient in transferring wealth than in sparing the lives of women with breast cancer. Some of the most aggressive treatments, such as high-dose chemotherapy plus stem-cell transplants, have been shown to be useless, but only after thousands of women were subjected to this treatment. However, if I take on the oncology shibboleths, I digress from my service to women who are well. Once a woman, occasionally a man, starts down this high-tech treatment path, they can only hope to be a "survivor" of their breast cancer rather than a survivor of the heuristic.

So our brief is the well woman coming to grips with the specter of breast cancer. Our brief relates to the credo of "early detection hence early cure." The credo seems sensible, even incontrovertible. But there are provisos, important provisos.

Death with, Not from, Breast Cancer

The ten-year and twenty-five-year data from the American trial comparing simple versus radical mastectomy trial need to be examined closely. By ten years, actually by five years, the evil from breast cancer had largely played out. After ten years, there was very little likelihood that any of the surviving women, node negative or positive, would experience recurrence of breast cancer or die from it. But there was a very high likelihood that they would die before the twenty-five years played out. The original group who volunteered for the trial, the inception cohort, was rich in fifty- to sixty-five-year-old women. The average life expectancy for a woman who was sixty-five years old in 1979 was less than twenty years. If this cohort never had demonstrable breast cancer, most would have died of something else by the end of twenty-five years. The "something else" is the other diseases vying for mortal primacy. They are termed comorbidities in epidemiology-speak. If you are approaching your ripe old age, or you are young but already burdened with diseases actively assaulting your longevity, breast cancer is less malignant a specter, probably the least of your problems.

TABLE 4. Survival of the Women of Ontario

Age	Still Alive	Incident Breast Cancers	Breast Cancer Deaths	Cardiovascular Deaths	Deaths from Other Causes
30–34	988	1	0	0	2
35–39	986	3	0	0	3
40–44	983	5	1	1	4
45–49	977	8	2	1	6
50–54	968	11	3	2	11
55–59	952	12	3	5	15
60–64	929	12	3	9	25
65–69	892	14	4	16	36
70–74	836	13	5	28	51
75–79	752	11	6	52	70
80–84	624	9	6	89	95
>85	434	5	7	224	203

Source: Adapted from Phillips et al. (1999).

In an essay published in the *New England Journal of Medicine* in 1999, Kelly-Anne Phillips and her colleagues from Toronto made this point eloquently and reinforced it with a life table (Table 4). If we start with a modern birth cohort of 1,000 Ontario girls, this table presents data as to their fate each five years over the course of their adult lives.

So the first proviso appended to the credo of "early detection hence early cure" relates to whether early cure will affect your longevity or your quality of life. It may be true, as the lay literature is wont to trumpet, that 1 in 9 women will "get" breast cancer if they live to eighty-five. The lay literature forgets to trumpet the fact that far less than 1 in 9 will die from breast cancer, or even know that they "have" it when they die. The proviso to the credo is that early detection can advantage only those women whose breast cancer is a threat to their longevity. Early detection makes less sense the older the woman, or the more morbidities she suffers. In such a circumstance, breast cancer is but one of the processes vying for the proximate cause of death, and not the most likely to win.

However, do not assume, based on the Fisher and Veronesi trials, that the converse holds that detecting tiny "early" cancers will necessarily advantage younger well women. The participants in these trials were selected because they had a palpable breast cancer but no palpable nodes in their armpit (axillary adenopathy). This is a population at "high" risk for death from breast cancer. To wit, 20 percent died from their breast cancer despite the various primary and adjuvant interventions. These are tragic losses. However, that doesn't mean that 20 percent of women with other presentations will suffer this fate. And remember that 80 percent of this "high"-risk population fared well. We do not know if a 20 percent fatality rate stalks women whose breast mass went unnoticed either by herself or her physician. Perhaps they are more like the 80 percent in the trials who did well. We do know that both the self-examination and the clinical examination are highly unreliable and inefficient in detecting lumps, and that most lumps that are detected are not cancerous. Nonetheless, it is reasonable to postulate that the malignancy would have been nipped in the bud if the cancerous lumps in the 20 percent who had fatal disease had been detected earlier and removed. The challenge is to distinguish the tiny lumps that are likely to metastasize from the benign breast disorders that become nearly ubiquitous with aging and that are best ignored.

Not All Breast Cancers Are Evil

Our discussion of colorectal cancer screening in chapter 5 was facilitated by the predictable nature of colonic neoplasia. The rate of transformation from polyp to metastatic cancer is still to be defined, but it is clearly both low in likelihood and slow in evolution. Polyps stay polyps (dwell time) for many years before they start to turn ugly, if they ever do. The same pertains to prostate cancer, as we will discuss in the next chapter. Unfortunately, the story with breast cancer is not so straightforward. I pointed out that the women with palpable cancers are at greater risk of death from breast cancer, particularly those whose disease has metastasized to their axillary lymph nodes. But their fate is not sealed. As many as 40 percent of women with positive axillary nodes survive ten years, and metastatic disease develops within ten years in 20 to 30 percent of women with palpable breast cancers but negative nodes.

Breast cancer is a very heterogeneous disease. It probably is more than one disease. There is the subset that behaves as if the cancer is metastatic very early on, perhaps at the oncogenic event, the event that altered the normal cell so that its life-cycle and near-neighbor interactions were cancerous. Some breast cancers behave as if the oncogenic event occurred at multiple foci nearly simultaneously. There are parallels with lung cancer. However, unlike lung cancer, the clinical course of the patient with metastatic breast disease can be very unpredictable, sometimes seeming to find a stable plateau for years before marching on. Some breast cancers have very little in the way of malignant potential, certainly little that is relevant to the longevity of most women. The breasts of a significant minority of elderly woman harbor several such foci of cancer.

"So what?" you might say. "Who cares if it's unnecessary to assault breast cancer more often than not? It's cancer and rid me of it before I find out if I'm the unlucky one." I'm not sure you would say that, but many would. The enthusiasm for cancer screening in the United States outstrips reason. But the enthusiasm for finding early breast cancer can only be justified if the finding actually benefits the patient. Otherwise, all we are offering women diagnosed with "early breast cancer" is a predictable year of anxiety or depression or both.

The Grail of "Early Detection" May Not Be Holy

The challenge becomes much more than the early detection of breast cancer. The challenge is the early detection of breast cancer that threatens the well-being and longevity of the woman. This goal demands a screening tool that can detect cancers accurately and with such great sensitivity as to distinguish the more evil of the subsets that are still amenable to resection. The extent to which the screening instrument falls short in these characteristics is the extent to which we subject a well woman to anxiety and the iatrogenicity of unnecessary biopsies. The goal to screen this efficiently and effectively may be unattainable. In that event, we must hope for the advances in science that thwart the oncogenic event or redress the consequent pathobiology.

Enter the mammogram. To this day, mammography is the best screening tool we have. But it is a blunt instrument, to say the least. I doubt anyone would argue with that assessment. Many, however, would disagree with my real opinion that its use approaches travesty. Furthermore, mammographic screening has become an article of faith, a cause célèbre, and an industry for various constituencies in the United States and nearly so elsewhere. Many countries with national health-insurance schemes have funded mammographic screening programs: Australia, Canada, Denmark, New Zealand, Norway, Sweden, and the United Kingdom.

To be useful, mammography must overcome two biological variables: the extraordinary variability in the eyes of the beholders and the extraordinary variability in the radiodensity of normal breast tissue. A well woman must decide if mammography overcomes either sufficient to the goal of sensible screening.

Radiologists vary, sometimes dramatically, when they read the same mammograms. In a study nearly a decade ago, a panel of ten radiologists read the same 150 mammograms with no knowledge of the clinical course. For the mammograms from women who turned out to have cancer, the radiologists got the correct diagnosis between 74 and 96 percent of the time. For the mammograms from women who did not have cancer, cancer was highly suspected between 11 and 65 percent of the time. The false-negative rate is moderate, and moderately variable. The false-positive rate is considerable and also quite variable.

While there has been improvement in the training of mammographers and standardization of their machines and techniques over the past decade, it is doubtful if this has led to improved interobserver reliability. More likely, it has led to increasing hesitancy on the part of the mammography community to read a mammogram as negative, a hesitancy that is fueled by the fear of legal liability for false-negative readings — but never for false-positive readings. The most prevalent Type I Medical Malpractice case in the United States seeks remedy for a false-negative reading of a mammogram. I am aware of one prominent senior mammographer who informed a sixty-year-old patient that he would feel compelled to recommend biopsies every year given the radiological appearance of her breast tissue. Rather than choose to eschew mammography, she chose bilateral simple mastectomies (no cancer was found). The false-positive rate escalated, so that by the 1990s over a third of women in screening programs had been faced with false-positive results. That translated into one negative biopsy per woman screened per decade. The recall and negative open surgical biopsy rates are twice as high in the United States as in the United Kingdom with no trade-off in cancer detection rates. The screening experience was worrisome for many women a decade ago. It should be even more so today; this is not a pleasant rite of passage. It is why I said at the outset that the best-case analysis of the Malmö experience would not generalize to the United States; our rate of overdiagnosis and overtreatment is beyond the pale.

Even if the interpretation of the mammographic image could be rendered reliable, screening would still be highly inaccurate. All radiographic images reflect the ability of the tissue to interfere with the passage of the X-rays to the detector. The more dense the tissue, the less the detector is exposed. The images are developed so that the denser the tissue, the more white the image. The image of a breast with a predominance of fatty tissue is black, allowing fibrous strands and glandular elements to stand out. Cancers, which are usually dense, sometimes with speculations or white flecks of calcified tissue, stand out better on images of fatty breasts. However, fatty breasts are anything but the rule at any age. Younger women tend to have less fatty breasts, as the tissue is rich in glandular elements and their supporting connective tissue. Menopausal status, number of live births, post-menopausal estrogen therapy, and body mass index all influence breast density. Most importantly, breast density is a familial trait. Furthermore, there is an increase in risk for breast cancer in women with dense breasts, a risk that is not entirely a result of the compromise in mammographic sensitivity and may reflect the quantity of glandular tissue that can turn cancerous. The upshot is that the denser breast is at greater risk for breast cancer but unfortunately also for a breast cancer that escapes detection by mammography.

There is much effort to improve the sensitivity and specificity of mammography by using higher-resolution imaging techniques, some employing other modalities such as ultrasound and MRI. If the mammographic images are digitized rather than visualized on film, there is some improvement in the accuracy of the detection of cancers in women under age fifty and in women with particularly dense breasts, but not enough of an increase in accuracy to consider digital mammography an important advance. Unfortunately, we are still waiting for compelling evidence of improvement in detection; the cancers remain nearly as stealthy regardless of the technique. We seem to be asking more of anatomical imaging technology than it can possibly deliver. Glance back at the life table above. Given the issues in reliability and accuracy, can you imagine that mammography can find the twelve new breast cancers that will occur in 929 women screened annually from age sixty to sixty-four? All it will do is give the mammographers license to recommend a biopsy in 150 of these women, including many of the twelve with breast cancer but not necessarily the few whose cancer is life threatening.

Many Women Are Better Off If Their Breast Cancer Is Never Detected

Not all breast cancers need to be cured. If nothing else, mammographic screening causes a lot of women to undergo breast biopsy. The results are predictable once you learn of the earlier experience with breast self-examination and breast clinical examination.

Early in the twentieth century, pathologists described small growths comprised of the cell type that lines the ducts from the milk glands. The cells look normal and did not seem to extend across the basement membrane that delineates the duct from surrounding tissue. These small growths were thought to be "precancers." By midcentury labels such as "lobular carcinoma in situ," "intraductal carcinoma," and "ductal carcinoma in situ" (DCIS) appeared in the literature. "Carcinoma" is another term for cancer, and "in situ" suggests that there is no discernible evidence for spread. No alarm was sounded. After all, these lesions were not palpable and were generally discovered incidentally in the proximity of benign nodules that were removed because they were palpable.

With the growing emphasis on biopsying lesions discovered at self-examination, DCIS was a frequent incidental finding by the mid-1970s. It's about this time that the notion of a "precancer" really took hold. Powerful surgeons writing in powerful journals were advocating mastectomy to expunge the risk, whatever its magnitude. Some went so far as to recommend random biopsies of the other breast, which revealed one or more foci of DCIS in 50 percent and which therefore led to a recommendation of bilateral mastectomies. The "precancer" notion evolved to denote one focus of DCIS as indicative of a predisposition to developing breast cancer. After all, as many as 70 percent of breasts removed for a single lesion were found to have multiple foci of DCIS. If the label "precancer" is allowed such weight, mastectomy seems sensible, particularly given the surgical hubris of the day.

DCIS is not a variation of normal; it's not a growth of normal cells. The cells of DCIS have abnormalities of their chromosomes and often display molecular markers that are associated with evil breast cancers. There are no particular common features, just much biological heterogeneity. Nonetheless, it is likely that DCIS is a stage in the development of breast cancer, or one subtype of breast cancer. The detection of any proliferative breast lesion is associated with risk for cancer somewhere in the breast.

So, DCIS may be a "precancer," but how often is it a precursor to the palpable adenocarcinomas that were targeted in the Fisher and Veronesi trials or to metastatic disease? DCIS can grow to be sizable; can be extensive, involving ducts out to the nipple (called Paget's disease of the breast); can be anaplastic (the cells can take on a more malignant appearance); and can be necrotic (the cells in the center die, producing so-called comedo carcinomas). All of these features are associated with recurrence at the site of excision if DCIS is not completely excised. DCIS can also be invasive and is more likely to be invasive if it manifests the features just mentioned. However, the low-grade, tiny DCIS lesions take their time to become invasive and even more time to become metastatic. As is true with many other low-grade cancers, pathologists are hard-pressed to define when the lesion crosses over to microinvasive disease and then to invasive ductal carcinoma. And there remains even greater uncertainty as to the timing of these transitions, but the conceptualization countenances decades. It is defensible to excise DCIS if it is discovered in a younger patient. That's not the issue. The issues are what are the yield and the iatrogenicity of trying hard to discover DCIS in the first place?

We are witnessing an epidemic of DCIS. In 1980 DCIS accounted for only 2 percent of breast cancers. Between 1973 and 1992, the age-adjusted incidence rate of DCIS increased nearly six-fold; the age-adjusted rise in the incidence of invasive ductal cancer was only 34 percent. Women are not getting more cancers. Rather, U.S. women are getting more breast biopsies thanks to mammography. DCIS is the incidental finding of this exercise. However, DCIS is another New Age shibboleth: local excision is always recommended, often with some adjuvant radiation therapy, chemotherapy (usually tamoxifen), or surgical exploration of the nodes. And "local excision" can be extensive, to assure both "clean margins" and an opting for painful, expensive breast reconstruction.

I have more than grave doubts about this therapeutic posture. I suspect that little of importance, perhaps nothing, would be lost if all these women with tiny lesions, only detected on mammography, never knew they had DCIS. The lesion can be found in the breasts of as many as 18 percent of women who die of unrelated causes. To me the current approach to DCIS is an exercise in circular reasoning. After all, you don't do anything for longevity by curing nonlethal lesions.

Mammography Has Become a Rite of Passage

So there you have it. Mammography is a technique with compromised reliability, limited sensitivity, and troubling specificity. It is a technique that is far more likely to lead to the extirpation of lesions that are best ignored than to the extirpation of lesions that are lethal, and it will miss many of the latter. Were it any screening test other than mammography, it would be relegated to the false-start category. But it's mammography. And breast cancer is the prototype for Susan Sontag's *Illness as Metaphor*. Breast cancer is viewed as a plague. A "war" on breast cancer is viewed as a crusade. Mammography is Excalibur. Blunt or not, it's the best we have.

But mammography is not just blunt; it's so terribly blunt it approaches useless. If a woman's life was saved because of early detection of an evil breast cancer, she should thank her lucky stars rather than her mammographer.

That's not just a proclamation of a man of the academy. There are three randomized controlled trials that test whether mammography detects breast cancer in a fashion that advantages the women in the screening program — that increases the likelihood that something else will carry them off at a ripe old age. Not surprisingly, none of these trials was American. One was Canadian, the other two were Swedish. All were sizable and lengthy. The Canadian randomized controlled trial tested whether adding mammography to an annual clinical breast examination improved any relevant outcome. The Stockholm and Malmö trials add screening mammography to usual care. There are at least four other scientific studies testing the same hypothesis that are less compelling because of less powerful designs (e.g., comparing outcomes between cities or between counties). These trials are of interest, but the randomized controlled trials supersede.

The Canadian trial enrolled some 50,000 women age forty to forty-nine and 39,000 women age fifty to fifty-nine. The enrollment occurred between 1980 and 1985. All these women were examined at inception of the cohort and received instruction on breast self-examination. They were randomized to a group subjected to screening with annual mammography and a group not so screened. There were three telling observations:

1. After eleven to sixteen years of follow-up, 213 of the 50,000 women who were forty to forty-nine years of age at inception of the cohort had died of breast cancer. These cancer deaths, and incident cancers that were not (yet) fatal, distributed equally between the mammography group and the usual care group.
2. After thirteen years of follow-up of the almost 40,000 women that were fifty to fifty-nine at inception of the cohort, 622 invasive and 71 in situ cancers had been detected in the group afforded mammography, as opposed to 610 and 16 in the group screened without mammography. There were 107 deaths from breast cancer among the women subjected to mammographic screening and 105 among the women not so screened.
3. Based on these data, several — but not all — North American bodies have backed down from recommending mammographic screening in women between age forty and forty-nine. None has backed down from mammographic screening over age fifty. Several have waffled, including the U.S. Preventive Services Task Force, which, in its 2002 iteration, recommends "screening mammography, with or without clinical breast examination, every 1 to 2 years for women aged 40 and older." The American College of Physicians doesn't waffle. We all agree that breast cancer is one of the most common causes of that most uncommon event, death of women in their forties. However, the American College of Physicians opine that the

risks of unnecessary biopsies far outweighs the likelihood of saving a life and therefore does not recommend mammography before age fifty.

Don't for one moment think that any of these august professional bodies operates free of sociopolitical constraints. Two stouthearted participants published the saga of the "consensus conference" convened by the National Institutes of Health in January 1997 in *JAMA*. The "consensus" was to equivocate regarding screening mammography in women age forty to forty-nine. However, this "consensus" was born of acrimony and was met with acrimony. Not only did the American Cancer Society disagree, but the U.S. Senate passed a resolution repudiating the consensus, demanding revised guidelines and convening investigative hearings. Woolf and Lawrence describe a climate and a response that was an assault on intellectual freedom. Three months after the "consensus panel" published its report, the National Cancer Institute reversed its stand and recommended mammographic screening for women forty to forty-nine years old. For those of us who are students of Karl Popper, this saga is dramatic but predictable. There are many, in many constituencies, committed to inculcating mammography into American life. This is the stand of the American news media in the 1990s, as documented by a published analysis of the coverage. Science is no match for such advocacy. The science and its messengers are not viewed as refuting the hypothesis that screening mammography is a solution to the specter of a woman dying of breast cancer. Rather, the messengers are viewed as callously refuting the problem. The messengers can be vilified, not just by those with vested and invested interests in promulgating mammography, but by the women on whose behalf the science is designed. Again, for students of Popper, this is a predictable dialectic.

I discussed the follow-up to the Malmö trial at the outset of this chapter. The Malmö trial enrolled over 40,000 residents age forty-five to seventy between 1976 and 1978. The Stockholm trials enrolled 60,000 residents in 1981. Both studies monitored their cohorts for at least eleven years. There was not a hint that the women of Stockholm were spared death by breast cancer thanks to the mammography. There was such a hint in the Malmö cohort. These trials have been reviewed and meta-analyzed ad nauseam. Because of methodological subtleties, the Stockholm trial is considered more lacking than the Malmö trial.

In 2001 two Danish investigators, Olsen and Gøetzsche, brandishing the impressive imprimatur of the Cochrane Collaboration (an international collaborative effort to offer "evidence-based" appraisals for many clinical challenges), published a series of papers examining the literature supporting the recommendations for screening mammography. They consider, not surprisingly, the Malmö and Canadian trials as the only trials of sufficient quality to hold sway. Their interpretation is similar to mine: mammography offers very little if anything of value to the women screened. To the contrary, mammography causes the screened women to undergo a dramatic excess of surgical procedures and adjuvant therapies to no demonstrable avail.

There is a counterargument, which is based on a secondary analysis and therefore is inherently suspect. However, the Finnish scholar, epidemiologist, and statistician Olli Miettinen launched the argument. The world of epidemiology has no more fertile, critical, or inventive mind. I will address Miettinen's alternative interpretation in the supplementary readings to this chapter because it is worthy of consideration.

But the argument does not hold sway with me. Harold Sox, the current editor of the *Annals of Internal Medicine*, has had a long-standing interest in evidence-based medicine and in mammography in particular. His comment on the U.S. Preventive Services Task Force recommendations, and the state of the art in 2002, concludes with a mandate to keep women informed as to the nuances of the debate. Fletcher and Elmore argue along the same lines for screening in women younger than fifty (whose close relatives have been spared breast or ovarian cancer early in life), although these authors still recommend screening for women fifty to sixty-nine. Steven Goodman, writing a companion editorial to Hal Sox, points out how Swiftian the debate has become. If we take the most optimistic approach to these data as they relate to women aged forty to forty-nine, this is much ado about almost nothing of value. Much the same perspective applies to mammography in women fifty years of age or older.

I have been emphasizing the randomized controlled trials, as they are the only way we can speak to efficacy. However, one can argue that "life" has variables that cannot be captured in such trials. Perhaps mammography in practice is more effective than one would predict from the trials because of factors that we have yet to define. In this regard, there are a number of "ecological" experiments, happenstances that can be informative.

The Australians have weighed in. They statistically modeled the data from "BreastScreen Australia," a monitoring data set of considerable size and duration. In this analysis, "Benefits and harms of screening mammography are relatively finely balanced." Norway, Sweden, and Denmark introduced screening programs in a fashion that allowed them to compare the effectiveness with historical experience or with regions without the programs. In Norway and

Sweden there was an increase in detection but no effect on outcome in terms of all-cause mortality. In Copenhagen, there were restraints on the diagnosis of DCIS and on the need for biopsy. Nonetheless, there was a decrease in breast cancer mortality, but not in all-cause mortality. If there is a benefit to screening even in countries where there is caution as to overdiagnosis, it is marginal.

The debate in the United Kingdom has been particularly instructive. Its national mammographic screening program is under scrutiny. Speaking as a "consultant breast surgeon," J. Michael Dixon is convinced that despite limitations, breast-cancer screening saves lives. Dixon is convinced that the newer machines with their technical improvements render the older trials irrelevant. He estimates that for every 400 women screened for ten years, one will be spared death from breast cancer. As you learned in chapter 2, this low level of effectiveness is beyond scientific determination, though certainly not beyond polemic or marketing. Because of this, the Nordic Cochrane Centre is arguing that women should be apprised of this level of effectiveness and afforded an opportunity for informed consent.

In 2007 the Clinical Efficacy Assessment Subcommittee of the American College of Physicians weighed in with a similar statement, but only for women forty to forty-nine years of age. I suspect they shied away from a more general statement for fear of revisiting the anger and controversy engendered by the National Cancer Institute Panel in 1997. Few in America will stand by silently with a similar recommendation for older women. That's a sad state of affairs. Schwartz and Woloshin took another stab at calculating the benefit that accrues to women over fifty who are taking advantage of mammographic screening programs. If 1,000 women enter into mammographic screening programs for the next ten years, 994 will not have died from breast cancer. If these 1,000 women avoided mammographic screening, 991 would not have died from breast cancer after ten years. Big deal? Measurable? Worth it? Those are questions that should be addressed to every woman before mammograms are ordered — as long as we are going to indemnify the procedure (see chapter 14).

In the supplementary reading for this chapter, additional data sets are discussed and illuminating elements of the scientific debate displayed.

chapter seven

The Beleaguered Prostate

Interspersed between all the direct-to-consumer drug advertisements, the hawking of the latest procedures and gimmicks by providers, and the boasting of the prowess of the local or not-so-local hospital are the announcements of health-promotion, disease-prevention, public-service programs. Your friendly health insurer is inducing you to check your cholesterol and blood sugar so that you can be treated early. Someone is urging colonoscopy, others newfangled mammography or total body CT scans, or the like. Blood-pressure cuffs dot the landscape. Health fairs abound. After reading the prior chapters, you will appreciate how much this activity serves purveyors far more effectively than the public, if the public is served at all. The "not-for-profit" health insurers are as damnable as the others in this regard, and much more (see chapter 14).

Tucked into this rush to preserve your health are the screening programs for prostate cancer. As a public service, blood is assayed for Prostate Specific Antigen (PSA). Urologists may offer to insert a gloved index finger in your rectum seeking telltale bumps on your prostate. Undergoing such screening starting at age fifty is advised by the American Cancer Society and the American Urological Association. It is considered a standard of care in the United States (though PSA-screening programs are not universal; the United Kingdom has no such undertaking, for example). PSA and digital rectal screening is hotly debated for reasons that will become clear shortly. However, don't assume that all this is a national hypocrisy. Almost 90 percent of male physicians aged fifty and older have had a PSA, and nearly all urologists have had one. I am one of the male physicians over age fifty who will not submit to having a PSA, let alone a rectal examination. Here's why.

Screening is defensible if most, if not all, of the following goals are met. First, the screening must detect something that is meaningful to me, some important disease or high likelihood of an important disease. Second, the screening must be efficient; it must have few false positives and few false negatives. And finally, if a true positive is detected, something meaningful can be done about it, something that provides much more benefit to me than harm. Screening for prostate cancer fails on all counts.

The Prostate and Its Cancer

The prostate is a walnut-sized gland that wraps itself around the male urethra as it travels from the bladder toward the base of the penis. It is far more important for its role in disease than its function in health. In the aging male it grows unevenly, and its glandular elements form lumps, or nodules. Lurking in this aging gland is the high likelihood of one of these nodules being comprised of cells with biology that is so altered as to qualify as cancer. Prostate cells produce many substances, some of which are peculiar to these cells, and one of which is now commonly measured in the blood — the PSA. PSA testing is frequently used in early detection programs because in general the higher the level, the more likely a cancer is lurking among the nodules.

Bob Dole, Arnold Palmer, Norman Schwarzkopf, and Rudy Giuliani have trumpeted their triumph over prostate cancer. All learned of their blight thanks to PSA screening. All suffered through the definition of their plight: the prostate biopsies, blood tests, and imaging studies designed to prove that they have prostate cancer and discern whether it is still confined to the gland. Then they met the enemy and it was vanquished. It was vanquished by a surgical procedure, the radical prostatectomy, that is designed to remove the entire gland but spare the urethra and the nerves that course through the region — the latter responsible for bladder control and erectile function. All bear scars of the battle, more than surgical scars. Some are worse for wear, some maybe not. Dole, for one, has been seen on television hawking the pharmaceutical he takes to treat his erectile dysfunction. All these men, and many others of similar or lesser repute, feel that engaging this enemy was tactically sound. They feel brave in their battling and justify any untoward consequences by the assurance that death by prostate cancer will not be their fate. They have won this war on cancer.

Today, the majority of men over age fifty in the United States have had a PSA level determined. Most with elevated PSAs undergo prostate biopsy. Even those with a negative biopsy pay a price in worry that lingers long after they are informed of the negative result. Each year, some 200,000 American men learn they are blighted by prostate cancer; half will choose the cure promised by removing their prostates. Others will choose less-radical procedures involving radiation therapy, either from an external source or from radioactive pellets implanted in the prostate. Such procedures are obviously less invasive, but they are also less certain to expunge the "crab." Less-invasive treatments are a little less likely to result in erectile dysfunction and urinary incontinence, although not that much less likely. Their spouses, their peers, and the public at large applaud these men who incisively confront their cancer. They have overcome anxiety, withstood indignity and pain, and subjugated morbidity in order to reap this benefit of modern medicine. Their triumph in the war on cancer lights the path so that others will follow.

It is no surprise that most physicians suggest PSA screening for prostate cancer. If the screening is negative, the physician and the patient sigh in relief. If the screening is positive, the enemy is revealed, hopefully in time. Screening awareness is everywhere, from the lay press to the U.S. Postal Service, which chimed in several years ago with a 33-cent stamp that called for "Prostate Cancer Awareness" and "Annual Checkups and Tests." William Catalona of Washington University and Patrick Walsh of Johns Hopkins Hospital are two urologists who attained near celebrity status as proponents of screening and the algorithm it engenders, particularly the algorithm that leads to radical prostatectomy.

American men expect to be screened. Any physician who advises otherwise has much to explain. Any physician who foregoes offering screening is ripe for a malpractice suit. Prostate screening is a rite of passage. It makes sense. It is common sense.

If only it worked.

Case-Control Studies

Case-control studies are generally considered the first crack at probing for an association between an exposure and a health effect, in this case between PSA screening and metastatic prostate cancer (prostate cancer that had spread widely). One study identifies a group of men with metastatic cancer and age-matched men who did not have metastatic cancer to see if one or the other group had undergone PSA screening more frequently. When this was done by surveying the experience in the Toronto community, it turned out that only 25 percent of men over age forty-five had ever been screened — a bit more in the controls than in those who went on to metastatic cancer. When a case-control study was performed in ten Veterans Affairs medical centers in the United States, among 72,000 patients there were 501 cases between 1991 and

1995. About 85 percent of these veterans had not undergone PSA screening regardless of whether they ended up cases or controls. The upshot of these case-control studies is that if there is a benefit to be derived from PSA screening, it is small and may pertain only to a subset of the population at risk. In these two case-control studies, the investigators attempted to discern characteristics such as coincident diseases (comorbidities), socioeconomic status, race, etc., that would denote a subset for whom screening was clearly more effective. Such an exploratory analysis is seldom a match for subtle differences in effectiveness; these studies are no exception.

The Scandinavian Trial at Five Years and at Ten Years

Prostate screening has never made good sense, if it has made sense at all. I will explain its flaws shortly. Since the proof is in the pudding, to paraphrase Karl Popper, let me take you through a landmark randomized controlled trial from Scandinavia. In 1988 a group of Scandinavian investigators started recruiting healthy men under age seventy-five with untreated and newly diagnosed prostate cancers. The tumor had to be early stage: confined to the prostate, not appearing too evil under the microscope, and not secreting an extreme amount of PSA into the blood. By 1999, 695 men were enrolled. At enrollment these volunteers were randomized so that half underwent a radical prostatectomy. For the other half, there was "watchful waiting."

The results after some five years were published in the *New England Journal of Medicine* in the fall of 2002. A second paper appeared in 2005, when the average follow-up approached ten years. The critical result at five years is in Table 5. Because men of different ages entered the cohort at different times, the analysis of these outcomes requires demanding statistics. Some were followed longer than others, and some were older and less likely to survive to 2000 even if they didn't have prostate cancer. The table demonstrates that if the volunteer was assigned to undergo radical prostatectomy, he was 50 percent less likely to die of prostate cancer. But he was as likely to be dead by the year 2000 from some other cause (the relative hazard of 83 percent was too likely to occur by chance for the 17 percent reduction in hazard to be meaningful). Prostatectomy does not change the date of death; it only changes the likelihood that prostate cancer will be the reaper.

There's another daunting message in this table. True, the men treated by "watchful waiting" were twice as likely to die of prostate cancer, but the men who underwent the procedure were not spared that fate. Six years after radical

TABLE 5. Five-Year Mortality Rates in the Scandinavian Trial Comparing Radical Prostatectomy with Watchful Waiting

	Watchful Waiting	Prostatectomy	Relative Hazard (percentage)
Deaths from prostate cancer	31	16	50
Overall mortality	62	53	83

Source: Adapted from Holmberg et al. (2002).

prostatectomy, 16 of the 347 men died of prostate cancer — a crude mortality rate of 5 percent. That means that even though their disease was defined as "early," it wasn't, or that "radical" prostatectomy was not radical enough. Regardless, no one should think that surgery will vanquish their risk of death from prostate cancer; it will only reduce it by half. And no one should think that surgery will increase his time on this earth; it will only change the likelihood of the mode of demise, the proximate cause of death.

The Scandinavian study probed the personal cost of radical prostatectomy. Sexual, urinary, and bowel function were monitored along with certain aspects of the quality of life. Notable results are presented in Table 6. Remember that this is an elderly and aging cohort. The "watchful waiting" group is not spared urological disorders. In fact, they suffer more from obstructive symptoms than the prostatectomy group. The aging male prostate enlarges, mainly reflecting the disordered growth of the glandular tissue, which creates multiple benign nodules that may impinge on the urethra as it passes through the gland. This "benign prostatic hypertrophy" (BPH) is a normal part of the aging process and is the cause of prostatism. Prostatism is the name given to the various symptoms engendered by the prostate's enlargement: increased urinary frequency, decreased forcefulness of the urinary stream, and dribbling. Radical prostatectomy, by removing the impinging nodules, decreases the likelihood of prostatism.

However, the trade-off also is documented in the table. Nearly 15 percent of the patients who undergo radical prostatectomy will have to cope with incontinence by wearing a diaper. That's a catastrophe for most. Nearly as many men will be afflicted with greatly distressful erectile dysfunction consequent to the surgery. For these men, that is a catastrophe.

Interestingly, there is no discernible difference between the groups in overall physical and psychological functioning. Nearly half of all these aging men

TABLE 6. Adverse Effects in the Scandinavian Trial Comparing Radical Prostatectomy with Watchful Waiting (All Figures Percentages)

Function	Prostatectomy	Watchful Waiting
Erectile Function		
Greatly distressful dysfunction	30	17
Greatly distressful decreased intercourse	28	16
Urinary Leakage		
Moderately or greatly distressed by	29	9
Regular dependence on diaper or bag	14	1

Source: Adapted from Steineck et al. (2002).

describe themselves as suffering decreased physical capacity, a moderate or high degree of worry, and low or moderate subjective quality of life. That's true whether they were subjected to radical prostatectomy or just observed. The burdens of urinary incontinence and erectile dysfunction are subsumed in this alarming universe of pall.

The inferences that can be derived from the fate of this cohort some five years later are not quite the same. Here's the outcome at ten years: after a median follow-up of 8.2 years, 8.6 percent of the men assigned to surgery had died of prostate cancer, compared with 14.4 percent waiting watchfully as one would expect from the earlier end point. However, the overall mortality that had been about 10 percent in both groups at five years increased differentially, so that 24 percent in the surgery group died as opposed to 30 percent in the watchful waiting group. Of course, there was more progression, short of disease-specific fatality, in the watchful waiting group, and more use of chemotherapy. Attempts to look at subsets are compromised by the small numbers. However, there is the suggestion of meaningful survival benefit of surgery in men younger than sixty-five.

The possibility that early prostatectomy will prolong the patient's life is also raised by two observational studies that were contemporaneous with the study above. One is a twenty-year cohort study of men in Connecticut with localized prostate cancer at the inception of the cohort who were treated with watchful waiting, sometimes with hormone manipulation therapy, but not with surgery. The annual mortality rate from prostate cancer was stable (33 per 1,000 person-years) for fifteen years and then escalated. A similar observation derived from a Swedish cohort. Were it not for the trade-offs, one would recommend early surgery, particularly in the younger man. But the trade-offs are substantial, particularly in the younger man. Besides, I'm not even certain the putative benefit pertains to the situation today.

Today, nearly all prostate cancer is detected by PSA screening. This was not the case when the three studies discussed above were undertaken since there were no PSA-screening programs. In those cohorts, cancer was discovered incidentally during a procedure designed to improve urinary flow by removing nodules that impinged on the urethra. Others were discovered when a physician, yet unaware of the dismal accuracy of examining the prostate for cancer, determined that a nodule felt ominous and arranged for a biopsy. Today all a man, middle-aged or older, has to do is go before most primary-care physicians and screening will result. The results are causing vast numbers of men to undergo biopsy, so that far more men who are otherwise well learn that they have prostate cancer. One should not assume that the results of radical prostatectomy in this New Age cohort will have anything in common with those outlined above. The New Age cohort is dripping "lead-time bias" by virtue of the earlier detection. It is possible that the consequent surgery will advantage more of the younger men with localized disease. It is more likely that we will be operating on younger men for no good reason.

An otherwise well man has much to consider before opting for screening for prostate cancer. If the digital rectal exam and/or the PSA is positive, and a biopsy is positive, then a radical prostatectomy might effect a 15 percent decrease in the likelihood he will die of prostate cancer and, if he's younger than sixty-five, a chance of a meaningful delay in the timing of his death. The quantity of life to be gained is indeterminate, but almost certainly small. The trade-off is in overall quality of life. The procedure is likely to produce a major insult in erectile and urinary function in well over 15 percent of men. For me, prostatectomy is no choice, nor is the gentler options that have no more favorable a benefit/ risk ratio.

As for men over sixty-five, there is additional science to bolster my convictions.

The Prostates of Seattle vs. the Prostates of Connecticut

The 1990s witnessed the flowering of the PSA-screening agenda. However, its implementation was not uniform across the United States. The Medicare beneficiaries aged sixty-five to seventy-nine residing in the Seattle area between 1987 and 1997 were five times more likely to be screened, and twice as likely to be biopsied, than the Medicare cohort residing in Connecticut. It follows that the Seattle cohort was more likely to be "helped" by early treatment of their cancers. Nearly 3 percent of the Seattle cohort underwent radical prostatectomy, and another 4 percent had radiation therapy. The respective numbers in Connecticut were 0.5 percent and 3 percent. However, there was no difference between the two groups in the likelihood of dying from prostate cancer! In fact, there was no difference in prostate-specific cancer mortality if you were biopsied at age sixty-five to sixty-nine, seventy to seventy-four, or seventy-five to seventy-nine. These are the ages at which nearly all prostate-specific deaths occur. Death from prostate cancer earlier than sixty-five is exceedingly rare.

The Seattle-Connecticut comparison is an observational, so-called ecological, cohort study. As such, it is not as powerful as the randomized controlled trial for testing hypotheses regarding the utility of PSA screening. Nonetheless, the take-home messages of these studies and the Scandinavian experiment are consonant. I don't envy the prostates of Puget Sound in the 1990s.

Why PSA Screening Is Disappointing at Best and Probably Harmful

The reader could probably write this section at this point. It will echo the lessons of the prior two chapters. Here are the facts.

1. After midlife, the normal prostate grows in a disorganized fashion so that the gland is riddled with nodules of glandular tissue. It normally grows large and lumpy. Furthermore, the lumps that are benign are exceedingly difficult to distinguish by palpation from a malignant lump in their midst. Hence, the time-honored tradition of the "digital rectal exam" to palpate the prostate for cancer turns out to be as nonspecific and insensitive as it is unpleasant and indelicate.

2. Starting at midlife, the likelihood is that some of the cells that comprise the benign nodules will lose the microscopic and biological features of their mature compatriots. They take on the characteristics of cancerous cells, a localized cluster of cancer cells (i.e., carcinoma in situ). In fact, given the glandular elements they populate, they are another example of ductal carcinoma in situ (see chapter 6). Nearly every man will have carcinoma in situ by age eighty, and probably most in midlife. Obviously, most never are aware of the cancer they harbor. These cells are generally slow to grow and slow to metastasize. Death supervenes long before the prostate cancer harbored by the vast majority of men is ever heard from.

3. The biology of these cancer cells is different, including their propensity to secrete prostate specific antigen (PSA). When their number is small, the serum PSA is not discernibly or consistently elevated. Normal prostate cells also secrete PSA. Inflammation and trauma can cause nonmalignant prostate cells to secrete more PSA than ductal carcinoma in situ cells. Hence, PSA is not "cancer specific." The higher the blood level and the more persistent the elevation, the more likely it derives from cancer, and the more likely the cancer burden is larger. There is a suggestion that the faster the PSA rises, the more likely one is faced with a prostate cancer with a malignant biology. PSA is a flawed screening tool. Not as flawed as the digital rectal exam, but a very blunt tool nonetheless. It offers an excuse to perform biopsies, which in turn offer some likelihood that we will stumble on some cancerous cells lurking among the glandular elements. This is a fallacy that echoes the mammography story.

4. The "biopsy" is really a number of sticks of nodules with a needle that cuts out a core of tissue. Who can hear that cancer was seen under the microscope without a sinking feeling? How many can turn away from the possibility of cure? The urologist recites probabilities based on PSA level and the "Gleason score." The Gleason score is a measure of how invasive and distorted the cells look under the microscope. Cancers that appear most disordered are exceptional, a few percent of positive biopsies, and may represent a biologically distinctive form of the disease. Most biopsies run a range of histology that bears little on the probability of the cancer spreading, as was the case in the Scandinavian study. Perhaps the benefit/risk ratio would be compelling if radical prostatectomy were reserved for the rare individuals whose PSA and "Gleason scores" were both extremely high and who still had no evidence of metastatic spread beyond the prostate. That is a hypothesis ripe for testing — if the testing did not require so many low-yield biopsies to find one high score sample. I wouldn't be surprised to learn that the surgery does not advantage even this subset. It is possible that such tumors spread very early, rendering any surgery after the fact.

All this is missing the forest for the trees. We saw the forest in the Scandinavian trial and the ecological Medicare data. No elderly man should undergo prostate cancer screening. Elderly is generally accepted as seventy or greater. Nonetheless, in a recent analysis, half of a cohort of nearly 600,000 U.S. veterans over age seventy were still undergoing PSA screening despite the data that suggests all they will be afforded is a likelihood of iatrogenicity. Furthermore, no man younger than seventy should be led to believe that PSA screening is clearly sensible. In one British survey of patients with suspected or confirmed prostate cancer, few men were aware that the evidence of benefit from screening was so tenuous. Those who became aware regretted having been screened.

I am writing this book in the hopes of arming others with the "hard" questions to ask before they submit to any screening program. If they rely on the currently available educational sources, including those on the Internet, those generally found in doctors' offices, and those that decorate health fairs, they will be misled.

chapter eight

Disease Mongering

We are a country of obese, hypercholesterolemic, hypertensive, diabetic, osteopenic, depressed, pitiful creatures perched on the edge of a cliff staring at condors: cancer, heart attacks, strokes, dementia, fractures, and worse. We fear for our future. We teach our children that they, too, must live in fear for their futures.

We mobilize all of our courage when faced with creakiness, achiness, heartburn and heartache, headache and bellyache, constipation or diarrhea, impotence, sleeplessness, and even restless legs. No infant can simply be fussy, and no child can simply be fidgety, obstreperous, or below average in performance. We are told that all these are symptoms, or at least harbingers, of disease. We are a vigilant society.

We are also a modern people blessed by remedies. For us, mortality is an abstraction, a formless beast that we can bring to heel by the determined application of the latest and most convincing scientific insights. All daunting, unpredictable challenges to our sense of well-being can yield to a canny choice of ministration. We exalt our modern scientific medicine; our forefathers had but sages, often religious sages, pointing to the path to a good life, if not a longer life. Today we wait, breath bated, for the next pronouncements of the biomedical establishment. Nearly all in our personal, intimate life that is untoward is now under their purview. Maladies beware.

How are we to know if we are well? We are bombarded by the print and broadcast media with the scare of the week. We are bombarded by purveyors with the cure of the weekend. Can we ignore these helpful people? They have taught us to be proactive. Can we ignore our body whenever it seems the slightest bit awry?

What's not a disease?

Something will go awry, and do so repeatedly, some alteration in our body that makes us question our wellness and that challenges our sense of invincibility. And each of us will die, usually carried off by one of several diseases standing between us and our eighty-fifth birthday. To be human is to be challenged in the course of living and to have it all come to an end.

To be well is not the absence of disease. To be well is to have some sense of invincibility: nothing, or nothing more, will happen to me that I can't overcome. Rare is the person whose sense of invincibility cannot be rattled, if not pulverized, by the voice of authority. When the authority is medical, and there's little or no valid reason for alarm, it's called medicalization (as opposed to chiropracterization, or physical therapistization, or naturopathization, or . . .). When you should be reassured but instead are taught to fear, that's disease mongering.

None of this is new. Your parents and grandparents confronted medicalization and disease mongering. For these past generations, orgasm and thinness were medicalized. Today, both are normal, while lack of orgasm and chunkiness are medicalized. As you will learn in chapter 13, at the turn of the twentieth century Sylvester Graham had invented his cracker, John Harvey Kellogg his corn flakes, Franz Mesmer his magnets and hypnotism, A. T. Still the osteopathy, D. D. Palmer the chiropractic, Mary Baker Eddy Christian Science, and so much more. All of this, and the Pentecostal movement, played on fear of illness and death. Today, the vernacular is riddled with scientific inferences spewed by physicians and metaphysicians. There is no better scientific support that screening you for high cholesterol, diabetes, osteoporosis, or breast and prostate cancer will advantage you than there is for neutraceuticals, Asian cures, poking and prodding, echinacea and garlic, glucosamine, vitamin E, and the like. Sectarian gobbledegook competes with the medical gobbledegook for your vulnerabilities. Neither camp is above disease mongering.

How about some reality testing? The death rate is one per person and the time of death is set near to your eighty-fifth birthday. Any claim to a science that offers a path to longevity beyond eighty-five years is fatuous. The best we can expect is to arrive at our eighty-fifth birthday feeling reasonably well, even healthful, regardless of our burden of disease. Modern medicine has something to contribute to our quest for longevity thus defined, but not much and certainly not as much as we are told. This reality is discussed in detail in chapter 1. If we fall victim to diseases that threaten and damage our tissues and organs, modern medicine offers cures for some and important comfort for others. However, most personal predicaments are more disconcerting than damaging.

Appropriate recourse and appropriateness of recourse are less certain, even contentious.

One choice is to try to "deal with it." From every side, from family members, from the lay press, from purveyors of sundries, we will hear of options in conceptualizing the predicament and in palliation. All this fuels our common sense. We have only prior experience and conviction to comfort us until we are better, or our conviction yields to all the advice.

Then we can choose to seek care. For most personal predicaments, there is a menu of providers. Each proclaims a theoretical underpinning. Each has a privileged language. Each offers an assortment of modalities that are applied with a skill said to reflect specialized training. For most of the predicaments of life, from fatigue to back pain, nearly all the modalities are ineffective, a few are minimally effective. What may be effective is the act of being treated rather than the treatment. We will learn the language and conceptualizations of the professional into whose hands we have consigned ourselves. Our self-image will change, as will our idioms of distress and of wellness. We will be different.

If you have chosen to entrust your care to a physician, you will be medicalized. Not all physicians are comfortable with this process. Many would rather reassure you than diagnose you and prescribe something that "might" work. These are the physicians who would like to tell you, "It's miserable, but it's not evil. Get on with life as best you can. It, too, shall pass." Can you countenance such? Or would you rather be medicalized?

The Enigma of Health

We care little as to how many diseases we have or which of our diseases carries us off as octogenarians. We care little as long as we can cope readily with whatever challenges our diseases present, as long as our passing is swift, and as long as our time is ripe. The pregnant phrase is "as long as we can cope readily with whatever challenges our diseases present." To be well is not to be free of physical and emotional symptoms or to be spared physical and emotional challenges. If that were the definition of "well," there never would be a well person, at least not one who was well for long. Life, normal life and its living, is replete with intermittent and remittent morbidity. To be well is to be able to cope efficiently and effectively with the challenges.

Hans-George Gadamer lived to a ripe old age and earned his place in the Pantheon of twentieth-century philosophers. Gadamer held medicine in highest regard when it would stare into "the face of illness . . . to discover the great enigma of health." Gadamer realized that to be well was not simply to be free of disease:

> The fundamental fact remains that it is illness and not health which "objectifies" itself, which confronts us as something opposed to us and which forces itself on us. . . . [T]he real mystery lies in the hidden character of health. Health does not actually present itself to us. Of course one can also attempt to establish standard values for health. But the attempt to impose these standard values on a healthy individual would only result in making that person ill. It lies in the nature of health that it sustains its own proper balance and proportion. The appeal to standard values which are derived by averaging out different empirical data and then simply applied to particular cases is inappropriate to determining health and cannot be forced upon it. (Gadamer 1996)

The discussion of the Metabolic Syndrome in chapter 3 illustrates the fashion in which the imposing of "standard values on a healthy individual" results in labeling many as ill, thereby medicalizing "healthy individuals" so that they grasp at unproven remedies for contrived diseases that are said to be life threatening.

Gadamer first penned his insight as to the enigma of health in 1991. By 1991 there was a literature, a science if you prefer, that could have informed this insight. However, it resided in corners of the clinical and epidemiological literatures, corners seldom visited by twentieth-century philosophers. In 1991 that literature was scant; today it is the product of a mature science. That literature will inform our discussion in the chapters that follow and in the supplementary readings for this chapter. It is a literature that attempts to define and quantify health. It is the counterbalance to the traditional epidemiological literature that attempts to define and quantify illness. The traditional literature takes the patient as its reference point. The epidemiology of health takes the experience of morbidity in community-dwelling people as its reference point. It is the scientific analysis of well-being.

The assertion that coping with intermittent and remittent morbidities is "normal" is on firm scientific grounds. None of us will live long without headache or backache or bellyache, heartache or heartburn, sadness or malaise, diarrhea or constipation, and on and on. When we pause in recognition of any such challenge to our sense of well-being, we are faced with a *predicament*. "Predicament" is a convenient term for my purposes, as it captures the challenge without casting aspersions or assuming causation. I can find no such word in a language other than English. We all have personal predicaments that often challenge our sense of well-being. Some are catastrophic: overwhelming chest or abdominal pain, acute neurological symptoms, broken bones, etc. For these events, choosing to be a patient of someone licensed to practice medicine or surgery is more than sensible; it's mandatory. Modern medicine has much to offer if we fall victim to such events. Most personal predicaments are less threatening to our physical well-being. That they are less than catastrophic gives us an opportunity to pause and consider what to do. Some have been medicalized to such good effect that it is as sensible to seek medical care for them as for the catastrophic events: burning on urination, fever and a productive cough, abnormal vaginal bleeding, for example. However, for many other personal predicaments appropriate recourse is less certain, even contentious. There is a science that informs our choosing among the options. Everyone must choose.

We can choose to remain a person with a predicament for as long as the morbidity persists. Or we can choose to seek care. The pressure to choose any option or any particular option reflects your common sense, just as choosing to remain a person with a predicament does. If you choose to seek the care of someone licensed to practice medicine or surgery, you move from a person with a predicament to a patient with an illness. This particular transition is a form of medicalization. Medicalization has a pejorative connotation, which is appropriate if you are not better off for the choice. Before choosing to be a patient, one would be wise to consider the ramifications: How will you fare as a patient with an illness? Is this an option that advantages you?

Medicalization has no corollary terms. If we choose to be the patient of a chiropractor, do we hear of chiropractorization? Physical therapization? Herbalization? Why not?

The next five chapters are object lessons in medicalization and disease mongering. They are not meant to be a reproach to our personal strengths, or a condemnation of those who play off our weaknesses. They are meant to illustrate that dynamic, and arm the reader with the perspective that maintains a level playing field. The supplementary readings for this chapter are supplementary, indeed. The notion of a dynamic between our fears regarding our health and the remedies of the day is further explored.

chapter
Creakiness
nine

We live in a time when science seems to be bursting with promise. Details of the very latest in diagnosis and treatment find their way into the headlines of print media and the feature stories of broadcast media. We are told to expect cures. All of us respond with great anticipation, some with speculative investing. Hidden in the bluster is another realm of advancement where contemporary science offers more than promise. We are witness to a revolution in our understanding of the aspects of life in "advanced" societies that foster or compromise our sense of well-being and thereby our sense of invincibility. There are many important examples, many that are surprising, even counterintuitive, and challenging to an establishment vested in the status quo. Backache is an object lesson. The following is the current evidence-based understanding of the commonest form of low back pain — the backache that bedevils working-age adults who are otherwise totally well. This is a pain that does not involve the legs and that comes on with no unusual precipitant. Years ago, I coined the term "regional back pain" to capture this circumstance.

It's abnormal to go long without experiencing regional back pain. Low back pain is one of many recurring predicaments of life, like heartburn and heartache. To be well is not to be spared. To be well is to have the wherewithal to cope until the pain goes away, cope so well that the episode is not even memorable.

Low back pain relates to posture and movement. It hurts less when lying down. It hurts more when slouched forward in a chair or propped up on pillows, let alone bending over. One is forced to choose between less pain and more invalidity. Compelling science says less pain is not worth it. Feeling useless just enhances the suffering without enhancing the rate of healing. Take an over-the-counter analgesic and get on with life as best you can.

Low back pain will go away, but seldom overnight. Weeks are more like it, and months for a few. One should never despair. Nor should one feel so desperate that one grasps at straws. And there are many offering straws, many who will gird your loins, push, pull, and poke you, offer you potions and pills, and attempt to excise the evil. Realize that despite all the jargon, there is no one who can reliably pinpoint the cause of your plight. Realize that despite all their theories and all you hear on the street, no one has a "modality" they can apply to you that can be shown to benefit you. All these helpful people are engulfing you and your pain in their frame of reference, in their belief system. You will no longer suffer alone. But your narrative of illness will change, as will your self-image, permanently. Despite these ministrations, you will not return to your prior state of well-being any more rapidly. If you return at all, you will greet any recurrence of the back pain with idioms that were taught to you. If all this is a pleasing prospect, go for it. But do so informed.

For some of us, coping is overwhelmed. Certainly, that could reflect the severity of the pain. But science informs us that another explanation is far more likely. It is not the pain but other aspects of life that blunt our coping skills. Leading the list of confounders are adverse aspects of life at home or at work (see chapter 12). If you cannot cope any longer, find someone trustworthy to discuss the possibility that the pain is surrogate for some assault on your coping skills. In all likelihood, you coped with similar predicaments in the past. If you are unwilling to countenance the possibility that something in life is more a pain than the pain in the back, you run the risk of feeling so desperate that you submit to pills, potions, magical thinking, or ineffective surgery before you come to grips with your psychosocial adversity. Surgery cannot excise an intolerable job, nor can an intolerable home situation yield to manual therapy. Don't let the pain cloud your thinking. Don't let preconceived notions lead you astray.

That's regional low back pain. It is but one of the regional musculoskeletal disorders that afflict working-age people who are otherwise well, who have no complicating major neurological deficits, and who have suffered no violent or even specific precipitant. A region of their musculoskeletal system hurts, particularly when that region is used. Most episodes of backache, neck pain, knee pain, shoulder pain, and the like are regional musculoskeletal disorders. These disorders are common. They rank second as the reason anyone seeks primary medical care. They rank first as the reason workers suffer long-term disability. They are *raison d'être* for entire professions, such as the chiropractic, osteopathy, and various manual therapies. They have left an indelible mark on language. Suppositions about the regional musculoskeletal disorders, about their cause and cure, are as powerful a contemporary social construction as suppositions about the sanctity of marriage or the goals of union movements or the ethics of academic health centers.

The regional musculoskeletal disorders support a great number of helpful people of many a therapeutic ilk utilizing myriad therapeutic facilities (see chapter 13). For the sake of the regional musculoskeletal disorders, factories spew forth putatively palliative pills and widgets. There are burgeoning bureaucracies contending with the sources for funding of all this activity. And there are entrenched bureaucracies operating public and private indemnity schemes to provide recourse for any who are not advantaged as a result of all the care afforded those whose backache or the like is insurmountable. No wonder regional musculoskeletal morbidity, and all of the response it engenders, has managed to avoid much perturbation by the science that finds the social construction fatally flawed and harmful.

Many of us have grown weary, even jaded, by the claim of yet another revolutionary biomedical advance. The science may not be prosaic, but the claim that our world will never be the same because of it rings hollow. This chapter, however, is advantaged by some of the most dramatic clinical advances in the past fifty years. The advances challenge the very being of a large clinical establishment and a powerful insurance industry. The advances may be making inroads into the behavior of both, painfully and slowly, but they have barely a foothold in the common sense. Given the predictable lag time, I am urging the reader to be proactive. This chapter celebrates these advances. If you have an open mind, your preconceptions are highly vulnerable.

The following are ten state-of-the-science tenets about the regional musculoskeletal disorders. They are Popperian "truths" (chapter 1) yet to be disproved. All have been largely ignored by society and by the medical and insurance institutions that are meant to service us. These tenets demand close attention if any one of us is to stand a chance of either fending for ourselves or fending off harmful notions and interventions.

1. The regional musculoskeletal disorders are ubiquitous intermittent and remittent predicaments of life. It is distinctly abnormal to live two years without an important backache, or three years without important neck and arm pain, or five years without important knee pain. By important, I mean pain that lasts weeks, even months, and causes one to alter customary life activities. By important, I mean likely to be memorable.

2. Less-"important" episodes are far more common, more fleeting, and less memorable, but nonetheless important predicaments when we have them. If we were to keep a diary of every morbid aspect of each day for six weeks, well over

half of us would have something to record. The commonest morbidity relates to upper respiratory symptoms. However, half of us would record regional musculoskeletal pain, most frequently low back pain that is likely to last one week out of the six. Few would feel the need to make more than minor alterations in lifestyle.

3. The majority of us manage with these predicaments without seeking care from medical or other providers. That holds for both the fleeting and for the prolonged episodes. Most manage to cope so effectively that the episode is not even memorable. How we cope varies from person to person and place to place according to prior experiences and cultural presuppositions. How we cope is far from immutable. For example, the consumption of analgesic pharmaceuticals (and of particular analgesic pharmaceuticals) is a predilection that can be enhanced by the marketing of over-the-counter and prescription drugs. Science cannot discern much effectiveness, or any differences in benefit, or in the likelihood of toxicity, but marketing can (see below). The proclivity to consume so-called neutriceuticals such as chondroitin and glucosamine is driven mostly by rumors promulgated by lay publications. Compounds of this nature can be sold without scientific or regulatory scrutiny. There will always be those with disposable cash who feel compelled to cast about for offbeat remedies.

4. Prior experiences and cultural presuppositions also play into whether one is likely to seek professional assistance in coping. This choice is subject to an influence far more powerful than the marketing by providers. If your life is not in order, the regional musculoskeletal disorder will seem more severe and the need for professional care more pressing. Family discord, psychosocial stresses, financial insecurity, and job dissatisfactions are prime movers in this regard. Which flavor of provider you choose reflects prior experiences, experiences of others you know, and marketing by the providers themselves. But the need to choose a provider is driven at least as much by psychosocial confounders that impede coping on your own as by the regional pain itself.

5. It follows that in choosing to be a patient with a regional musculoskeletal disorder, one is voicing a surrogate complaint. The presenting complaint may be something like, "My back (or shoulder, or knee) hurts," which is surrogate for, "My back (or shoulder, or knee) hurts but I can't cope with this episode." If that was the stated complaint, and/or the complaint inferred by the provider, interventions could be fashioned that address the painful anatomy *and* the compromised coping. Addressing just the first is inadequate.

6. When workers find their back or arm pain disabling, seldom is the content of their tasks as limiting (if it is limiting at all) as the negative context in

which they labor (see chapter 12). For the elderly woman with knee pain, the limiting lesion is far more likely to be psychosocial — often loneliness — than anatomical.

7. It is normal to have degenerative changes of the musculoskeletal system. If you have a pristine spine at midlife, that is distinctly "abnormal." Our ability to define which abnormality is the cause of a particular episode of backache or neck pain is small, too small to justify any imaging study. It isn't much better for "pinched nerve" pain, so-called radicular pain that shoots down the arm or leg (sciatica). Whatever we see on the MRI is likely to have been present before you started to hurt and likely to persist when you heal. The discal hypothesis, the idea promulgated seventy years ago that a "ruptured disc" is the culprit, has withstood scientific scrutiny very poorly. It is largely untenable for axial pain (backache and neck pain) and marginal for radicular (nerve root) pain. Most asymptomatic adults have impressive degenerative changes in their spinal discs by age fifty, as do all of us who manage to make it to eighty-five. Regardless of whether this discal pathology occurred suddenly or was painful, it caused no particularly memorable predicament. "Ruptured disc" and "bad back" are two terms in the lexicon that deserve to be relegated to the historical archives.

8. Knee pain is another intermittent and remittent predicament of life. Memorable knee pain will afflict up to 20 percent of us each year, whether we are twenty years old or seventy. As with the axial skeleton, the episodes of pain are nearly totally discordant from any demonstrable anatomical abnormality at all ages. Most that hurt have no demonstrable pathology, and most with demonstrable pathology don't hurt. That holds for damaged menisci, cruciate ligaments, and cartilage surfaces. We have learned that the knees of persons whose lifestyles incorporate much weight bearing are more likely to have more and better cartilage despite spur formation (osteophytes), one of the classical changes of osteoarthritis. It is as if there are good and bad spurs, good spurs forming around healthy, well-used joints and bad spurs forming around joints that are suffering the loss of cartilage and biomechanical integrity we call osteoarthritis. Osteoarthritis or not, knee pain is an intermittent and remittent predicament.

9. The common denominator of the myriad interventions purveyed as specific treatments for the regional disorders is lack of effectiveness. There are hundreds of randomized controlled trials of treatment modalities for low back pain, and nearly as many for the other regional musculoskeletal disorders. None of the various forms of poking, prodding, injecting, exercising, yanking, girding, needling, and the like can be shown to consistently and robustly offer advantages

over placebo events. None of the various pharmaceuticals have effectiveness, efficacy, risk/benefit ratios, or cost/benefit ratios that exceed that of low doses of aspirin or acetaminophen. There is not a hint that surgery for regional back pain is helpful. There is barely a hint that surgery for radicular pain might be helpful. Total hip replacement is a solution to biomechanical compromise as well as hip pain. But there is not a hint that surgery for knee *pain* is helpful. Reconstruction for knee instability may help with gait, but knee pain is a tenuous indication. So too for shoulder, elbow, and wrist pain. Surgery for nearly all regional musculoskeletal pain has earned its place in the historical archives next to tonsillectomies, hysterectomies for retroverted uteruses, radical mastectomies (chapter 6), coronary artery bypass grafts (chapter 2), and other misguided empiricisms. Unfortunately and sadly, surgery for the regional musculoskeletal disorders has yet to be relegated to the archives. To the contrary, it is a booming industry.

10. We do not know what causes particular episodes of regional musculoskeletal pain. The risk that can be attributed to particular tasks on or off the job is trivial. That means we have no more reason to label a regional backache an injury than we have to label a spontaneous headache an injury. We must decry the semantic that the motion that causes the back to hurt more is the motion that caused the back to hurt in the first place. For example, labeling your lateral elbow pain "tennis elbow," even if you don't play tennis, should sound like the nonsense it is. That label is no more sensible than calling angina "stair-climber's chest." These are more than semantic issues; they are semiotic issues. The changes I am suggesting have serious ramifications for workers' compensation indemnity schemes (see chapter 12). The state of the science is such that when a person complains of regional knee pain, the most valid diagnosis is likely "a painful knee." Such is the case for regional shoulder pain, back pain, and neck pain. When a patient with a regional disorder complains of neck pain, the most valid diagnosis today is a "painful neck." Someday, maybe soon, we will have a handle on the microanatomy and biochemistry that is at play. That will suggest new diagnostic labels whose validity is worthy of testing. But the traditional labels that infer pathoanatomy or causation are no longer tenable.

Those are the tenets that can arm us to cope with our next episode of regional musculoskeletal pain. They are well supported by the literature, as I document in the extensive supplementary readings that accompany this chapter. Let me present five circumstances of regional musculoskeletal pain, circumstances that each of us is likely to suffer during our lives and that demonstrate how a person informed by these tenets might cope.

A prototypical episode of acute regional backache. It started midmorning, suddenly, when you bent over to tie your shoelace. The pain was searing, low in the back, such that you could barely stand up. It has settled slightly since onset, though you still can't stand erect. You can walk, listing, with great difficulty. Sitting at your desk offers some relief, which is where we find you, contemplating your options. Aside from difficulty getting to the bathroom, bowel and bladder function are intact. You have no lower extremity symptoms . . . no weakness or loss of sensation. You're just miserably uncomfortable, particularly when you move. You recognize your plight as an acute backache, just like you might recognize that you were faced with the "flu." You are not alarmed but disconcerted that for the next few days, if not weeks, discomfort will compromise your normal activities. That will take some understanding on the part of your family, employer, and coworkers. There has been some friction at work, of late, but your boss should be willing to cut you some slack if you are diplomatic in approaching her. Perhaps that business trip could be postponed, and you could focus on desk work instead. The acetaminophen you took an hour ago is taking the edge off. You'll remember to repeat that dosage a few times a day. Several house chores can also be postponed, and your spouse can empathize, having had a similar episode last year. You'll make the best of it and get on with life. This too shall pass.

Subacute regional shoulder pain. It has been insidiously getting worse for a week now. At this point, reaching behind to fasten a brassiere is too painful to accomplish. Brushing your hair with the right hand is impossible. Fortunately, there are front-fastening bras to circumvent the first disability and the left hand to circumvent the second. That does not make this circumstance any less disconcerting. It's particularly annoying at night; rolling over onto the right shoulder can awaken you with pain. You are no match for your weekly tennis game. The good news is that aside from compromise in reach, dexterity is preserved. The bad news is that you know that such regional shoulder pain often takes several months to run its course. You might as well hunker down for this longer haul. Acetaminophen and a warm shower at bedtime help get you through the night, most nights. Your fitness should not suffer if you switch to jogging or another aerobic lower-extremity routine, although your tennis game might. You bemoan the fact that modern medicine is no match for this predicament. Doctors might demonstrate some anatomical abnormality at the right shoulder, perhaps of the rotator cuff, but there is a high likelihood that they'd find the same pathology at the other cuff. So who knows what's really hurting? Maybe a steroid shot would help, maybe not. Certainly there is no surgical solution, not even an arthroscopic solution. It's annoying, to say the least. But this too shall pass.

Regional knee pain at age twenty-five. You're a fit, recreational athlete. At least you thought so until the past month. Intermittently at first, and now more persistently, your left knee hurts. It seems a bit swollen and tight. If it weren't for this knee, you'd feel fine. But the knee is hard to ignore. You tried jogging but didn't get too far before the knee felt unstable and caused you to limp. You paid a price for the next few days with increased swelling, discomfort, and limping. You have a friend who had a similar experience last year. He saw Dr. Jones, a local orthopedist who obtained an MRI of the knee followed by arthroscopy to remove a torn meniscus. That was a year ago, followed by several months of physical therapy, then progressive exercises. Only now is he back to speed. You're tempted to pursue the same recourse, particularly since your health insurance will pay nearly all the fees. But you read *Worried Sick* and learned that there is no data to refute the idea that your friend would be as well even sooner had he let the knee heal spontaneously. You also became aware of the long-term follow-up data on the open meniscectomy, the "answer" twenty years ago. The knees are not spared damage. Newer data with the "less-invasive" arthroscopic meniscectomy is pointing in the same direction. No, you'd rather opt for spontaneous healing. You want to maintain the muscular tone of your leg since that is essential for normal knee function. So, you'll alter your fitness regimen to avoid activities that unduly impact the knee; cycling for a couple of months sounds reasonable, maybe swimming a little. This too shall pass.

Regional knee pain at age fifty-five. Maybe it was the abuse from playing football in high school, although you don't remember any severe injuries. You have been a recreational jogger since college, but that's no explanation; there are studies of people like you and they do fine, better than most. You are fit and enjoy the fact that your lifestyle, on and off the job, is far from sedentary. Yet you are faced with weeks of episodes of nagging left knee pain, limping and being cautious descending stairs, and a stiff knee when you wake up in the morning. Your knee feels tight and unstable, and although it has never given way, you feel too insecure to jog, let alone play tennis. This has all proven quite anxiety provoking. Is your fate to be similar to that of your father's who, by the time he was your age, was hobbled by awful knees? At least today a "total knee replacement" might save you from that fate. But isn't there something to do short of that? Arthroscopic surgery is not an option, not since the randomized controlled trial published in the *New England Journal of Medicine* suggesting you would be worse off for that effort. You suppose you could join the glucosamine–chondroitin sulfate bandwagon, even though the data that these concoctions are useful is marginal — particularly unimpressive since the purveyors underwrote the slightly positive studies. You decide you have better things to do with your money than advantage tainted arthroscopists or shameless hawkers. You'll just have to figure out some way to make the best of it. Non-weight-bearing sports like cycling and swimming will become the mainstay of your fitness regimen. And you'll try to keep slim so as to ask as little as you can of the knee when it is hurting. This may not pass, but if it does not progress that's good enough. "Total knee replacement" is neither a replacement, nor an appealing option. Few enjoy the dramatic relief that those with total hip replacements often revel in.

Chronic neck pain with radiculopathy at age sixty. It seems diabolical. For months, maybe six or more, there is this nagging pain in the neck that comes and goes. Of late, it is coming more than it is going. And it is more than just a nuisance. You have to be careful backing out of the driveway since your neck won't rotate sufficiently to see over your shoulder. Sleeping is no mean task, either. You can find a comfortable position and fall asleep, but one turn and you're up and hurting. Yes, taking acetaminophen at bedtime along with a warm shower helps, but that's no panacea. About four months ago, this nagging neck pain was joined by a pain that ran down the outside of the right arm toward the wrist associated with numbness, tingling, and some loss of sensation in the middle fingers. You could cope with the neck pain, had even done so with less pervasive neck pain in the past. But this arm symptom was too uncomfortable, too unfamiliar, and too disconcerting to tackle alone. Your family doctor referred you to a neurosurgeon who found your physical examination reassuring in that there was no weakness, but she did note a loss of a reflex in the arm. Because of that and the fact that your neck symptoms had been present for six weeks or more, you experienced the height of claustrophobia in the quest for Magnetic Resonance images. The neurosurgeon explained that there was a lot of degenerative disease — spurs and disc-space narrowing — at multiple levels and on both sides. The neurosurgeon couldn't be certain as to which abnormality was pinching the nerve provoking the arm symptoms. However, the particular arm symptoms, the radiculopathy, pointed to the problem being at or near a particular nerve root. She offered you surgery to remove any spur or the like from the neighborhood of that root and then "stabilize" that region of the neck with hardware so that it couldn't move and pinch the nerve again. You demurred. You were aware that this surgical approach was based on a theory that had never been put to the test. The neurosurgeon was extrapolating studies for radiculopathy at the low back (sciatica). Those studies suggest that the radiculopathy responded somewhat to the surgery, although the natural rate of healing did not lag by much. That was not a good enough reason for you to submit to the wielding of the knife. As long as the neurological symptoms do not progress, you'll take your chances with the natural history. You're not even tempted to try a neck collar or accept the referral to physical therapy. Soft neck collars do little more than remind you to sit erect so as not to unduly stress whatever is hurting by flexing your neck forward. You have adjusted the height of your computer and the like to accomplish as much. And what do physical therapists, or other manual therapists, have to offer that has been shown to be effective? You'll trust the natural history, even though you may have residual symptoms for months to come.

Are these vignettes contrived? If you ask members of the treating professions, most would doubt that there are very many people in the United States who can cope with these predicaments in this fashion. It takes more than self-assurance; it requires empathy, support, and encouragement from family, friends, coworkers, employers, and community. Without such support, it takes extraordinary fortitude and certitude to withstand the advice of neighbors who are beneficiaries (survivors) of modern treatments and the phalanx of professional practitioners whose pronouncements in purchased advertisements and in the lay press would seem to suggest that anyone who copes in this fashion is a short-sighted, self-destructive Luddite — or, worse yet, a student of Hadler. However, truth be known, community-based epidemiology suggests that there are many who cope in this fashion, perhaps the majority with these particular predicaments. Furthermore, they do so by relying much more on their personal and community resources than on having any comprehensive grasp of the relevant science that supports their approach. Those who seek professional assistance in coping do so either because they are lacking in supportive community, are faced with elements in their community that interfere with their coping, or are overwhelmed by the seductive pronouncements of the purveyors of help and the people who are convinced they were beneficiaries of such help. And once so seduced, they are prone to make the same choice come the next episode of a regional musculoskeletal disorder. Alas. We have the science to bolster the self-assurance of those who feel they lack control and to inform their community as to their critical influence. Unfortunately, as I said at the outset of the chapter, we are barely making progress in that regard.

To summarize, if you are faced with the predicament of a regional musculoskeletal disorder, there are only a few sensible reasons for abandoning your personhood for the patient-client role and no sensible reasons for abandoning your control over your fate.

If you are not comfortable with your assessment that you are suffering from a regional disorder, you should seek reassurance from an appropriately trained professional. If you feel generally poorly, have fevers or are losing weight, you need to seek reassurance. If the pain is not clearly "mechanical" — relieved by rest and exacerbated by usage — you need to seek reassurance. If you have back or neck pain and important neurological symptoms such as weakness in a limb or difficulty with bladder or bowel function, you need to seek reassurance. If you have a red, warm, painfully swollen joint (knee or any other joint), see your physician. Otherwise, it is sensible to remain a person and try to cope until your predicament resolves.

If you are comfortable that your predicament is a regional disorder but there seem to be insurmountable barriers to coping, then you should seek assistance from an appropriately astute professional. Be prepared to engage in a discourse as to psychosocial influences that might be the critical confounders. Discussions of troubles in life at home or at work should not be taken as irrelevant or offensive; such troubles are responsible for impairing your ability to cope with the pain. Airing them is sensible. At the very least, you'll learn to recognize the enemy.

If you do succumb to the blandishments of treatment, at least be certain every step of the way that you are benefited by the concepts you are expected to assimilate, and that the modalities you are offered are appropriate. If you are comfortable with the metaphysics of pressure points, unstable segments, discal herniations, subluxations, vital forces, and on and on . . . fine. If you find comfort in being stretched, poked, girded, injected, arthroscoped, or even fused, so be it. That is your choice. I would hope you are paying out-of-pocket. I, for one, would be resentful if I am sharing the expense of many of these treatment acts by virtue of the magnitude of my health-insurance premiums. If you want to participate in therapeutic metaphysics, you pay for it. I return to this argument in chapter 14.

Such is the state of the science. It is possible that great progress is just around the corner. After all, many people are coping with painful and limiting predicaments for which no anatomical explanation holds up to scrutiny, but this does not preclude that a more fertile explanation, likely at the biochemical level, will someday be found. There are novel agents in development that are worthy of testing, and a vast market awaits any such success. Many a drug will be touted as effective and some will pass muster with the FDA, but "all that glitters is not gold" — unless you're an investor, and even investors need be wary. The recent history of the development and introduction of the COXIBS is an object lesson as to why one should be sophisticated about the process and wary of the hype that too often masquerades as "progress." COXIBS are a class of aspirin-like drugs that includes such brands Vioxx, Celebrex, and Bextra. The lead-up to the COXIB debacle was long and colorful, dripping the familiar and the unfamiliar and worthy of summary.

The COXIB Canard

The first multinational pharmaceutical firm was the Jesuit order. The miracle drug of the seventeenth century was "Peruvian bark," also known as "Jesuit bark" because it was imported from South America by the Jesuits. It was harvested from the chincona tree by indigenous South Americans who had been converted both to Catholicism and to the task of harvesting. Chincona was the name of the duchess who was the wife of the Spanish governor of Peru. "Jesuit tea" was an antipyretic, an agent that could reduce the fevers and agues that plagued Europeans. For Western medicine of the day, fever was a disease, as was the agues. Jesuit tea was an effective antipyretic, perhaps more effective than just an antipyretic. After all, the active ingredient is quinine, which is also an antimalarial, and malaria was a scourge in England and the Continent. The Western physician had no remedy that compared favorably with Jesuit tea. Not surprisingly, the medical establishment was very receptive when the Reverend Edward Stone wrote to the Royal Society of Medicine in London in 1763 that the bark of the willow tree, the "sallow" tree of the species *Salix*, was a match for Peruvian bark. This battle of the barks, which played out until the end of the nineteenth century, was the first skirmish of the NSAID wars. NSAID is the commonly used acronym for nonsteroidal anti-inflammatory drugs, agents other than the cortisone family that abrogate any or all of the symptoms of inflammation regardless the cause: swelling, warmth, redness, and painfulness. NSAIDs can provide a modicum of relief for myriad conditions, from a dental abscess before or after extraction to inflamed joints, whether from trauma or rheumatoid arthritis. The ongoing competition between the various NSAIDs has, with good reason, been described as a war.

The end of the nineteenth century saw the flowering of Prussian organic chemistry. The active principle of willow bark was isolated, labeled salicin, and chemically modified to produce a number of congeners (chemically related substances), some of which were found to be pharmacologically active. I mean *found*. The randomized controlled drug trial was an invention of the mid-twentieth century. Prior to that, chemists were likely to swallow their own concoctions or give them to physicians who had the temerity to give them to the ill. Effectiveness was left to the eyes of the beholder and toxicity easily overlooked by the same eyes. At the turn of the twentieth century, salicylic acid was used to "burn" warts, while sodium salicylate was a widely used antipyretic (fever-reducing agent), despite the fact that it induced nausea more frequently than quinine-containing potions. Other salicylates remained on chemists' shelves. Acetyl salicylic acid had been synthesized by Karl Löwig and labeled aspirin ("a" for acetyl and "spir" for the spiraea or spirsäure plant from which he isolated the salicylic acid). It remained on the shelf of the I. G. Farbenfabriken company in Bayer-Eberfeld until Felix Hofmann, a chemist, had the temerity to treat his father with that compound. Papa Hofmann declared it effective for his arthritis and tolerable. This event was not lost on Friedrich Carl Duisberg Jr. The Western world would never be the same.

Duisberg, as a young chemist, took a job with Friedrich Bayer & Co., a minor player in the dye-chemistry industry, and by virtue of cunning and genius transformed it into the enormous Prussian industrial powerhouse known as I. G. Farbenindustrie A. G. — or I. G. Farben. Duisberg was one of the larger-than-life barons of industry in the early twentieth century, strutting the world with the likes of John D. Rockefeller and Andrew Carnegie. He left a complex legacy, including his firm, whose successor directors took their place in the dock at Nuremburg alongside the likes of Himmler and Goering.

Duisberg understood that chemistry could produce more than industrial compounds; it could produce compounds that would supplant biologicals in the pharmacopoeia and in medicine chests around the world. Aspirin was a natural, since the market was vast and his company its leading manufacturer. The modern pharmaceutical industry was born in Prussia, but it was not to remain provincial for long. Duisberg traveled to Rensselaer, New York, in 1903 and built a factory. But he didn't simply want to produce aspirin — he wanted to make it part of the fabric of life. He was the marketing genius who emblazoned the "Bayer Cross" on more than pills. Bayer *was* aspirin. The Rensselaer factory came under American ownership during World War I, sold to a patent-medicine firm, which evolved into Sterling Products. Sterling purveyed "Bayer aspirin" until a decade ago, when corporate reshuffling returned the name and the brand to Germany. While aspirin was still under patent, infringers thrived. When the patent expired in 1917, competitors thrived. This was the heyday of the American patent-medicine industry hawking unctions and potions, often very profitably. But aspirin found an unprecedented market around the world, including the developing world. Bristol-Myers, American Home, and Miles Laboratories (Alka-Seltzer) joined Sterling in evolving from patent-medicine firms into lucrative industrial powerhouses competing among themselves and with I. G. Farben for the sale of aspirin and aspirin-containing preparations. Aspirin sales grew unchallenged until the 1960s. Tons were consumed each day in the United States. For most of the twentieth century, aspirin overdose was a leading cause of emergency-room visits and drug-induced fatality.

In the 1930s, another product of the nineteenth-century Prussian chemists, long collecting dust, started a tortuous journey to commercial success, emerging in the British marketplace in the 1950s and then in the United States as acetaminophen, which was marketed as Tylenol by McNeil Pharmaceuticals. Johnson & Johnson, already an enormous purveyor of consumer-health products, purchased McNeil. Tylenol would soon do battle with Datril, Bristol-Myers's version. Both made important inroads into the aspirin market as an analgesic (painkiller) and antipyretic (lowers fever). Acetaminophen has little of aspirin's effect on the swelling, redness, and warmth that characterizes inflammatory lesions, just the tenderness and painfulness. Acetaminophen does not cause gastropathy, or shallow erosions of the lining of the stomach. Nonetheless, this was the start of the erosion of aspirin's dominance.

The Boots Company is a venerable British retail drug chain. In midcentury Boots added a small research division to seek a new anti-inflammatory agent as powerful as corticosteroids (steroids) but without the toxicities of steroids or aspirin. A young pharmacologist, Stewart Adams, was screening agents for this purpose. He took advantage of animal models of inflammation, initially using a sunburned guinea pig model he developed. A biochemist, John Nicholson, produced the chemicals for screening. They were lucky. They discovered a new NSAID, ibuprofen, which was patented in the late 1960s and marketed shortly thereafter as Brufen in Britain and as Motrin under license to Upjohn in the United States. The floodgates to NSAID development were opened and marketing became ever more vicious.

Motrin was the first New Age NSAID, the first anti-inflammatory agent to undergo scrutiny by the modern FDA. The FDA was born as a bureau within the Department of Agriculture in 1906 and was charged with expunging misbranded and adulterated drugs from interstate commerce. In 1912 the Shirley Amendment added the prohibition of fraudulent therapeutic claims, although it was never clear how "fraud" could be proved. So it remained caveat emptor until 1937, when the Massengill Company of Bristol, Tennessee, began shipping gallons of elixir of sulfanilamide. Sulfanilamide was an early "miracle" antibiotic, a sulfa drug that was insoluble in water. Massengill's chief chemist found it to be highly soluble in ethylene glycol ("antifreeze" today), but he didn't realize that ethylene glycol was a poison until many people died. The chemist, not Mr. Massengill, committed suicide. Senator Royal S. Copeland, a homeopathic physician, shepherded his revised Federal Food, Drug, and Cosmetic Act through Congress in 1938. It stipulated that no drug could be marketed until safety was demonstrated. However, there was no mandate for efficacy, just safety. A mandate for efficacy awaited another disaster, the thalidomide tragedy, following which the Kefauver-Harris Amendments were passed in 1962 demanding "substantial evidence" of benefit as well as safety and purity before any new drug could be licensed for sale in the United States. And so the modern FDA came into being, charged with designing and revising the process by which this mandate can be served. That was a watershed for consumer safety. It also marks the modern age of biostatistics and epidemiology: methodologies had to be devised to serve this mandate and revised repeatedly. Every NSAID since has had to pass FDA muster. The following is true about every NSAID that has been approved:

1. Every approved NSAID has been shown to be more effective than placebo.
2. No approved NSAID has been shown to be less effective than aspirin.
3. No approved NSAID has been shown to be more effective than aspirin.
4. No approved NSAID has been shown to be safer than aspirin.

There is one more element of the story before we are ready to tackle the COXIB debacle. Generations of scientists have sought the mechanism by which aspirin is anti-inflammatory. Many a theory has proven untenable. One has stood the test of time, and clearly explains some, maybe most, of the action. In 1971 Sir John Vane, working for Burroughs Wellcome in Britain, discovered that aspirin (and all NSAIDs) inhibited the enzyme cyclooxygenase (COX) that is critical in the biosynthesis of prostaglandins, known chemical mediators of inflammation. No doubt this is a major insight, even though the story is far from over. Vane was awarded a Nobel Prize. Prostaglandins are also involved in maintaining the integrity of the stomach lining, so that inhibition is the explanation for the shallow erosions that come and go in everyone who ingests NSAIDs, so-called NSAID gastropathy.

In the early 1990s, it was shown that there were two forms of COX: COX-1, which is present in many cells, and COX-2, which could be induced in certain cells. Experimental studies suggested that COX-1 was active both in inflammatory processes and in the stomach, whereas COX-2 was more exclusive to inflammatory processes. The race was on for a new NSAID that inhibited only COX-2 and therefore might be an effective anti-inflammatory agent that spared the stomach — the putatively perfect aspirin. Many were discovered in the laboratories of many pharmaceutical firms, much to the glee of their stockholders. These new NSAIDs were called COXIBs, to denote that they were specific COX-2 cyclooxygenase inhibitors. Two, marketed as Celebrex and Vioxx, were the first to be tested in trials and to pass muster with the FDA. The trials recruited patients with rheumatoid arthritis or with regional musculoskeletal disorders, usually knee pain in the setting of osteoarthritis. These are demanding and expensive undertakings, which, more and more, are outsourced to contracted research organizations (CROs). CROs are private-sector enterprises that service the pharmaceutical industry by managing the clinical trials, data analysis, and application process before the FDA. CROs, or another specialized contracted organization, recruit physicians, who in turn recruit subjects from their practices. The CROs, the recruited physicians, and usually the patients all receive remuneration for their participation. Long gone are the days when drug trials were free of vested interests, conflicts of interest, marketing undercurrents, and fraud. There are scandals that have made national press involving "paper patients" and data massaging and that have forced regulatory agencies to monitor the quality of the trials. The COXIB cozenage is subtler.

Pharmacia (the Swedish pharmaceutical firm that was to be swallowed by Pfizer) and Merck were breaking new ground in the escalating tendency of the pharmaceutical industry to market at the very edge of veracity. This is the impression one gets from the content of their numerous sponsored professional symposia, the dinner talks by "thought leaders," their advertising in professional journals, and their direct-to-consumer advertising.

Direct-to-consumer (DTC) advertising has an interesting history. The Kefauver-Harris Amendments to the Food, Drug and Cosmetic Act in 1962 did more than mandate assessments of efficacy. The jurisdiction over prescription-drug advertising (not over-the-counter drug advertising) was transferred from the Federal Trade Commission to the FDA. The FDA met the mandate by a series of regulations that evolved to require detailed disclosure of benefits, risks, indications, and contraindications in package inserts and to call for this level of detail if the pharmaceutical firm was to directly market to physicians or consumers. That explains all the fine print in all print advertisements for pharmaceuticals to this day. Boots Pharmaceuticals was the first to test the DTC waters with advertisements for its brand of ibuprofen in 1981, causing the FDA to call for a voluntary moratorium on all DTC advertisements until 1985, when the moratorium was lifted — but not the mandate for detailed disclosures, which were prohibitively cumbersome in broadcast marketing. The matter smoldered for a decade until it was enflamed by a report from Scott-Levin, a consulting firm that conducted a survey and concluded that physicians would prescribe or consider prescribing specific drugs at the suggestion of patients. In 1995 the FDA conducted public hearings, at which representatives of pharmaceutical firms urged a relaxation of the regulations on DTC advertisements. The argument hinged on the advantages for patients in becoming informed consumers rather than on volume of sales. In August 1997 the FDA relaxed the regulations for DTC on broadcast media; the advertisement must disclose major risks along with "adequate provision for" dissemination of the approved package insert information. As to the latter, the FDA offered "guidance": a toll-free number, referral to a health-care provider, a website, or referral to a print advertisement.

Spending on direct-to-consumer advertising of prescription drugs has tripled between 1996 and 2000 to $2.5 billion (which is only 15 percent of the pharmaceutical marketing budget) and reached $4 billion by 2004. Vioxx led the charge. In short order Celebrex and Vioxx each accounted for revenues that exceeded $3 billion per year. Merck and Pfizer convinced consumers and prescribers that their COXIBs are worth the considerable extra expense compared to inexpensive over-the-counter aspirin and other NSAIDs. The advertising campaigns suggested that a sufferer could enjoy relief with diminished risk of gastrointestinal toxicity, as was predicted by the test-tube studies of the cox-2 inhibitors. They convinced patients and physicians alike, though they had never generated data that convinced the FDA — or me. One has to wonder what possessed the FDA to license COXIBs in the first place, given that the agency was not convinced of either any advance in effectiveness or in safety over available drugs with long-term track records. I suspect outside influences were at play. After all, the FDA is not immune from congressional pressures, an influence dramatically displayed when the agency considered regulating tobacco as a drug. Furthermore, members of the FDA "advisory panels" are not barred from financial arrangements with pharmaceutical firms, and many are so entwined. Much was at stake when COXIBs came under FDA scrutiny.

Once licensed, the enormous success of the new cox-2 agents was a testimony to the power of rumor, to the gullibility of the lay press, and to a slick approach to marketing to physicians and patients. For example, shortly after Celebrex was released, Jerome Groopman wrote an essay in the *New Yorker* that relied on attestations and enthusiasm of the principal scientist of Pharmacia's pharmaceutical subsidiary that developed the agent. I have never prescribed a COXIB and warned against anyone doing so in the second edition of my monograph, *Occupational Musculoskeletal Disorders*, published in 1999.

I am barely inclined to be charitable toward Groopman as a journalist; he was seduced by the enthusiasm of a respected senior pharmaceutical scientist who was self-deluding. However, I do not applaud the behavior of the members of the medical profession who are "thought leaders" with manifest conflicts of interest. For example, the American College of Rheumatology convened a "subcommittee" to "update" the "recommendations for the medical management of osteoarthritis of the hip and knee." In 1998 the college's recommendation leaned toward acetaminophen. It's not that acetaminophen is impressively effective. It's just that it is as effective as any NSAID without the risk of gastrointestinal toxicity. The "update" argued that the risk/benefit ratio favored COXIBs for patients over sixty-five years old. Because of the increasing wariness regarding vested and conflicted interests of authors, many journals now require that the authors of articles declare any potential bias. Similarly, the members of the subcommittee were asked to list their "relationships," such as paid consultancies or speaking contracts, with pharmaceutical or biotechnology companies. The four members of this subcommittee listed four, nine, eleven, and seventeen such arrangements, respectively, mainly to companies in the COXIB business. Perhaps, the college and the authors feel cleansed by such a declaration. I would hope readers would share my outrage that four men with such clearly stated personal ties to companies marketing COXIBs should be asked to advise the membership of a specialty college. This practice is now commonplace.

In spite of the exorbitant profits, sufficient to underwrite predatory marketing and still cause stock values to soar, neither Pfizer nor Merck nor their stockholders were content sharing the market. Both sponsored large clinical trials attempting to demonstrate safety to the satisfaction of the FDA so that the "serious gastrointestinal toxicity" forewarning could be expunged from the labeling, thereby unbridling marketing. Pfizer's "CLASS" trial appeared in *JAMA* in 2000 comparing Celebrex with ibuprofen or diclofenac (Voltaren) in patients with rheumatoid arthritis (RA) and with regional musculoskeletal pain in the setting of osteoarthritis (mostly regional knee pain). Merck's "VIGOR" trial appeared in the *New England Journal of Medicine*. It compared Vioxx with naproxen in RA. So armed, the pharmaceutical firms and their hired CROs petitioned the FDA to expunge the warning.

Neither the FDA's advisory panel nor its in-house reviewers were convinced by the CLASS trial data. When the statistical analysis offered by Pfizer was scrutinized, there was no demonstrable advantage to Celebrex. However, the FDA's reviewers and the advisory panel differed on whether there was a discernible margin of gastrointestinal safety when Vioxx was compared with naproxen. The FDA's in-house reviewers were not impressed; the advisory panel thought there might be an edge but not enough to assume an edge over all NSAIDS. Merck's quasi-victory proved Pyrrhic. An unanticipated finding of the VIGOR trial was apparent to all reviewers of the actual data provided the FDA. There were more cardiovascular deaths in the patients on Vioxx than on naproxen, several more than had been revealed in the version of the VIGOR trial published in 2000 in the *New England Journal of Medicine*. The editors published an "expression of concern" in 2005.

Celebrex is still on the market, still marketed aggressively, and still selling well. This reflects the rumor that it spares the stomach from grief, a rumor bolstered by the conclusions from the CLASS trial that was published in JAMA. The published version convinced the "peer reviewers" that Celebrex was gentler on the stomach. But a separate review of the results of the CLASS trial did not convince the FDA to lift the stomach warning, although there seemed no need for a cardiac warning. There is another side to the CLASS trial that is as outrageous as that regarding the display of data in the VIGOR trial. It was learned and widely publicized by investigative reporters that the CLASS trial was published with incomplete data. The completed data that was presented to the FDA later contradicted the published conclusions. The FDA reviewers were correct in their conclusion that Celebrex offered no benefit/risk advantage whatsoever. It was later learned that the complete data was available at the time the paper was submitted, but somehow someone decided to publish the incomplete data and the analysis that appeared to favor Celebrex. Subsequent marketing was based on the publication; 30,000 reprints of the JAMA paper were purchased for distribution. Celebrex sales increased from $2.6 billion in 2000 to $3.1 billion in 2001. I don't know if any of the authorship knew any of this. The CLASS trial masthead listed sixteen authors; six were employees of Pharmacia and the rest had academic affiliations but were paid consultants for Pharmacia, which funded the study. One of the academic-affiliated authors had a long-standing financial relationship with Pharmacia and other drug firms, was the lead author of earlier Celebrex trials, and went on to a stint directing the division of the FDA responsible for reviewing applications to license new anti-inflammatory drugs.

The VIGOR trial proved a "smoking gun." True, Merck was able to eke the acknowledgment of gastrointestinal safety from some observers. I'm not one of the convinced, since the acknowledgment is based on a trivial difference, too small to measure reliably. But Merck had a greater market in sight. In chapter 5, I discussed the hypothesis that NSAIDS might decrease the likelihood of colonic polyps. I also detailed the tenuous basis for someone to think polyps are meaningful harbingers of colon cancer. Nonetheless, Americans are told as much. It would follow that if NSAIDS blocked polyp formation, they would banish colon cancer from the aging population. If NSAIDS were safer, everyone would take them regardless of the cost. So the purveyors of COXIBs were busily conducting trials to see if their cash cows could become fixtures in the lives of our colons, like fluoride for our teeth. That's when the smoking gun blew up in the faces of Pfizer, Merck, and many of their fellow travelers.

COXIBs lead to a small dose-related increase in cardiovascular events. For example, Celebrex at a dose of 400 mg per day does not significantly increase the hazard for death or other cardiovascular events. But at 800 mg per day, the hazard increased threefold. That observation gained the attention of the FDA, the mainstream medical journals, and the lay press. However, the reader of *Worried Sick* is wary of the expression of a result as a relative risk. Of the 671 patients on the 800 mg daily dose, twenty-three suffered death from cardiovascular causes or a nonfatal heart attack, stroke, or heart failure. That was the fate of seven of a similar number taking a placebo pill. So the additional absolute risk is slightly over 2 percent over the course of three years in a population with a mean age of about sixty. In other words, one would have to treat over forty people for three years to cause any one of these adverse events. One would have to treat 200 for three years to kill one. The former iatrogenic hazard is at the margins of believable for reasons I developed in chapter 1. The latter exceeds that. However, since there are no claims for effectiveness over the old standby NSAIDS, and since I find nothing about the claims of safety to be convincing, even a remote possibility of toxicity is unacceptable. This was my response to multiple requests from the press for my opinion. These drugs should never have been released.

Meanwhile, Merck and Pfizer found themselves in a maelstrom. Both withdrew their COXIBs from the market. In February of 2005, the FDA convened a panel of thirty-two arthritis and drug-safety experts, which listened to three days of testimony. The committee voted 31 to 1 that Celebrex should stay on the market, but 17 to 15 for Vioxx. The *New York Times* noted that ten members of the panel (at least) had overt ties to the pharmaceutical industry. These ten voted nearly to a person to keep COXIBS on the market. And so the FDA complied, stipulating that a "black box" warning be appended to the labeling. Merck felt vindicated and reintroduced Vioxx (though only briefly). Pfizer demurred. But the saga was far from over.

On 5 May 2005, the Government Reform Committee of the U.S. House of Representatives held a hearing. Realize that "Big Pharma" is a lobbying organization that had a hefty presence on Capital Hill for years. Coincidentally, Congress has had a gentle relationship with the pharmaceutical industry—until the COXIB canard forced their hand. Congress learned a good deal about what Congressman Henry Waxman termed the "hidden corner of the health care system." We all learned that in addition to the $4 billion spent in direct-to-consumer marketing, the industry spent more than $5.5 billion to promote drugs to doctors ($5.5 billion is more than all the U.S. medical schools spend yearly to educate medical students). The industry employed over 90,000 sales representatives —one for every 4.7 doctors—to "educate" doctors about new drugs and new indications. The committee uncovered a Merck bulletin sent to its 3,000 Vioxx sales representatives shortly after the FDA reviewed the VIGOR trial to the effect that they should "not initiate" discussion of these events with their customers. Furthermore, Merck trained its representatives to identify speakers for "educational events" who were "opinion leaders" with "favorable views" of Merck and of Vioxx.

And there's more. The fact that Vioxx increases the risk of adverse cardiovascular events has not gone unnoticed by the plaintiff's bar. Lawsuits are ongoing and will be for some time. The "discovery" process has revealed a zeal for marketing for which the schemes mentioned above are but symptoms. Furthermore, there is no honor among thieves. Eric Topol is a prominent cardiologist who was recruited from the University of Michigan to be chief of cardiology at the Cleveland Clinic. Topol has been the principal investigator on numerous trials of pharmaceuticals and widgets throughout his career and a major consultant to industry. No doubt he has "skills" in this regard that appealed to the Cleveland Clinic, a nonprofit foundation that generates nearly $4 billion in annual revenues and boasts a 15,000-square-foot "innovation center" to help its researchers with commercial development. Topol was chief academic officer and sat on the clinic's "conflict-of-interest" committee and board of governors. Topol made himself available to the plaintiff's bar in the pursuit of a remedy from Merck for purveying Vioxx without revealing its potential for cardiotoxicity. It turns out that Topol was advising a hedge fund that profited from the decline in Merck stock resulting from the Vioxx debacle. The clinic stripped Topol of his provost title and pulled from under him his seats on the conflict-of-interest committee and board of governors. I don't worry about Dr. Topol. He resigned from the clinic in February 2006 to go across town and join the medical faculty of Case Western Reserve University. *Sic transit gloria mundi*. Topol was succeeded at Cleveland Clinic by Steven Nissen, whose Avandia meta-analysis is discussed in the supplementary reading for chapter 3. Although the FDA houses many a committed and honorable staffer, it is clear that its approach to safeguarding the consumer is a blunt instrument in the current climate. Reeling from the COXIB canard, the FDA turned to the Institute of Medicine (IOM) in 2005. The IOM is the most politicized of the National Academies of Science in that members can be anointed based on academic power rather than scholarly accomplishment. The IOM formed a committee whose work product led to a "New Initiative" announced by the FDA in January 2007 (‹http://www.fda.gov›). The FDA is proposing an enormous effort that is aimed largely at process but offers little but circumlocution about two of the three pressing substantive challenges:

1. A program of systematic postmarketing surveillance (Phase IV) is proposed. This is long overdue. The current approach relies on voluntary reporting by physicians. The FDA is proposing developing some more systematic approach using the Veterans Administration as the test ground.

2. Lax definitions of effectiveness are the soft underbelly of the drug-evaluative process today, and little but promise can be found in the New Initiative. We, as a nation, must begin to understand this construct so that we might applaud setting a standard higher than just "evidence." There must be evidence of substantial benefit in Phase III randomized controlled trials to license any drug. Such a hurdle will do away with "me too" agents and the many, many good ideas that translate very marginally at the bedside. This would streamline the process of drug discovery and approval since discerning major benefit requires far less burdensome clinical trials. It would make it harder to massage and torture data to produce minor effects. And it would allow for a meaningful benefit/risk assessment.

3. The initiative largely avoids the third rail, the testing of devices. Let's finally do something about "devices." Our nation needs to demand that these widgets and gizmos be subjected to the same high standards of

effectiveness we would demand of pharmaceuticals. Today, devices face a high hurdle in terms of safety but a problematic hurdle in terms of effectiveness. That's why there are so many widgets competing in the same market.

If we can hold these three goals as primary, much that has sullied the FDA in the past would not do so in the future, and we'd all be better off in every way. Furthermore, it's time to take the testing of drugs out of the private sector. We could establish federally funded "clinimetrics" units at many medical schools, staffed by appropriately trained investigators who are prohibited from establishing fiscal relationships with pharmaceutical companies. The companies would still patent their drugs, test them in animal models, and carry out the early phases of clinical testing. But the industry would no longer perform the definitive randomized controlled trials. A panel of appropriately trained scientists would prioritize new drugs for trial based on the likelihood of an important advance. In a paper I published in 1983, I suggested a statistical methodology that would take advantage of enrolling a limited number of patients in each of a limited number of testing sites. "Me too" and "minor effect" drugs would disappear rapidly and cheaply in this process, as would much of the vested interest. So too would CROs and related industries disappear.

I am not holding my breath. There is much invested in perpetuating the current approach. The marketing of COXIBs is a window. There is so much at stake, and so much money in play, that the marketing minions that have come to dominate the executive suites of the pharmaceutical industry have marshaled forces that are a match for the FDA. The application process is underwritten by the applicant firms, placing the FDA into a client role. Advisory panels are riddled with "experts" with industry ties. The political appointees to the FDA and many senior staff are recruited from industry. An alarming number of physicians, including academicians, have assumed paid roles in the process of performing clinical trials and marketing drugs. There is a cogent argument that trials with FDA-approved drugs are marketing exercises rather than attempts to test hypotheses as to risk/benefit ratios. An alarming number of publications are written, even ghost written, and lectures delivered by individuals with pharmaceutical company income. An alarming number of papers describing trials are authored by physicians who had no direct control over the design or data analysis, and who then take to the hustings in sponsored lectures, workshops, and publications. None of this has escaped attention. Editorials decrying all this abound, but to little discernible effect.

The most diabolical aspect of the COXIB canard is that the entire enterprise is based on a misconception. NSAID gastropathy comes and goes while the patient is taking NSAIDs, is totally discordant from symptoms, and bodes no evil in most people. NSAIDs increase the likelihood of important gastrointestinal complications in very small, easily defined subpopulations: those with a prior history of ulcers, those on ulcerogenic drugs (steroids and alcohol lead the list), those who are taking anticoagulants (blood thinners), those with a prior history of clinically important ulcer complications, and the elderly, particularly elderly women. For the rest of us, nearly all of us, there is no important hazard (including the hint of a miniscule cardiovascular risk). For the subsets at risk, the sensible advice is to avoid exposure. NSAIDs are never mandatory agents. For the subsets at risk, acetaminophen is the sensible first-line alternative analgesic. COXIBS are simply never a sensible option.

I should point out that the marketing of NSAIDs over the past forty years has been very effective. Some 80 percent of U.S. adults report taking over-the-counter analgesics frequently during the course of a year, some very frequently. Physicians in the United States wrote more than 312 million prescriptions for analgesics in the year 2000, and 140 million prescriptions for narcotics in 2002. Talk about medicalization!

The supplementary reading for this chapter is extensive. It is truly a shadow chapter, detailing the science that underlies the narrative above and providing copious references.

chapter

It's in Your Mind

Nothing can pierce the soul as the uttermost sigh of the body. — George Santayana, *The Life of Reason* (1905–6)

In chapter 8, I reviewed the literature that supports my argument that to be well is not to be spared symptoms (morbidity) but to have the wherewithal to cope with intermittent and remittent morbid predicaments such as creakiness, heartache, heartburn, and much more. In this chapter I want to explore the process and consequences of having a "bad day," a day when we're indisposed. The reader is advantaged by the fact that I have been musing about this for decades, and my conceptualization has matured, if not ripened. In a monograph published fifteen years ago (*Occupational Musculoskeletal Disorders*, 1993), I suggested that a "bad day" was a syndrome, the Syndrome of Being Out-of-Sorts, which, in keeping with tradition, lends itself to the acronym soos. "Out-of-sorts" struck me as an appropriate image for a "bad day." It's a term that dates to the earliest days of the printing press. The printer would place the letters of a word in a restraining device, a sort, so that they would stay contiguous during printing. When the printer was out-of-sorts, letters could fly helter-skelter. So it is on a "bad day": we can't quite keep it together. soos has multiple manifestations, not always at the same time, but often so. I've listed these below.

I. Loss of the sense of well-being:
Decreased energy
Easy fatigability
Heaviness/achiness in the temples
Inexplicable anxiousness
Perception of a sleep debt
Vigilance as to unusual symptoms

II. Musculoskeletal symptoms:
   Diffuse achiness
   Disconcerting stiffness, often on awakening
   Sense of swelling, particularly in the hands
   Tenderness about the neck, shoulders, and low back
   Intermittent numbness of the fingers and/or toes
III. Gastrointestinal symptoms:
   Increased or decreased stool frequency
   Keen awareness of bowel function
IV. Peculiar associations of well-being with external events:
   Improvement with exercise
   Exacerbation with stress
   Exacerbation on gloomy, damp, or cold days

None of these manifestations are "specific." None stands out in our minds as the "problem." Those clustered under I and IV are the common denominator, but II and III are frequently present. Usually, we can identify no precipitant. Without rhyme or reason, it's a "bad day."

All of us have been faced with bad days, and we will be again. They often come out of the blue, pass, and are forgotten. Each of us has a threshold at which the number of components and the degree of their intensity causes us to be "under the weather." The variability in our tolerance is remarkable. For example, as many as a quarter of us frequently experience alternating diarrhea and constipation, but very few consider this worrisome. As many as 20 percent of us find our joints stiff for thirty minutes or more without finding that bothersome or worrisome. But if the day has features in cluster I, our sense of invincibility is bound to erode, so that features captured in II and III are more likely to be worrisome than they had been in the past, and those in IV more likely to be in play.

There are people in our communities who are more prone than others to experience soos and more prone to experience prolonged soos. We will explore this further shortly and in detail in the supplementary reading for this chapter. However, this is not a trivial segment of the population. In various surveys around the world, 5 to 15 percent of people are coping with soos at any moment, and many with some persistence. These are the chronically vulnerable; they are worried and forever grasping at information proffered as helpful by friends and the media. Most perceive themselves as no longer well people. They are particularly likely to seek medical care and do so repeatedly. The consequences of seeking medical care, or alternative care (see chapter 13), are predictable and predictably untoward.

Medicalizing the Syndrome of Being Out-of-Sorts

Someday a person will stand before a Western physician and say, "Doc, I feel awful. Could it be in my mind?" And that physician will reply, "I hope so. That's a lot better than leukemia, or renal failure, or lupus, or the like."

For most westerners, especially for most North Americans, such repartee is anathema. It is tantamount to an admission that one is whining, or feigning, or "crazy." A study from Edinburgh is illustrative. New patients attending a general neurology outpatient clinic were interviewed before they saw the doctor. The patients were asked how they would respond "if you had leg weakness, your tests were normal, and a doctor said you had . . . [X]." Table 7 is culled from this study, with some liberty. I am using less-vernacular responses (for example, the connotation "putting it on" is tabulated as "feigning"). For each presumptive diagnosis, the percentage of patients who impute a negative connotation is tabulated. The authors went on to compute the "number needed to offend" based on the idea that people are most offended if they think they are being accused all at once of malingering, of confabulating, and of being crazy. Telling patients their symptoms are "in your mind" will offend 50 percent to this degree. It will similarly offend about a third with any of the next four labels in the list. The four labels after those offend some 10 to 20 percent. A few percent are offended if the diagnosis is "stroke," and very few are offended by a diagnosis of multiple sclerosis.

This is an exercise in semiotics. The investigation is probing the symbolism in these labels. Hysterical weakness, psychosomatic weakness, depression-associated weakness, and stress-related weakness are not as offensive as "all in your mind," though all these are terms that imply the symptom is perceptual rather than a reflection of end-organ pathology. These terms are essentially synonymous with "in your mind." So is "functional weakness," but it carries less baggage in Scotland. Elsewhere, particularly in the United States, all these terms would be perceived as offensive.

When a person with SOOS chooses to be a patient, any diagnosis that implies it's "in your mind" is not comforting. The expectation on the part of the patient is that there is a "cause" that needs to be identified and vanquished. In *Medicine & Culture: Varieties of Treatment in the United States, England, West Germany, and France* (1988), Lynne Payer said it well: "The American regards himself as

TABLE 7. Offensive Diagnoses (All Figures Percentages)

Diagnosis	Connotation		
	Feigning	Crazy	Imagining
Symptoms all in your mind	83	31	87
Hysterical weakness	45	24	45
Psychosomatic weakness	24	12	20
Medically unexplained weakness	24	12	31
Depression associated weakness	21	7	20
Stress related weakness	9	6	14
Chronic fatigue	9	2	10
Functional weakness	7	2	8
Stroke	2	5	5
Multiple Sclerosis	0	1	3

Source: Adapted from Stone et al. (2002).

naturally healthy. It therefore stands to reason that if he becomes ill, there must be a cause for the illness, preferably one that comes from without and can be quickly dealt with. . . . Such a system gives primacy to the idea that disease is some wild and hairy monster that can be locked up with diagnosis."

The dialogue between the patient with soos and the diagnostician will focus on particulars of the syndrome. As a reflection of the patient's proclivities to focus, or more likely the diagnostician's preconceptions, an element or two will emerge that seem more significant. The fatigue, or the tenderness and achiness, or the headache, or the diarrhea becomes the most telling symptom. There follows a diagnostic "workup": blood tests, imaging studies, perhaps colonoscopy, and much more are to follow in due course. Time will pass. The patient anticipates that the next result is likely to uncover the culprit. Why else would they be put through this workup? Despite all the efforts, the disease remains elusive. What then? Overtly declaring uncertainty by offering a diagnosis of "medically unexplained" symptoms is more offensive than a label of uncertain clinical value, which has cachet in the public mind. Hence, the patient who entered the diagnostic exercise with soos is likely to emerge bearing such labels as "Chronic Fatigue Syndrome" (CFS), "Irritable Bowel Syndrome" (IBS), "fibromyalgia" (FM), and the like, to learn their respective acronyms, and to seek comfort among individuals similarly labeled.

Clearly the establishment of rapport in the medical treatment act plays out within well-circumscribed semantic boundaries, which reflect the culture of the day. In generations past, SOOS evoked labels such as hysteria, neurocirculatory asthenia, epidemic neuromyasthenia, and more from the medical establishment. There is a history to labeling by alternative practitioners that is as colorful and rarely grounded in the scientific inferences of the day. One does not seek the ministrations of a physician to hear magical thinking such as the invoking of some vitalistic forces to explain symptoms. Nor does one seek the ministrations of a physician to hear, let alone to learn, that one's symptoms are perceptual in nature. Rather, one seeks out a physician in order to learn the "scientific" cause of the symptoms with the expectation that the cause will be remedied and the symptoms regress pari passu.

This has not always been so. Michel Foucault, in his elegant monograph *The Birth of the Clinic: An Archaeology of Medical Perception* (1973), dates this conception of the contemporary treatment act to the turn of the nineteenth century. Earlier, symptoms were considered to be diseases. Fever was a disease, along with agues, rheumatism, lumbago, catarrh, and the like. If you sought medical care because you were coughing up phlegm (sputum), you would be treated for catarrh — that is, for coughing up phlegm. Unctions, potions, and worse would be plied along with pontifications as to prognosis. Some generations of physicians has produced an iconoclast or two who bludgeon the prevailing dogma until it is readied to yield to progress. The early eighteenth century was so blessed, most notably by Thomas Sydenham (1624–89) in London, who realized the fallacy of this diagnostic reasoning. Sydenham posited that symptoms were the illness, the presenting manifestation of an underlying causal disorder — a disease. This insight was a major intellectual achievement, truly a paradigm shift from illness as disease to illness as an indication of disease. Without it we would still be treating catarrh instead of pneumonias, rheumatism instead of rheumatic fever, and on and on. Without Sydenham's insight, scourges such as smallpox and polio would not be history. Modern medicine is anchored on this illness-disease paradigm and rightfully rejoices in its many successes. Unfortunately, this success has a downside.

The illness-disease paradigm has enjoyed nearly 300 years of acceptance and is firmly embedded in our culture. To question its essence is not just heresy; it is irrational. However, to assume this paradigm is without shortcomings is ignorance. What do we do when the disease that underlies the illness remains indeterminate despite modern diagnostics? What about the possibility of suffering illness in the absence of disease? Would the illness then qualify as a medicalization of a life event?

The disease is indeterminate. Despite an ancient tradition that decries hubris, the admission "I don't know" is not a regular feature of many treatment acts. Sometimes one hears "medically unexplainable symptoms," which is an assertion that the patient often interprets to signify that someday the symptoms will be explicable, not that the doctor is insinuating that the symptoms are "in the mind" of the patient. More often, the doctor's uncertainty is often camouflaged by the differential diagnosis, or as a "syndrome" diagnosis, which is nothing more than a New Age categorization of symptoms. My use of soos takes this tendency to its limit. The former has the virtue of structuring the clinical investigations, the latter of providing some basis for prognostication. Such labeling is little more than avoidance of admitting ignorance. It is not my style. However, my only qualm is when the labeling is not comforting to the patient.

But I get my hackles up when such labeling supports an unproved, often self-serving clinical heuristic. "In my experience" or "it is common practice" all too often takes iatrogenic license with the illness-disease paradigm in that it becomes the rationale for unproved remedies. This practice has left indelible and inexcusable marks on the history of medicine. It is a form of quackery that masquerades as science. It usually operates as follows. Given the belief that there must be a disease underlying every illness, it is seductive to assume that any demonstrable coincident abnormality, or difference, is the likely culprit. The twentieth century has witnessed the extirpation of countless tonsils to protect children from pharyngitis and of many a retroverted uterus for backache before prescient judgment and then the appropriate epidemiological studies took hold. There are many medically similar examples that remain in practice today, some in use without the backing of any scientific testing and some in direct contravention of science. Prior chapters bear witness.

Illness without disease. Payer's observation that Americans regard themselves as naturally healthy is telling. For that to be true, we Americans must be convinced of our invincibility. As discussed in chapter 8, life presents us with morbid challenges. Our sense of invincibility is repeatedly under attack by many intermittent and remittent predicaments of normal life. Feeling "well" demands the sense of invincibility that we can cope with our next musculoskeletal morbidity. Being "well" symbolizes our triumph that we had the wherewithal to cope with the last episode for as long as it took for that episode to remit, and often to cope so well that the episode is barely memorable if at all. Being "well" does not mean avoiding the challenges of soos, or the regional musculoskeletal disorders (chapter 9); that is not possible, for such challenges are as much a part of life as heartache, heartburn, headache, and the like.

I am wont to emphasize regional musculoskeletal disorders not simply because I've studied them for decades (though the maturity of the relevant science is another inducement), but also because they are the chief complaint of a sizable minority of people who choose to seek the ministrations of primary-care physicians and the vast majority who choose to seek the ministrations of chiropractors and other practitioners of manual medicine (see chapter 13). It has long been common sense that a press toward recourse, to potions or professions, is driven by the physical intensity of the person's predicament. The more severe the pain, the more likely it is memorable and the more likely the person is to consume analgesics, experience work incapacity, and seek professional care. Epidemiology has put this common sense to the test. It is not tenable. Compromise in the person's wherewithal to cope with the regional musculoskeletal disorder supersedes the severity of the pain and biomechanical compromise in driving our response.

This insight has great implications for the clinical treatment act. The narrative of distress of a patient with a regional musculoskeletal disorder is often delivered as a substitute for difficulties the person is having in coping with the demands of life that render the musculoskeletal disorder the last straw. For example, "My back hurts" is likely to mean, "My back hurts but I'm here because I can't cope with this episode," or, more particularly, "I'm here because I can't cope with this episode and the turmoil at home (or work) at the same time." Yet, treatment acts for back pain are wont to focus exclusively on the back. The same can be said of treatment acts for shoulder pain focusing on the shoulder, knee pain on the knee, and so on. Such is the patient's expectation in seeking care and the expertise purveyed by the chosen professional. The clinical contract demands specific treatment for the cause of the pain. Yet for nearly all the regional musculoskeletal disorders, such a treatment act rests on the shakiest of scientific grounds. It follows as no surprise that the response of these patients to primary care and other treatment acts cannot be shown to facilitate remission, though several render the patient less dissatisfied with the pace of the natural history. Perhaps this ineffectiveness reflects the inability to design specific treatment for discrete disorders. For back pain, there are over 300 randomized controlled trials testing pharmaceuticals, advice as to activity, various gadgets, and many physical "modalities" without a hint of benefit (with the exception of a hint for a single osteopathic back crack administered at two weeks to patients whose illness is not confounded by sociopolitical factors such as work incapacity). I suspect these treatment acts don't work because they focus on the pathoanatomy and not on the psychosocial confounders to coping. They miss the forest for the trees. Regardless of the fact that these treatment acts do not work, the patient is instructed as to the various clinical hypotheses upon which these treatments are based. Needless to say, such instruction will irretrievably alter the patient's conception of health and peoples' choice of idioms to describe current and future distress.

Persistent widespread pain. Hidden in all the community surveys of the people with discrete regional musculoskeletal disorders are people burdened with persistent pain at multiple sites. Their numbers are impressive, varying between 3 and 10 percent of the population depending on the community studied and the definition of "persistent widespread pain," but only recently has their plight been recognized. People with regional musculoskeletal pain at multiple sites are more likely to manifest psychological disturbance and to report other somatic symptoms than people who suffer from, or recall, discrete regional disorders. They have relentless SOOs. They are frequent consumers of medical care. They are often people bedeviled by life challenges that may render Sisyphean any quest for some sense of being well, let alone sense of invincibility. The intermittent and remittent morbid predicaments of life that well people find surmountable are insufferable and unforgettable setbacks for those living under this pall. Hence, they take note of and report other somatic symptoms. Variation in bowel habits looms large, and diminished vigor oppresses them. Joie de vivre is absent.

I suspect that few suffering with persistent chronic pain suffer in silence. I further suspect that their narrative of distress is very dependent on the listener. The idioms of distress that would enlist the empathy of a clergyperson are hardly the same as those that might enhance communication with a social worker, a sibling, or a physician. We have no data as to how these unhappy people select a confidante, but their cultural setting is likely to influence this decision. If they are seduced by the blandishment of "scientific," or pseudoscientific, medicine, they will choose a physician. As is the case for the discrete regional musculoskeletal disorders, the medical contract demands specific treatment for the cause of the pain, although again the treatment provided, seemingly rational or not, is unlikely to have a scientific grounding. Such putatively scientific treatment acts abound, generally predicated on a circularity of argument. The symptoms are ranked, a specific pathology is postulated, and a neologic diagnostic label is applied that reiterates the presenting symptoms. This labeling exercise is but "catarrh" redux. All the while, the treatment act is plying the patient with intimations as to the pathophysiology of his or her painfulness.

That is how the person suffering persistent widespread pain learns to be a patient with fibromyalgia. The clinician can find no specific cause for the complaint of persistent widespread pain. And the clinician feels compelled to discern that the patient dislikes being poked at particular bodily sites. Since fibromyalgia is defined as a state of chronic widespread pain and tenderness at certain body sites, the clinician pronounces, "You have fibromyalgia." Any clinician who applies the "fibromyalgia" label and promulgates a treatment act on that basis must disregard the observation that putatively diagnostic "tender points" are related to generalized pain and pain behavior in all clinical settings. Fibromyalgia denotes nothing more than persistent widespread pain. However, in the labeling, the patient is forever changed. As the patient learns more about fibromyalgia, the patient's narrative becomes laced with the new knowledge, which is then recited with objectivity that approaches dispassion.

The fate of patients with persistent widespread pain labeled as "fibromyalgia" stands in reproach to whatever theory underpins this labeling and subsequent treatment act. In the community, the majority of people with persistent wide-spread pain improve with time, but those labeled as "fibromyalgia" seldom do. Based on the science that pertains to the regional musculoskeletal disorders, I would suggest that this unhappy fate is not solely a reflection of the intensity of their symptoms or the pervasiveness of the psychosocial factors that confounded their coping so that they chose to be patients in the first place. I would suggest that the treatment acts, dripping with empty promises of elucidation and unproved promises of palliation, are iatrogenic; the treatment is causing more disease. I would further suggest that these circular treatment acts will exacerbate whatever mood or thought disorder is complicating the plight of these patients. Such are present in a large minority.

The proponents of the fibromyalgia construction are convinced that their pathophysiological insights and theories are valid, albeit as yet unproved, and their therapeutic approaches need but tweaking to produce the benefit that has eluded demonstration to date. They could, of course, be right, but undoubtedly their approach is causing harm today. I admit it is possible that a therapeutic triumph is but one scientific discovery away, rendering my psychosocial and sociocultural synthesis secondary, if not fatuous. After all, it would not have been far-fetched to have constructed sociocultural models for the pathogenesis of pulmonary tuberculosis and AIDS were it not for the superseding microbiology. That is why many an intrepid investigator has stalked the cause of fibromyalgia in the labyrinth of our neuroendocrine and immune systems, but clues are hard to come by and subtle changes prove unreliable, secondary, or nonspecific. Genetics plays a role, but it's slight and overwhelmed by the influences of the familial environment. Investigators have sought associations with unusual psychological or physical traumatic events, but the results are inconsistent at best. Testing biomedical theories is proving difficult but not insurmountable. To date, no such theories have survived formal testing. Furthermore, we are about to witness another wave of agents; nearly all are forms of antidepressant or antiseizure medicine said to improve the illness narrative of patients labeled as "fibromyalgia." The trials supporting this assertion, and that are likely to convince the trigger-happy FDA, are industry sponsored and executed by investigators with major ties to the purveying pharmaceutical firms. The improvement is anything but dramatic. I have no doubt that these agents will be popular for a year or so and then slip into ignominy, leaving behind disappointed patients and far wealthier entrepreneurs. I have said as much to reporters from the *Wall Street Journal* and *Los Angeles Times*, and was quoted for saying as much . . . to no avail.

Life under a pall. My psychosocial and sociocultural theory has not survived formal testing either, and indeed such testing is difficult to design and perform. I am suggesting that chronic persistent pain is an ideation, a somatization if you will, that some are inclined toward as a response to living life under a pall, and not vice versa. I am not defining "pall" further, as my theory countenances a wide range of individual differences in the tendency to somatize. I am further suggesting that these unfortunate people choose to be patients because they have exhausted their wherewithal to cope. If this is so, the complaint of persistent widespread pain should initiate a treatment act quite different from that leading to labeling as "fibromyalgia." The symptoms of persistent widespread pain should be heard as likely surrogate complaints for difficulties in coping with life's sometimes overwhelming problems. Months, often years, of poking, testing, pharmaceutical empiricisms, and the iatrogenicity of medicalization might be avoided by directly approaching the challenge to coping. Perhaps patients can be spared instruction in illness behaviors and contending with contrived neologisms such as "central sensitization," which connotes little more than the illness is in their mind. Then they might not need to attempt to unlearn illness behaviors with "cognitive behavior therapy" or the like.

Examining the prevalence of persistent widespread pain in populations living under psychosocially challenging circumstances offers an opportunity to seek associations that are inconsistent with my sociocultural theory. Many well people encounter challenging life events that offer an opportunity to examine the incidence of developing persistent widespread pain. My sociocultural theory of the pathogenesis of persistent widespread pain has yet to be buffeted by such data, as will become clear in the discussions to follow.

There is no more valid a diagnostic label for patients complaining of persistent widespread pain than "overwhelming persistent widespread pain." Certainly, "fibromyalgia" means nothing more. Leading investigators are promulgating two other labels: "functional somatic syndromes" and "medically unexplained symptoms." Their reasoning is worth consideration, but I doubt the clinical utility of either rubric. The former is difficult to define, even by its proponents, but it draws on the idea that there is a spectrum of degrees to which normal people feel compelled to focus on unpleasant bodily sensations. At one end of the spectrum, the focusing becomes severe enough to warrant a diagnosis of "functional somatic syndrome." The other label, "medically unexplained symptoms," implies that one would be better off if symptoms were medically explicable. That promise thwarts confronting the psychosocial issues that compromise coping and serve to render the pain intolerable. However, the label "functional somatic syndromes" derives from important observations.

The people in the community burdened with persistent widespread pain who have yet to avail themselves of a treatment act that labels them with fibromyalgia suffer more than just chronic pervasive pain. Other everyday symptoms become momentous. Unlike the invincible person, people who are succumbing to the challenges of life and use illness as a surrogate complaint seem easily to accumulate unpleasant and unexpected bodily events, turning them into mountains of concern. Something must be dreadfully wrong. Some of these unfortunate people quietly accept this sad state as their fate, but others vigorously cast about for an answer. The lay press and the Internet are at their service, as are many health-care professionals. Diagnostic banter such as Sjögren's, Raynaud's, lupus, Crohn's, fibromyalgia, chronic fatigue syndrome, TMJ syndrome, candida, EB virus, and many more are pressed into service. Many of these sufferers seem convinced that their condition was sudden in onset with a discrete cause rather than being the slow erosion of their coping until some critical level of reserve becomes depleted. Many generate a causal hypothesis that takes on a life of its own, an attributional ideation. Such ideas include "chemical imbalance," "virus," "stress," and "emotional confusion." According to a Canadian survey, most physiatrists, orthopedists, and general practitioners are not convinced that fibromyalgia can be a consequence of or "reactive" to discrete events, including discrete traumatic events. Only some Canadian rheumatologists are comfortable with that hypothesis. However, if one follows a cohort of well workers closely over time, those who develop persistent widespread pain are no more likely to experience any unusual event than those who remain well.

Functional somatic syndromes. It is on this background that a medical treatment act is initiated. If it is with a primary care or specialty physician, it will commence with a history of the present illness. In either case, a clinician predisposed to the hearing of certain complaints elicits the history. The primary-care physician is prepared by prior experiences, the specialist by training. That is why if you ask rheumatologists to examine the patients in a gastroenterology clinic, they will diagnose "fibromyalgia" in the majority of patients previously diagnosed as suffering "Irritable Bowel Syndrome" by the gastroenterologists. The gastroenterologists will return the favor if they examine the "fibromyalgia" patients in the rheumatology clinic. The symptoms of patients labeled as "Chronic Fatigue Syndrome" overlap those of patients with "fibromyalgia" (the tender points as well) so as to render the distinction untenable. Hence, there is the argument that all of these patients have a single "functional somatic syndrome" characterized by a spectrum of "medically unexplained symptoms." To my way of thinking, another way of looking at it is that these are people who are predisposed to somatize when under stress, and this predisposition takes over their lives when they are overwhelmed by life's difficulties. Unfortunately, they are then rendered more ill by the process of medicalization, which I will describe shortly.

All of us "somatize" to some degree. We have our bad days, days of soos. On such occasions we feel blue, or become aware of our bowels, or feel tired or stiff, as if we slept poorly. Sometimes we know why, for challenges at home, or at work, are all too obvious. If we are concerned that our aggravating knee pain or backache or headache has returned, or is worse and harder to deal with, we become even more out of sorts. Sometimes there is no certain association. It just happens. Fortunately, it just passes, too. A bit of good news, a beautiful day, or an invigorating jog is often salving.

For some of us, feeling out of sorts is all too familiar. Some of us may be predisposed to somatizing because we burden an unusual sense of vulnerability. That may be the result of our upbringing. Some parenting styles create "vulnerable children." These parents are not "bad" or psychologically disturbed, nor are their children disturbed. They are the kind of parents who, at the end of the day when they are tucking their child in, are inclined to the thought, "Thank God Johnny made it today." They infect their child with a subtle, subliminal sense of impending doom. Such a pessimistic view of the world sometimes seems to run in families. Parents raise children to see the world as they do. The "vulnerable child" has been the subject of considerable academic interest in pediatrics for the past decade. The vulnerable child grows up to be the vulnerable adult, for whom being out of sorts carries the weight of a self-fulfilling prophecy. Shaking off that sense of impending catastrophe is challenging, and the inability to do so has been labeled "catastrophizing." These are normal people, living life at one end of the spectrum of normal coping, and it is easy for them to trip up. The consequences of any such trip are easily modeled by the community in which they live or the community they seek out, depending on the recourse they choose. If it's medical recourse, medicalization and iatrogenicity is a specter.

If you have to prove you are ill, you can't get well. There are circumstances in life that predispose most if not all of us to somatize and catastrophize. Abusive relationships will do it. Job dissatisfaction and job insecurity will do it. A workers' compensation claim for a chronically disabling regional musculoskeletal disorder (back pain, arm pain, or fibromyalgia in particular) will do it. Being a plaintiff in a personal injury lawsuit, a tort, will do it. Many of these circumstances are discussed in chapter 12. In the settings where a person bases a claim for a disability indemnity award or legal settlement for a regional musculoskeletal disorder allegedly caused by a personal injury, the claimant is expected to prove illness. Traditionally, the proof of illness has been subjugated to the proof of disease — demonstrable tissue damage. If there is enough physical damage and undisputed culpability, the symptoms are considered credible and an award follows efficiently. However, in the absence of sufficient "damage" and culpability, a contest is joined that demands that the plaintiff or claimant prove illness. For all the regional musculoskeletal disorders, most demonstrable "damage" is incidental and correlates little if at all with symptoms and function. Furthermore, by definition, regional musculoskeletal pain occurs in the course of activities that are customary and customarily comfortable, so that culpability is seldom certain. These two features drive the claimant or plaintiff into a corner, beleaguered by adjusters and others who are demanding proof of specific damage and certain culpability.

Patients labeled with "fibromyalgia" are spared coincidental demonstrable specific damage by definition. These dreadfully ill people have to prove their illness in the absence of disease. The only way to do so depends on emotion and body language, levels of communication foreign to bureaucracies. The inevitable contest may be broached by the health insurer who must approve treatment or, more often, by an insurance carrier who needs to determine the magnitude of disability consequent to "fibromyalgia." Lawyers who serve the claimant recruit "experts" who find many "tender points" and espouse biomedical theories to explain the claimant's injury-related complaints. The insurer has a fiduciary responsibility to approve only effective treatments and to validate awards for "disability." Their lawyers recruit "experts" who find fewer "tender points" or invoke alternative interpretations of the symptomatology or of the medical literature. The most predictable outcome is that the patient with the pervasive illness labeled "fibromyalgia" will get sicker and less capable of performing in society. That patient will focus on all symptoms, recalling and often recording them at the instruction of legal counsel in a drive to document the magnitude of illness. Symptom magnification is predictable. Since the veracity of the symptoms is at stake, diminution in their intensity is made virtually impossible; regression in intensity is tantamount to yielding to the insinuations that their symptoms were feigned in the first place. Illness escalates predictably. The other predictable outcome is that considerable wealth will be transferred from those who pay premiums to all involved in this medicolegal process, with the exception often of the claimant for whom pathos is the reward and impoverishment the price to be paid.

Medicalization. The contest I've just outlined plays out in a public arena. A more private contest awaits the person with persistent widespread pain who chooses to seek medical recourse. While less violent than the medicolegal contest, it is as likely to inflame illness. This contest is joined when the physician and the patient set out to define the biological "cause" of the persistent widespread pain as prerequisite to treatment à la Sydenham, a process that is bound to recruit the patient's undivided attention. Their persistent widespread pain is medicalized. The contest remains subliminal until the diagnostic process has proven fruitless, a time-consuming and anxiety-provoking exercise in testing, consulting, and running down false clues. The diminishing return of the diagnostic exercise is met with increasing tension in the patient-physician interaction. Any suggestions the doctor now offers as to the value of psychological counseling are heard as accusations of "it's in your mind." The patient is placed in the position of proving to the physician that the pain is real, and proving the same to skeptics in their family, social network, and workplace. Such a patient often recalls and records symptoms in the course of the treatment act, just as they are likely to do in the course of a more public litigious contest. Their illness escalates. For these patients caught in this vortex, the label "fibromyalgia" is much more than a diagnosis; it is a symbol of self-actualization. For me, or anyone else, to discuss its semiotic or offer a sociocultural theory of pathogenesis is infuriating. That too is viewed as an assault on their veracity, an accusation that their symptoms are "in their mind."

One of the most dangerous acts physicians perform is to take the "history." Physicians cannot avoid doing so. The "history" provides the information needed to formulate a differential diagnosis, around which testing is structured. However, the history is stylized at its foundation and designed to pursue every positive responsive into a tree of cognition. Physicians query in a fashion such that symptoms long ignored are revealed. Inevitably, the history medicalizes the symptoms so that they become the illness. To what end? Certainly there are the occasions when crucial symptoms emerge from this process, which lead to a specific diagnosis, specific palliation, and even cure. In those instances, the medicalization of less crucial symptoms is subsumed by the triumph of scientific medicine — at least that is the hope and probably the myth. Being a patient is a hazardous process. A person may sensibly consult a doctor for the treatment of acute bronchitis only to learn during the course of healing that their PSA, or blood pressure, or blood glucose is elevated — or other labeling events we have considered previously. Both skill and responsibility are required if the doctor is to avoid unnecessarily keeping patients as patients, rather than facilitating their return to personhood.

For the patient with the complaint of persistent widespread pain, taking the history offers nothing but medicalization. Undoing the medicalization brings us full circle to the start of this chapter: "It's in your mind."

Mind-body duality. Why is this diagnosis so offensive? The answer relates to a social construction growing out of the sixteenth century. When William Harvey discovered the circulation of blood, medicine and society could finally cast off the intellectual constraints of Galen. Vital humors were not amenable to testing, but science could contend with phenomena that were concrete, even measurable, such as Harvey's discovery. The workings of the body were open to study. The mind-body relationship was a different matter. Even the greatest philosopher-scientists and philosopher-physicians of the day could not cast off the abstraction of a "soul," or its cogitating handmaiden, a "mind." The "body" was comprised of concrete, objective forms and structures, but the mind and the soul were beyond ken. Yet, somehow they must be connected. René Descartes and his contemporaries went to lengths to infer the connection, usually relying on models of pain. Descartes was fascinated by the phenomenon of the "phantom limb," in which pain is perceived in an amputated limb. Sensations were the purview of the body, the nerves in particular, but pain was a higher function, a purview of the soul. It followed that pain, unaccompanied by correlative sensations in the body, should be considered like a phantom limb—a pain in the mind that is imaginary.

Of course, for the sake of brevity, I am not doing justice to this historiography. Cartesian thinking was far more involved. Others also had their versions of the mind-body duality: Sydenham conceived of an "internal man"; Pascal posited that "the ills of the body are nothing more than punishment [for the] ills of the soul"; Henry Cabinis, a French physician, conceived of a balance between pleasure and pain. Others argued variously from religious, metaphysical, psychological, or physiological perspectives. Over the centuries, the nature of pain caused—and for that matter still causes—much scientific and philosophical confusion. Philosophers have contended with the idea that pain might not just be evil; it might be useful. Western medicine was taken to task more than once to justify the inflicting of pain for some putative good by a theological tradition of comforting, and it is still taken to task on this basis.

Woven into these centuries of discourse and debate was the concept of hypochondria. In the early nineteenth century, Xavier Bichat, another French physician imbued with Cabinis's pain-pleasure duality, postulated that there were two "lives"—one inherent to the viscera, a "vegetative" life, and the other interactive and conscious, an "animal" life. Hypochondria resulted when the normal painful vegetative sensations, thought to be seated in the upper quadrants of the abdomen (the hypochondrium), moved across the threshold into conscious suffering. All this sounds archaic, but modern psychology now terms this process "amplification" and recognizes Cabinis's "forces" as cognition, attention, context, and mood.

The label "hypochondriasis" is reserved for individuals with obsessive vigilance regarding bodily changes. These are the people who can't notice a mole without thinking melanoma, or note a palpitation without concluding heart disease. They establish a contract with medical providers calling for the repeated reassurance of the diagnostic process. Medicalization is less an issue; there is no sense of invincibility at risk. Modern psychiatry considers hypochondriasis at the extreme of a spectrum of "somatoform disorders" that afflict individuals who suffer from any physical symptom that defies medical explanation. If there are multiple such symptoms, the term "somatization disorder" applies. These are terms that supersede hysteria, conversion disorder, and a litany of discarded labels, such as neurocirculatory asthenia, neuromyasthenia, railway spine, and the like. However, all this labeling tends to belittle the symptoms and stigmatize the patient. It is but a New Age form of "in your mind."

This takes us back to Cartesian mind-body duality. As important as that paradigm was in pushing back the frontier of ignorance and metaphysical obfuscation in the seventeenth century, it is an impediment today. First, it is wrong. The "mind" is no longer an abstraction. Today we can probe it with PET scanning, forms of MR imaging, and neurochemistry. We are starting to peel back the veils that shrouded the molecular basis of learning and emotion and of nociception (the perception of pain beyond its sensation). The mind is no longer abstractly that which thinks. Nociception involves receptors and transmitters and modulating electrophysiology. There is an underlying commonality to pain that makes it unspeakable, inexpressible in language, reflexively aversive, and opiate responsive. The Cartesian mind-body duality no longer belongs in the clinic.

It is perhaps being superseded by another duality. Pain does not just involve injury and physical disease. Pain recruits memory and cognition, and suffering recruits the psychosocial context of the afflicted individual. Nothing in life is as idiosyncratic as the *experience* of pain as suffering. If the pain-suffering duality could supplant the mind-body duality as the social construction, a Western patient could ask a Western physician, "Is it in my mind?," without losing face.

The supplementary reading for this chapter is another shadow chapter that expands on these major points.

chapter eleven

Aging Is Not a Disease

We will all die. Dying is not a disease; it is as much a fact of life as being born. The process of dying can be a disease, and too often in the United States it is an iatrogenic disease. But die we must. Very, very few of us will get to die as nonagenarians, though many will come close (see chapter 1). The biological odyssey from birth to death is one of subtle incremental changes, punctuated with occasional drama: puberty, pregnancy, female menopause. Most of the changes we take in stride, even a proud strut. Some changes, like the bulging of a midline or the drooping of a buttock, we find less appealing and usually accept blame. Of course the reason we find a bulge or a droop less appealing is socially constructed. Past generations found such symbolic of robustness and success in life. But today, they are symbolic of sloth. The closer we come to the end of life, the more we run into socially constructed impediments to "strutting our stuff." We are taught antipathy toward our wrinkles, cellulite, superficial varicosities, and nocturia (waking to urinate). These ubiquitous changes of later life are far less dramatic than those of puberty, which we were taught to celebrate. Are these ubiquitous changes of later life diseases? Are wrinkles a disease? Should we consider a face lift a cure?

Is graying a disease? I am not being facetious. Graying is a consequence of biological senescence. The follicles that turn skin cells into hair lose the capacity to introduce pigment. These follicles have lost a normal biological function resulting in obvious biological consequence. Is the consequence pathologic? If so, graying is a disease. If the consequence is not pathologic, graying is "normal."

Is graying an illness? For some, gray hair is a symptom. For these people, it is a biological event that is a cause of concern and discomfiture. For these people, graying is an illness, often an illness for which recourse is sought. The recourse is symptomatic in that hair dyeing palliates the illness. The causal pathobiology of the follicle, the disease, is unchecked. Of course, for others graying is not an illness regardless of its underlying biology. These are folks who disregard graying or find it pleasing, even distinguished. For them it is one of many normal life transitions. They may find the underlying biology may be dramatic, but it is not pathologic. C'est la vie.

To consider graying an illness is to "medicalize" it. As we discussed in chapters 8 and 10, if the illness-disease paradigm is to be fulfilled, the underlying follicular biology must be pathologic. Graying is the illness one "gets" from diseased hair follicles. The syllogism calls for treatment of the disease to cure the graying. No doubt if a wayward antihypertensive drug happened to reinvigorate the production of pigment by hair follicles, as one happens to "cure" balding, its manufacturer would be quick to petition the FDA for licensing. The drug would be eagerly marketed as the "cure" for graying. It is even likely that new subsections of august dermatology societies would form to discuss the breakthrough. Competing pharmaceutical firms would race to synthesize "me too" drugs that would pass muster at the FDA at least in terms of convenience if not effectiveness. These firms would compete to underwrite educational programs for physicians and consumers. Advocacy organizations would seek to have the agents covered by Medicare.

Parody? Hardly.

We are already witness to one of the most effective and pervasive campaigns to medicalize aging: the assault on our aging skeleton. If I have my way, it will leave as legacy caveat emptor, its only redeeming feature.

Osteopenia

For a generation or two, a small cadre of clinical investigators from several disciplines has studied age-dependent changes in our bones. They enjoyed steady progress and a low profile—until recently. Today, the aging public lives in fear of painfully shrinking away from "osteoporosis." Screening programs are recommended. Pharmaceutical firms are marketing aggressively to convince prescribers and consumers that they offer a product, by prescription or over-the-counter, that is the best choice. This is an enormous enterprise bolstered by advocacy groups, professional societies, educational programs, and the like. Seldom does one hear an argument against screening, let alone chewing pills, often composed of ground oyster shells, or taking other potions. Almost no one is raising the issue of whether this entire enterprise is an egregious example of medicalization. This chapter is written to raise that issue.

THE AGE-DEPENDENCE OF MINERALIZATION

Bone is an extraordinary biological material. Shape and resilience are properties of its protein matrix, most of which is collagen. Mineral salts, mainly calcium salts incorporated into the matrix, give bone strength. Although the mineralized matrix is inert, bone is populated by cells specialized for its maintenance. The composition of the resident cell population and the fine structure of the mineralized matrix are not uniform across all bones. For example, the bones of the spine, the vertebrae, differ importantly from both the femur and the skull. Each bone is a living organ. All bones are preprogrammed as to shape and architecture. Long bones and vertebrae respond to the habitual application of physical forces by compensatory changes in architecture. As is true of all organs in the human body, bones are continuously renewing themselves. The adult skeleton turns over about every decade, though individual bones differ in this frequency. To achieve this "turnover," the bone cells must demineralize the collagen and then degrade the naked collagen while other cells are synchronized to replace the collagen in forms that facilitate remineralization with calcium salts. The tearing down is termed "resorption," and the rebuilding is "accretion." The entire process is termed "remodeling."

Sometime after puberty, all of our bones finish growing in length. However, they continue to "grow" in fine structure, gaining mineralized matrix well into our third or even fourth decade. This means that the remodeling results in a positive balance until we approach midlife, when there is neither net gain nor loss. The degree of mineralization at midlife is quite variable. On average, the plateau reached by women is less than that reached by men. Ancestral origin has a striking influence; bones of those with African roots are more mineralized than those with either Asian or European roots. There is a positive influence of moderate weight-bearing exercises on the degree of mineralization and a negative influence of thinness (a low BMI) and of tobacco abuse.

In our fifth decade, the balance turns negative; we slowly come to have less mineral-per-unit matrix and therefore less well-mineralized bone. In men, this negative balance is a gentle slope that continues until death. In women, the negative balance accelerates with menopause. There is much variability in the rate of demineralization both between people and within the skeleton. If the articulating ends of the bones (the joints) have osteoarthritis, the bones tend to be spared demineralization. The bones of individuals who have more fatty tissue, have avoided cigarette smoking, and/or exercise habitually are also relatively spared demineralization. But the sparing is relative; demineralization is "normal."

Bone that is less well mineralized is more fragile. Whether the fragility results in a clinically meaningful event depends on many more factors than just the degree of mineralization. Very few well people demineralize to the degree that important fractures are unavoidable; since our discussion is aimed at well people, I will not detail drugs and diseases that drive demineralization to this extreme. However, there are people who demineralize sufficiently to incur a measurable increase in risk for fracture. The jargon terms this status "osteopenia," meaning scant bone. If someone with osteopenia suffers a fracture without an extraordinary physical exposure, the fracture is termed a "pathological fracture" or a "fragility fracture" and the underlying disease is termed osteoporosis to denote a pathological degree of osteopenia. Extrapolating from our discussion of the plateaus of mineralization, the people most at such risk are found among thin women of European or Asian ancestry, but no one is spared some degree of risk.

FRAGILITY FRACTURES

Osteopenia is never an illness. No one knows that her or his bones are demineralizing. The issue is the disease manifest as pathological fractures. Reasonably, people might want to know if their osteopenia is severe enough to put them at sufficiently high risk of a pathological fracture to justify trying to restore mineralization. However, this assumes there is an intervention proven to be effective with a favorable benefit/risk ratio. If the intervention were effective with trivial risk, then perhaps it would be sensible for everyone to partake of its beneficence regardless of the degree of osteopenia. Such was the basis for the public-health policy of fluoridation of drinking water to prevent dental caries. However, if the intervention is of uncertain beneficence, or the benefit/risk ratio is indeterminate or marginal, should one be fooled into intervening simply because osteopenia imparts risk? Indeed, the interventions for osteopenia are of uncertain benefit across the board. For some the benefit/risk ratio is uncertain but likely unfavorable, while for others the interventions approach the trivial. I will examine the interventions below, but first there is much more to understand about the disease osteoporosis and its principle manifestation, pathological fractures.

Three regions of our skeleton carry this risk: the spine, the proximal femur (hip), and the distal forearm (near the wrist). Pathologic fractures from primary osteoporosis elsewhere are too rare to factor into the decision to screen and intervene for osteopenia.

Fragility fractures of the spine. Remarkably, the scientific, clinical, and lay literatures relating to osteoporotic pathological fractures of the spine treat the topic as if there were no other spine disorders affecting the elderly. The impression given is that banishing osteopenia would free the elderly of axial morbidity. Nothing could be further from the truth. All elderly have degenerative diseases of the spine. All elderly cope with backache frequently. There are many surveys suggesting that backache colors the year for as many as half of women over age sixty-five. Osteoporotic pathological fractures are a minor factor in all this morbidity.

Part of the degenerative process leads to the loss of discs, the soft tissue structures separating the vertebrae. Few over age sixty-five have not suffered this change at more than one spinal level, particularly at the low back and neck. As discussed in chapter 9, the presence of such degenerative changes correlates very poorly with symptoms. However, these changes always exact a penalty on the height of the individual as well as on suppleness. Inches are lost as we age because of loss of the disc spacing alone. Even if your spinal bones were pristine, you'd lose height.

The degenerative spine is the field upon which osteoporotic compression fractures play out. Most compression fractures occur in the thoracic (chest) portion of the spine, particularly affecting the vertebrae between the shoulder blades. The vertebrae normally are cylinders. If they are osteopenic, the end plates of the bony cylinder can collapse, creating "codfish" vertebrae, so called because they acquire the shape of fish vertebrae. This type of fracture has little consequence in terms of posture. However, if the anterior wall (the wall facing forward) collapses, the cylinder assumes a wedge shape, creating a forward-leaning curve to the thoracic spine — a kyphosis, or "dowager's hump." The result is additional loss in stature and some degree of deformity.

Both degenerative changes and backache are ubiquitous in the elderly, but compression fractures are comparatively rare. If you identify 1,000 women in their seventies who have no compression fractures on spine X-rays and follow them for a year, fifteen or so will develop a compression fracture. Women who develop a compression fracture are several times more likely to have a new compression fracture in the following year.

Is this all there is to it, analogous to graying? Because of degenerative changes, all of us lose stature, all of us lose flexibility, and all of us tend toward kyphosis. Some age in this fashion more than others. Some assume a distinctive posture.

Would it be absurd if the social construction held that all these alterations in stature and posture were distinguished and appealing concomitants of aging? Or is there more to this? Is there an illness consequent to these compression fractures?

This last rhetorical question might seem absurd at first. After all, this anatomical change is a "fracture." However, most patients can recall no distinctive episode of pain that might be ascribed to this compression fracture. Most compression fractures are incidental findings on chest X-rays. Occasionally a patient presents with acute severe back pain, often between the shoulder blades, associated with a coincident radiographically demonstrable compression fracture. That the association is likely to be causal is tenable since this presentation is unusual except in the elderly; most episodes of acute back pain from other causes are in the neck or low back. The syndrome of acute symptomatic compression fracture is a miserable experience, particularly since it can be prolonged and difficult to palliate. Fortunately, it is self-limited, though there is a tendency for a recurrence or two. However, this acute compression-fracture syndrome is an exceptional presentation for a disease that is not particularly prevalent in the first place. Population studies show very little or no association between an increase in back symptoms and an increase in the prevalence or incidence of compression fractures. Whatever suggestion exists probably reflects the occasional case of the acute syndrome. All this means that there would be very limited impact on the burden of spinal pain or pathoanatomy in the aging population even if we did manage to prevent spinal compression fractures.

Fragility fractures of the hip. No one will argue that hip fracture is much ado about nothing. Pathologic hip fractures are not the same as compression fractures. Both occur in the course of normal activities. Spinal compression fractures are generally asymptomatic, or the symptoms they engender are perceived as yet another of the intermittent and remittent axial pains that are common experience in the elderly. Pathologic hip fractures are never subsumed by the "background noise" of the musculoskeletal disorders. They are painful, and they halt weight bearing. Coping is not an option unless one wants to take to bed forever. It would seem that hip fractures should be a compelling argument for the treatment of osteopenia, but they are not.

Hip fractures are easy to fix. There are surgical options, the commonest of which, pinning, is straightforward and requires little postoperative rehabilitation. One of the paradoxes of the circumstance of osteoporotic hip fractures is that the "cure" is both ready and Pyrrhic. Most osteoporotic pathologic hip

fractures are the fate of the elderly, but only some of the elderly. If you follow 1,000 Dutch women in their eighth decade for a year, five will suffer a hip
fracture. If you follow a subset of Dutch women in their eighth decade who are
particularly osteopenic, the likelihood doubles or triples. This is not simply
a matter of chance. The women who suffer the fractures are frailer and more
likely to fall, which is the reason the longevity and functionality of women and
men who suffer an osteoporotic hip are severely decreased despite the fact that
their fractures are expeditiously and safely managed. That is why the most effective intervention to prevent osteoporotic hip fractures in the frail elderly is
to decrease the likelihood and severity of falls.

Colles fractures. Fragility fractures of the distal forearm are not really "pathological" in that they are always a consequence of trauma. The typical story is
that breaking a fall with the extended wrist breaks the distal forearm. As was
the case for osteoporotic hip fractures, the first principle of treatment is to avoid
falls. For the elderly, particularly the frail elderly, this often requires more than
advice. It is important that the living area be unencumbered by objects and surfaces likely to trip one up. Assistive devices might be necessary to stabilize gait
and transfers: canes, walkers, elevated seats, and the like. There is also evidence
that balance and stability of the elderly can be improved with training and
practice. The European Prospective Osteoporosis Study followed some 5,000
men and women over age fifty for three years. The study found that a history of
falling is far more predictive of Colles fractures than the degree to which bone
is mineralized.

To return to the "graying hair" analogy, pathological fractures are a disease
that becomes more likely as the degree of osteopenia increases. However, in
the case of spinal compression fractures, the illness that can be ascribed to
this disease is quite variable. Most often there is none. Sometimes the illness
is considerable but transient — an acute compression-fracture syndrome of the
spine. Sometimes there is an alteration in posture beyond that which one expects in the peer group and that some consider deformity. For spinal compression fractures, the benefit/risk ratio of proactively treating osteopenia must be
convincingly favorable. Nearly all well people who are fortunate to live long
enough to contend with the specter of spinal compression fractures will not
have to contend with the reality.

For osteoporotic hip and wrist fractures, a bit more leniency in the risk/
benefit ratio is acceptable, but not much. If attention is given to reducing the
risk of falling, there is little more to be gained. To gain that little more, little risk

should be tolerated. However, families and managers of residential facilities for the elderly need to be aware that interventions that are based on assessments of function can reduce falls. These should include behavioral interventions and modifications of environmental hazards.

Meddling with Osteopenia

Given these benefit/risk considerations, let's examine the marketed menu in order of acceptability.

DIETARY SUPPLEMENTS

Calcium and vitamin D supplements top this list. These are preparations that are offered over the counter. They are hawked aggressively in stores and in the media and form part of the enormous North American vitamin scam. The average person eating an average diet in any industrialized country has no need for vitamin or mineral supplements. For most well people, there is no discernible benefit, but there is little risk either. As you will learn in chapters 13 and 14, I have no argument with people who seek out and avail themselves of unproved remedies, or even those proven to be worthless, as long as the putative remedies are harmless, the consumers are informed, and I don't have to share the expense by virtue of my health-insurance premiums or tax dollar. I should mention that several vitamins are anything but harmless if taken in excess, notably vitamins D and A.

There is a reason why the average person receives no benefit from calcium and vitamin D supplements. Our endocrine system is highly committed to monitoring the blood level of calcium and maintaining it just at our personal set point, and our calcium absorption is tightly controlled to that end. The mechanism is elegant. If the blood-calcium level trends down, vitamin D is converted to an active metabolite, which makes the intestinal absorption of calcium more efficient, and vice versa. No matter how much calcium you ingest, the fraction absorbed will be controlled to reflect the blood-calcium level. The same holds for the activation of most forms of vitamin D, including the form produced by our skin after sunlight exposure. It is estimated that about an hour in the midday sun will generate our daily requirement.

I hasten to add that there may be subsets of well people in advanced countries who are at risk for dietary insufficiency of calcium or vitamin D. In theory at least, people who avoid dairy products and thereby have a lower calcium intake and less vitamin D supplementation should be at risk for a special form of osteopenia called osteomalacia. (Osteomalacia occurs when the collagen is not well mineralized; in osteoporosis the collagen is well mineralized but there's less total bone.) However, such a subset is difficult to tease out of the general population, even among postmenopausal women. The data to support a public-health recommendation as to calcium and vitamin D supplementation of a normal diet or as to dairy-food consumption are quite inconsistent and any such recommendation is controversial. However, there is one subset of well people for whom a diet deficient in calcium or vitamin D is a risk for osteopenia. That subset is the elderly, particularly the institutionalized elderly and most particularly institutionalized or homebound elderly women. This is the only subset in which there is scientific support for supplementing the diet with calcium and vitamin D. The support is tenuous and speaks to supplementing twice the customary 400 IU (international units) of vitamin D each day.

HORMONE REPLACEMENT THERAPY

Hormone Replacement Therapy (HRT) is next in our hierarchy of acceptability for meddling with osteopenia. It is next in spite of the ongoing brouhaha. Menopause is a biological passage. For a generation of women, it has been followed by a rite of passage: the decision to continue menstruating in the absence of ovulation. I have not seen it argued that this decision is ever prejudiced by some need to continue menstruating. Rather, HRT was foisted on the postmenopausal woman under the widely advertised banner of prolonging youthfulness. The medicalization of menopause was a gold mine both for gynecologists and the pharmaceutical firms that manufacture and market estrogen-containing compounds. Undoubtedly, HRT can have beneficial effects both on vaginal dryness and perimenopausal symptoms, which can occasionally be quite challenging. However, the former responds to topical estrogen, and the latter to brief exposure to low-dose estrogen. Nonetheless, the benefits of long-term HRT became a social construction that continues to sway as many as 40 percent of postmenopausal women. They were swayed initially by the promise of an improved quality of life and later by the promise of a lessened risk of osteoporosis and its disabling consequences. The latter follows from the observation by Fuller Albright, a pioneer of modern endocrinology, in 1941 that menopause was associated with spinal osteoporosis, for which he recommended estrogen therapy.

The promise of HRT did not stop there. After all, there are many diseases that spare premenopausal women and afflict postmenopausal women for which HRT might prove the salve. Heart disease was suggested, to name one. Albright had very few lapses in logic during a stellar career that was all the more remarkable for his perseverance into later life despite severe Parkinson's disease. However, assuming a causal association between estrogen lack and osteoporosis was one serious lapse. It's an example of the fallacy of *post hoc, ergo propter hoc*, or affirming the consequent. It's like inferring that since every time the rooster crows, the sun rises; therefore, the rooster's crowing causes the sun to rise. But Albright was a giant, and eminence-based medicine carried the day.

For nearly thirty years, epidemiology has picked away at the associations between HRT and clinical outcomes. The quality-of-life myth has proved unsupportable except for perimenopausal symptoms. One study suggests that HRT increases the risk of back pain. Although HRT had been shown to decrease the rate of bone mineral loss, no compelling effect on the fracture rate has been demonstrated. Multiple trials examining cardiovascular outcomes have yielded inconsistent results, perhaps an increased risk that is transient with the institution of HRT. Some increased risk of thrombophlebitis and pulmonary embolism seemed to emerge, along with an increased risk of breast and uterine cancer with prolonged exposure to HRT. However, the many studies on all these associations had inconsistencies and small effects.

Despite little or no evidence in its favor, HRT consumption probably would have continued at much the same levels, but then along came the results of the randomized controlled trial of the risks and benefits of estrogen plus progestin (the combination HRT most commonly prescribed) from the Women's Health Initiative. Between 1993 and 1998, the initiative recruited some 162,000 postmenopausal women into a set of clinical trials sponsored and monitored by the NIH and conducted at forty centers across the United States. The HRT component involved 16,000 of these women, selected because they had escaped having their uteruses surgically removed. They were randomly assigned to take HRT or not. After 5.2 years, the investigators charged to monitor the trial outcomes considered the results to be so dramatic, if not horrifying, that they felt duty bound to stop the trial early. The health risks exceeded health benefits. The media likes medical miracles, but it revels in medical disasters. In the summer of 2002, the world press trumpeted this result. The powerful HRT social construction has been tottering ever since.

Table 8 displays the principal results. Of course, much of the trumpeting was of the relative risks. It sounds awful that HRT causes a 41 percent increased risk of stroke, doesn't it? We visited this form of propagandizing science in several earlier chapters. This is a particularly egregious example. HRT sounds less awful if I say that 8 out of 10,000 women will suffer a stroke because they took HRT for

TABLE 8. Women's Health Initiative HRT Randomized Controlled Trial

Health Outcome	Relative Risk	Absolute Risk (events per 10,000 people per year)
Heart disease	29 percent increase	7 more
Invasive breast cancer	26 percent increase	8 more
Stroke	41 percent increase	8 more
Pulmonary embolism	113 percent increase	8 more
Hip fracture	34 percent decrease	5 less
Colorectal cancer	37 percent decrease	6 less

Source: Adapted from the Writing Group for the Women's Health Initiative Investigators (2002) and Fletcher and Colditz (2002).

a year. That is a gamble many might take if they believed their youthfulness and vitality were at stake. Some might argue that the trade-off with hip fractures and colorectal cancer makes the hazards more tolerable. After all, there were no extra deaths ascribable to HRT; most sailed through their cardiac event, recovered from their stroke, or were "cured" of their breast cancer. At least that's what one would predict on rereading chapters 2 and 6. Add to that my cynicism regarding the reliability and validity of such small differences detected in a huge trial, also belabored in those chapters, and you understand why I find this saga disconcerting. The benefit/risk assessment of HRT remains imponderable. Benefits are trivial. Risks are trivial. Therefore, why should anyone ingest such an agent? Why should anyone prescribe such an agent? Even the U.S. Preventive Services Task Force, which held up releasing their updated recommendations until they could be revised in light of these results, can find no justification for the routine use of HRT. As recently as 2005, the Task Force concluded that "the harmful effects of combined estrogen and progestin are likely to exceed the chronic disease prevention benefits in most women." However, who is looking at Table 8 and proclaiming "much ado about nothing" in risk *and* in benefit? Rather, the race is on to convince physicians and patients that the HRT social construction is incorrect. Further analyses of the results of the Women's Health Initiative have reinforced the finding that there is a slight, arguably measurable increase in the absolute risks for stroke, cognitive impairment, venous thrombosis, and gall bladder disease. At the same time that postmenopausal women taking HRT are being pummeled by these statistically significant albeit tiny hazards, they are aggressively marketed as to putatively less-concerning pharmaceutical alternatives for meddling with osteopenia. I have no doubt that the HRT brouhaha has advantaged pharmaceutical firms that market drugs other than HRT far more than it has advantaged women taking HRT.

Standing in the wings, actually in the pharmacy, is a New Age estrogen, a SERM. That's an acronym for "Selective Estrogen-Receptor Modulator." There are two forms of receptors to which estrogen binds to initiate its biological effects. Pharmaceutical firms have been busy synthesizing molecules that compete with estrogen for these receptors. Two flavors are available. One, Tamoxifen, effectively blocks the receptor. Tamoxifen is an agent used to treat breast cancer and has been studied in large trials on the prevention of breast cancer (which discerned marginal and balancing risks and benefits). One concern in these trials was that blocking the estrogen receptor would predispose to osteopenia, if not osteoporosis. That concern did not materialize, surprisingly. There is another compound, raloxifene (marketed as Evista), which is structurally similar to Tamoxifen and also binds estrogen receptors. However, raloxifene preferentially targets receptors in the cells in bone, and rather than blocking, it effectively activates those receptors. The hope is that a SERM of this type might prevent osteopenia by estrogen effects on bone without stimulating the uterine endometrium. Thus, both menstruation and any increased risk of uterine cancer might be avoided. The manufacturer underwrote a multicenter randomized controlled trial, first recruiting lead investigators (many of whom avowed financial arrangements within the pharmaceutical industry) and then recruiting over 7,000 women. After three years, the women on raloxifene had less osteopenia. Those women who had no vertebral fractures at the beginning of the trial had no meaningful reduction in new vertebral compression fractures after three years (there was a significant difference but it was tiny — a couple of percentage points of absolute reduction). However, for women who had fractures at inception, the reduction was over 5 percent. There was no reduction in hip fractures. There was a trade-off in leg cramps, hot flashes, edema, and flu-like symptoms. There was no trade-off in terms of cardiovascular events. Much ado about nothing? The FDA didn't think so. However, I never prescribe a novel compound unless the benefit/risk ratio is compelling and, as I explained above, there are too few benefits to justify much risk, or unknown risks. I am unwilling to expose my patients to uncertainties regarding long-term consequences unless there is a compelling trade-off with short-term benefits. Revisit the earlier discussion and decide if a reduction in incident spinal compression fractures is a compelling benefit.

Those who argue for treating osteopenia with a SERM reserve therapy for

people at higher risk for spinal compression fractures. This subset can be identified either because they already have a spinal compression fracture or they
have a greater degree of osteopenia. This argument has been better developed
for another class of agents: the bisphosphonates.

PIPE CLEANERS

In the 1960s, chemical engineers at Procter & Gamble solved a problem that
had long plagued the manufacture of soap. The effluent from the process of saponification was rich in calcium salts, which formed concretions in the plumbing. The engineers came across a class of small calcium-binding molecules, the
bisphosphonates, which could keep the pipes clear.

There is a rare hereditary disorder, myositis ossificans, which causes muscle
to turn to bone. In the 1960s, before such an initiative could bring the wrath
of the FDA if not the plaintiff's bar on one's head, a well-read clinician treated
a patient devastated by this disease with a bisphosphonate. He published a
promising anecdote. Unfortunately for that patient and others with this rare
disease, the anecdote does not reproduce. However, the fact that this class of
agent was not intrinsically toxic opened the door to inventive chemistry and
clinical investigation. The pharmaceutical division of Procter & Gamble has
been a leader.

It was soon discovered that bisphosphonates had totally different effects on
human biology than on industrial plumbing. They did not bind calcium in
the body. However, they did have interesting and varied effects on the resident
populations of cells in bone. Etidronate was one of the earliest bisphosphonates to find a place in clinical medicine when it was used in the treatment of
Paget's disease of bone, a condition in which the unbridled resorption of bone
outstrips the formation of proper new bone so that remodeling is disorganized.
Etidronate slows the resorption, thereby improving remodeling. It also slows
resorption of normal bone, thwarting postmenopausal osteopenia. However,
use for that purpose is not straightforward because at higher doses it also interferes with the renewal process, leading to osteopenic bone by another mechanism. In practice today, the agent is prescribed for two weeks out of every two
months for two years. Trials suggest that this regimen is about as effective as the
SERM we just discussed; the incidence of vertebral fractures is reduced by about
5 percent over two years of treatment. That's an absolute reduction of 5 percent.
There is no demonstrable effect on the incidence of hip or other nonvertebral
fractures. However, more intense or more prolonged dosing causes, rather than
thwarts, osteopenia. In fact, one has to be wary of all bisphosphonates as double-

edged swords. For example, there was one agent that was withdrawn from the market because leukemia was a side effect.

The experience with etidronate was favorable enough for Procter & Gamble and its competitors to pursue new bisphosphonates for the prevention of osteopenia. Two bisphosphonates were introduced in the late 1990s and now compete to dominate the market. They were recently joined by ibandronate, which is taken monthly. I will not discuss this agent further; my philosophy will not countenance prescribing any "me too" drug until I'm sure that the long-term consequences do not tarnish the advertising hype. The competition plays out in advertising campaigns aimed at professionals and direct to consumers. All these marketing dollars are highly visible in "continuing education" programs and sponsorship of professional meetings. If anything is shoring up the osteoporosis social construction, it is this effort coupled with industry-sponsored research protocols that are far more effective in inserting these agents into medical practice styles than in pushing back the frontier of medical ignorance. Women are increasingly aware of and fret about the fate of their skeletons. Machines designed to measure their degree of osteopenia (vide infra) abound. And many, many women who feel well and are well are consuming these expensive bisphosphonates because their bone mineral density (BMD) is said to offer them no better choice.

Alendronate (marketed by Merck as Fosamax) barely preceded risedronate (marketed by Procter & Gamble as Actonel) in passing muster at the FDA. The randomized placebo-controlled trials that convinced the FDA to license these two agents were similar in design: multicenter, inception cohorts of thousands of postmenopausal women and follow-up for several years while monitoring BMD and the incidence of fractures. Both agents have a measurable therapeutic effect on BMD. For women with prior vertebral fractures or a relatively low BMD, both agents decrease the incidence of vertebral fractures to the same degree, an absolute reduction in incidence of about 5 percent over three or so years of observation. Not surprisingly, the publications and the marketing emphasize the *relative* reductions, which get up to 40 percent or so because the incidence in the placebo groups is only around 10 percent. *These fractures are defined as a 15 percent decrease in the height of a vertebra for risedronate and 20 percent for alendronate — not as a decrease in the incidence of acute pain or likelihood of an important alteration in posture.* Risedronate is reasonably safe and well tolerated in the short run. Alendronate ran into problems with irritation of the esophagus. Merck has partially circumvented this toxicity by altering the dosing schedule from daily to weekly, but that was done after licensing by the FDA.

TABLE 9. Number of Fractures in the "VERT" Trial

Treatment	Wrist	Hip	Arm	Leg	Clavicle
Risedronate	14	12	4	4	3
Placebo	22	15	10	8	0

Source: Adapted from Harris et al. (1999).

Both agents are also marketed as effective in the prevention of nonvertebral fractures. Pshaw. Table 9 contains the incidence data from the pivotal 1999 risedronate trial, the "VERT" trial. This is the number of fractures that occurred at each site over the course of three years. Realize this was a three-year study randomizing 1,600 postmenopausal women. The risk of nonvertebral fracture is small in the placebo group, an incidence of 3 percent for wrist fractures and 2 percent for hip fractures. It is difficult to measure a meaningful reduction with such a low incidence. The claim is for an overall reduction in nonvertebral fractures: thirty-seven incurred by women taking risedronate and fifty-five on placebo. But there is no statistical difference in hip fractures. Osteoporotic fractures of the arm and leg are far less frequent than hip fractures in the population; this placebo population is not representative. In that regard, they were unlucky. I have combed the published trial data that tests the assertion that treatment with alendronate or risedronate for several years reduces the hip-fracture rate, even in women with moderately severe osteopenia. It is not impressive. In fact, it is hard to justify the enterprise that identifies women with osteopenia to treat them prophylactically with any agent, let alone a bisphosphonate. As for the women with clinical osteoporosis who already have asymptomatic vertebral compression fractures or have suffered symptomatic spinal or other osteoporotic fractures, the argument to treat is more compelling. However, even in this circumstance, the clinical context is our master. In the frail elderly, what is to be gained?

Measuring BMD

I have postponed discussing the measurement of BMD in order to first inform the reader as to its tenuous rationale. Measuring BMD has become another rite of passage for women of all ages. Even young, menstruating, recreational athletes are now made to worry about osteopenia. Screening is advertised, promoted, urged, and advised in print, voice, and broadcast media, in health clubs and health magazines, and in many a professional office. Determining BMD is big business and largely bogus. Here's why. *No one should be screened for any disease, ever, unless*:

1. The test is accurate.
2. The result has meaningful predictive value.
3. There is something meaningful to be done if the test is positive.

BMD measurement fails on all accounts.

Most "storefront" BMD measurements are performed by DEXA scanning, or dual-energy X-ray absorptiometry. This is a technique that is both difficult to standardize and subject to many technical errors. There are other kinds of measurements on the market and many discussions about which anatomical site is most predictive. Most of the data we have discussed was based on DEXA scans at the hip and spine. One can do better using variations on computerized tomography (CT), but that assumes one can justify devoting such expensive hardware to this exercise.

As one might infer from our discussions of the hazards of osteopenia and the response to treatment, any measured value short of the extremes of osteopenia has very little predictive value in those under the age of sixty. No well woman under the age of sixty should even consider this test. The U.S. Preventive Services Task Force ducked this population, unwilling to recommend for or against in their 2002 recommendations, as did the authors of a recent influential review in *JAMA* in 2002 — authors who have a relationship with Merck in that they have been leading investigators on the alendronate trials. These authors suggested that a trade-off in "changes in behaviors that might decrease fracture risk" might justify rendering a young woman "unnecessarily anxious about a low result." That's a slippery slope. Should they exercise more to increase bone density or exercise less to gain in BMI since that too correlates with increased BMD? Both the Task Force and the alendronate investigators favor screening after age sixty-five and between sixty and sixty-five for women with "risk factors," such as a low BMI in white women. Anyone with a low BMD should be treated. This recommendation is echoed by all kinds of professional organizations, from the "National Osteoporosis Foundation" to the professional bodies for orthopedics, endocrinology, geriatrics, and more. It departs from the recommendation against such universal screening of a consensus conference sponsored by the NIH and published in 2000.

Am I wrong in doubting? These august bodies supported by their comparably august experts are convinced that universal screening of BMD meets the criteria above. While we all agree with those criteria, the differences hinge on the distinction between clinically significant and statistically significant. The pro-measurement experts base their recommendations on the latter. I base mine on the former. Universal screening at age sixty-five cannot be defended because its predictive value is marginal. I will go further. Based on the trivial magnitude of benefit that has been demonstrated in the wealth of therapeutic trials, even if it were possible to predict risk accurately, the clinical benefit would be tenuous. I am not alone in my skepticism. The U.S. Agency for Healthcare Research and Quality convened a panel to write guidelines, which were published in 2001 and justified my skepticism. The charge to this government agency was to perform analytic literature reviews in the name of evidence-based medicine. It is now defunct, subsumed into a larger agency with a different agenda (see chapter 9). However, its deliberations are precious.

Osteopenia: A Social Construction

I have yet to see a research paper on this topic that doesn't commence with a statement to the effect that "osteoporosis is important because it is common and often occult, yet it causes substantial morbidity and costs over $14 billion per year" or some such assertion. I can find very few authors who wonder if this construction is medicalization of aging and if this price tag is part of the unconscionable American process of dying. Many Americans, particularly the more-advantaged American women, have bought into this construct. Further-more, they have bought into the notion that screening and treatment makes sense. This is more than just buying into an idea; the construction has become a commonly and tightly held tenet. It is a social construction.

Many wait with bated breath for the next breakthrough. With the announce-ment that zoledronic acid, a bisphosphonate, could be given intravenously once a year for the prevention of osteopenia, the press and Novartis stockholders took notice. The fact that bisphosphonates, particularly long-acting bisphos-phonates, can cause catastrophic death of the jawbone has hardly squelched the zeal. When Eli Lilly's novel pharmaceutical, a parathyroid hormone fragment, was shown to prevent osteopenia and even diminish the incidence of osteo-porotic fractures, medicine and Wall Street took notice. It seems sensible that all this effort be expended. It seems sensible that all white women and maybe others, at age sixty-five and maybe younger, should rejoice at the progress of science. That it seems sensible is a social construction.

Social constructions are not "bad." Daily life abounds in social construc-tions, in belief systems that have yet to be refuted. For many such social constructions, the idea that they are refutable seems absurd. Each culture, each era, has operational social constructions and always will. Prior chapters of this book are replete with exercises in the testing of contemporary social constructions that relate to health. There are social constructions that relate to behaviors, "race," income distribution, and much more. Many social constructions seem to have had a finite life expectancy. History marks some that passed quietly and others that left scars. Some have a life of their own. Some are resilient in spite of the assault of science. The concept of "race" is an example, surviving for over a century in spite of its tragic history and the recent scientific pummeling.

Osteopenia is an example of a New Age social construction, propelled to its status in a decade by aggressive marketing and vested interests. It has been tested and is being tested, and it has proven marginal if not untenable. It has also proven resilient. There is much invested in that resilience on the part of all the providers of recourse for all the women who have come to adhere to the tenet. It may even become a "meme" (rhymes with "beam"). A meme is a recent term to describe an idée fixe that is infectious. The proponents of the concept of a meme even postulate some biological reality, some infectious unit of knowledge or of memory. I'll settle for a more psychological conceptualization. "Fibromyalgia," for example, is a meme for the susceptible (see chapter 10). Memes insert themselves into the very being of the infected.

It is very difficult to alter a social construction. It is more difficult to ablate a meme. There is much at stake whenever either is up to no good. Has osteopenia, along with fibromyalgia and other fashionable illnesses, become a meme?

In the supplementary reading for this chapter, many of the critical concepts are revisited with expanded analyses.

chapter twelve

Working to Death

Chapter 1 introduced the notion that longevity in a resource-advantaged country is largely predicated on socioeconomic status and employment. The most powerful life-course hazards relate to impediments to the pursuit of nurturing, gainful employment.

That such is true for any who have no gainful employment is obvious. A lifetime of poverty, even tottering on the edge of poverty, is a lifetime likely to be base, mean, often discouraging, sometimes desperate — and short. Poverty is defined as a disposable income less than three times what is necessary for subsistence in your community. Some living in poverty are so desperately poor that inadequate shelter and nutrition are mortal threats. But not all are quite so desperately poor. What is it about a lowly socioeconomic status (SES) that is so malevolent? The clues derive from studies that explore life in poverty, or on its edge, for elements most closely associated with compromised longevity. Multiple psychosocial factors have emerged. Some factors operate from conception. There is no reason to think that a small number of such factors will emerge. Something about the loss of self-respect and the resentment, if not hostility, that results from the sense of abject vulnerability associated with and imposed by poverty is clearly detrimental. There are hints of other associations from life-course studies of nutrition, life-stage maturation, and more. Much remains unknown, but it is clear that the array of psychosocial challenges to be faced in poverty day by day, and that prove insurmountable day after day, levy a toll on health and longevity like none other in the "advanced" world. Poverty in nations that are not resource-challenged is a reproach to both their political systems and public-health agendas.

However, the dreadful consequences of the psychosocial milieu that is poverty can be dissociated from "poverty level" or other measures of disposable wealth. Employment is no generic solution. There are aspects to life in "modern" workforces that rival the psychosocial aspects of poverty in extracting a toll on healthfulness and longevity. For example, downsizing and outsourcing may warm the hearts of stockholders, but they assault the happiness, health, and longevity of the targeted workforce. A consistent story is emerging with major implications for the health of the public.

Working Well
  Do you like your job?
  Are you valued at work?
  Do you feel justly served?
  Is your job secure?

These four questions deserve a prominent place in whatever caring community life affords us, let alone in clinical history gathering. They should anchor a major public-health initiative. They demand a prominent place in the body politic. Untoward answers associate with much personal pain and clinical morbidity. Untoward answers harbor crucial secrets to longevity, even for those who could change jobs. For growing numbers of workers whose answers are untoward, job mobility is not an option or leads to less acceptable alternatives. For growing numbers of the aging workforce who commenced their career assuming a meritocracy and expecting job security, this reality comes as a surprise with awful personal consequences.

Most of us are all too aware when employment is such that it would elicit a negative response to any or all of these questions. Most of us could verbalize our awareness. Very few of us, if any, can leave this awareness in the workplace at the end of a workday. Very few of us realize how such adverse circumstances play on the other aspects of life. Interpersonal relationships outside of work are strained. Tendencies toward substance abuse are unbridled to various degrees. I am not downplaying these aspects in the least. However, in keeping with the thesis "worried sick," I am going to focus on another predictable adverse consequence: the culturally facilitated tendency to somatize. If the psychosocial context of working is adverse, your sense of invincibility will be compromised and you are at risk of feeling ill.

As illustrated in chapters 8 through 10, life for all of us presents challenges to coping with unusual and unpleasant symptoms — morbidities. We will all experience variations in mood, intermittent musculoskeletal discomfort, occasional headaches, episodic respiratory symptoms, and much more in the way of intermittent and remittent physical distress. To be well, to feel invincible, is to have the personal wherewithal to cope with both the physical and the psychosocial challenges that cannot be wholly avoided, if avoided at all. When overwhelmed, we express our distress in narratives that are culturally constrained. If life is fine and we experience low back pain, we likely will cope the best we can with as little compromise in function as we can muster. Rarely are we so overwhelmed by the intensity of the backache that we even seek professional assistance.

If life is not so rosy, inside or outside the workplace, we are likely to recognize the challenge, even verbalize the challenge, as psychosocial. If the psychosocial challenge is a feature of our life outside the workplace, we might seek professional help if we are overwhelmed and insightful. If the psychosocial challenge is in the workplace, we might have access to assistance from a human resources department or an astute supervisor; we might seek alternative employment or we might grouse thereby answering several of the critical questions in the negative.

What happens if your next backache finds you coping with psychosocial turmoil in your life? Backache happens frequently enough so that coinciding with a vulnerable time in your life is not unlikely. There are cultures — that of Yemen, for example — that treat backache as no more than a serious annoyance, even if it coincided with stressful challenges. In our culture the common cold might be considered to be but an annoyance, even if it coincided with other stressful challenges. But we are not culturally conditioned or constrained to frame backache as a coincident annoyance when it coincides with psychosocial stress. We are conditioned to meld the morbidities in such a way that they are synergistic. We are not likely to question whether it is the pain in the back or the pain in the psyche that is the "last straw," the "straw that broke the camel's back." Rather, we are likely to assume that the pain in the back is so intense as to interfere with our ability to cope with the psychosocial stress. The converse narrative is akin to the idiom "it's in your mind," which we dissected in chapter 10. Sometimes we're correct; it is the pain in the back that is interfering with coping with the psychosocial turmoil. More often, we are resolute in our misconception that in this episode the physical distress is primary; the physical is confounding the psychosocial challenges, not vice versa, and therefore should commandeer narrative. So it is in the workforce where misconceptions about the physical cause of regional musculoskeletal disorders have misled the occupational health and safety agenda for over sixty years.

Occupational musculoskeletal disorders are a window for understanding why employment that is not nurturing can be harmful, if not lethal.

Backache as a Compensable "Injury"

After World War II, disabling regional musculoskeletal disorders became the bane of the workforce. Today, they account for the preponderance of long-term disability. Regional backache is now joined by regional arm pain as a scourge of the Western workforce. Remember (chapter 9), regional musculoskeletal disorders are an affliction of working-age adults who are otherwise well and who have suffered no overt trauma. Since motion can exacerbate these symptoms, the contemporary industrialized world is quick to ascribe any associated work incapacity to the physical content of tasks at work. This was not always so. Understanding how it came to be, and the semiotic it represents, is prerequisite to understanding why disabling regional musculoskeletal disorders are a window into the quality of life in the workforce and pari passu the hazards to healthfulness and longevity that emerge when that quality is compromised.

Why me? This plaint pertains to all illness, not just backache. In the less-enlightened and even more convoluted times long past, the sufferer was likely to light on such answers as fate or, if one was inclined to believe in an even-handed world, retribution for ill-advised behaviors. The Elizabethan answers for backache included retribution for dissipation, if Shakespeare's *Measure for Measure* (act 1, scene 2) bears fair witness. Attribution superseded retribution as a comfortable explanation only during the past century. Before then, tasks had to be "back breaking" before it seemed reasonable to attribute backache to them. It is still more customary to ascribe a "pain in the neck" to the behavior of another person than to one's own activities. To "shoulder a burden" remains less a condemnation than a designation of fortitude.

It required new social constructions for attribution to supersede retribution as the ready answer for the lament of the backache sufferer, "Why me?" These came late in the nineteenth century. First was the invention of "railway spine" and its promulgation as a Victorian contribution to the history of medicalization by John Eric Erichsen, professor of surgery in University College London and surgeon to the Queen. The railroad was one of the engines of industrialization. Building railroads was dangerous work, too often maiming or lethal work. Even riding the rails was dangerous; collisions and derailments were so commonplace that Queen Victoria herself refused to allow her private train to travel beyond a snail's pace. However, the hue and cry as to the carnage on the early railroad did not hold sway until after the turn of the century. What first captured the mass psyche was the illness that befell passengers who were spared violent events but were exposed to the jostling and vibrations of a ride in a railroad coach. Passengers developed a pervasive debilitating illness notable for axial myalgias and fatigue and ascribed by Erichsen to "concussion of the spine from slight injury." Victorian England reeled from condemnation and litigation as a consequence of this social construction, from which even Erichsen withdrew support near the end of his life. "Railway spine" disappeared, but it left as legacy the common belief that one can be "injured" during the course of customary activities and without unusual trauma. More particularly, it left that legacy in the context of backache. Backache was firmly established as a medical problem.

At the time of the demise of "railway spine" a century ago, Europe was in the throes of social reformation. Nearly 15 percent of the population of a city such as London eked out a living on the streets to support a lifestyle that was notable for meanness, fecundity, and brevity. Nearly all workers feared such a fate for themselves or their families should they develop incapacitating illness, suffer a disabling injury, or die. All agreed that people who suffered such a fate are deserving of our charity. Such are the Judeo-Christian and Islamic creeds. All agreed, as well, that among the people who seek such assistance are some who could do well enough on their own if only they set to the task. Are they deserving of our assistance nonetheless? Or, as Cotton Mather opined, "As for the sturdy beggar, let him starve."

Distinguishing the worthy from the unworthy poor has bedeviled Western society for millennia. Historically, the task fell to families and religious orders by default and with uneven results. "Poor Laws" were statutes first drafted in the sixteenth century but still in effect in the American colonies and in Britain early in the twentieth century. In effect, these statutes charged the gentry with the obligation to care for whoever was deemed worthy poor. Various forms of almshouses were constructed to shelter those deemed deserving. This was an uneven remedy in an agrarian society with its creed of noblesse oblige. It was no match for an industrialized society.

As a young man, in his socialist phase, Jack London dressed in rags and attempted to survive on the streets of east London, petitioning for shelter in one of these "Poor Houses" on a cold night. He captured the experience in *People of the Abyss*, published in 1902.

> The unfit and the unneeded! The miserable and despised and forgotten, dying in the social shambles. The progeny of prostitution — of the prostitution of men and women and children, of flesh and blood, and sparkle and spirit; in brief the prostitution of labor. If this is the best that civili-

zation can do for the human, then give us howling and naked savagery. Far better to be a people of the wilderness and desert, of the cave and the squatting-place, than to be a people of the machine and the Abyss.

No wonder the end of the nineteenth century found the industrial West roiling in demands for social reformation. The union movement came into being, and the plaintiff's bar gained footing. Karl Marx, Ferdinand Lassalle, and others found audiences. Legislature after legislature followed the Prussian precedent to craft programs that pension the elderly and care for the ill and disabled. The United States of America was to participate reluctantly and piecemeal in a dialectic that has yet to fully play out. In the early decades of the twentieth century, only "workmen's compensation insurance" was to make landfall, and not gracefully; each state legislated a version in its fashion and in its time. All American schemes, however, are "no fault" and indemnify medical costs and lost wages consequent to personal injuries that "arise out of and in the course of employment," the language of most statutes. The intent is to minimize the financial toll that compounds such injuries. When it became clear that workers could be harmed by more than physical force, such as by mercury and lead exposure or anthrax, new legislation provided a remedy for occupational diseases. Even so, the notion of "injury" was contentious from the outset.

"Writer's cramp" and "telegraphist's wrist" were rallying cries of the early union movement in Britain, with the result that they were added to the British schedule for occupational diseases in 1908, but not without medical debate that culminated a decade later in the rubric "occupational neurosis." If you first notice your inguinal hernia at work, is that a compensable injury? It became so when "rupture" became parlance. Regional back pain is the backache that afflicts working-age adults who are otherwise well and who experienced no unusual, let alone violent, precipitant. Regional back pain was not considered an injury until the mid-1930s when W. J. Mixter, a senior neurosurgeon working at the Massachusetts General Hospital, ascribed cauda equina syndrome, if not all backache, to disc herniation and described a surgical remedy. In the titles of his seminal contributions, Mixter chose to term the pathobiology a discal "rupture," symbolizing the rending of normal structure. One of Mixter's coauthors, the young orthopedist Joseph Barr, lamented this semiotic twenty years later. "Rupture" captured the attention of all workers' compensation administrators and adjudicators, as well as others involved in workplace safety and in providing remedy whenever safeguards failed. If the outcome is a "rupture," even if the precipitant is an activity that is customary and customarily comfortable, the worker has suffered a compensable back "injury." It is this inference that informs our suffering and tests our coping with our next episode of back pain. Not only do we cope with the pain, we also cope with the notion of trauma. That's why our narrative of distress for backache can include the idiom, "I injured my back." That's why we physicians feel compelled to query a patient presenting with backache, "What were you doing when it started?" Neither the patient nor the physician would countenance such discourse for headache.

Rutherford Johnstone describes the social construction of the "industrial back" in his 1941 monograph, *Occupational Diseases: Diagnosis, Medicolegal Aspects and Treatment*:

> In complete disregard of the multiple causes of backache, the tendency in industrial medicine is to "mass-group" all these cases under the diagnosis of back sprain. This error seems to be predicated upon the "locale" of the onset of pain. If it ensues while a man is cutting his own lawn, the term "lumbago" is invariably applied and the condition attributed to causes within the man. But pain arising while stooping, bending, or lifting at the plant is called "back sprain" and considered the result of motion while working for someone else. The situation assumes added import when it is appreciated that this disability is becoming one of the most frequent causes of claims for compensation. (Johnstone 1941)

So for seventy years, back "injury" has hung like Damocles' sword over the resource-advantaged world, inside and outside the workplace. It can wreak havoc on the lives of workers with disabling backache for whom workers' compensation insurance is designed to provide a remedy. Over the past few decades, the construct, the diagnosis, and many of its ramifications have been put to the test. We have learned why discal "rupture" is a flawed pathogenetic theory and compensable back "injury" an iatrogenic sophism. These are object lessons that can inform a social reformation redux. First, the object lessons.

Regional back pain has little if anything to do with ruptured discs or any other form of spinal pathology (chapter 9). The causes of regional back pain continue to elude scientific inquiry. The degenerative changes that characterize spinal pathoanatomy escalate in incidence with each passing decade until they are ubiquitous. But they have almost nothing to do with what we do in life. The age of onset and the degree of change are largely genetically determined; the contributions of environmental influences are barely discernable. Our aging spines, however hoary, do not bear witness to a life of damaging trauma, nor do they offer anatomical clues as to the cause of our backache. They mark longevity, not decrepitude.

Back "injury" is a social construction, not a valid clinical diagnosis. Traumatic amputations, fractures, and crush injuries can "arise out of and in the course of working." The "common cold" can also arise in the course of working and, in all likelihood, out of the course of working, since so much of our exposure to droplet infections occurs in the workplace. But we don't consider the "common cold" an injury or even an occupational disease, although it may well be a transiently disabling illness. Certainly regional backache can occur in the course of working. But can backache also "arise out of the course of working," as an injury? Can biomechanical stressors that are usually comfortable turn pathogenic? That seems intuitively appealing. After all, regional back pain is always mechanical; it hurts more when we place biomechanical strain across the hurting back simply by leaning forward. Tasks that were always comfortable at work and at home are now more daunting, if not prohibitive. The back "injury" construction holds that the physical demands that exacerbate the pain are the proximate cause of putative damage rather than an influence on the degree of discomfort. We need to liberate our medical and social-welfare systems from this damaging misconception. Multiple cohort studies in the contemporary workplace can discern little if any influence of the physical demands of tasks on the incidence of disabling backache. As is true of spinal pathoanatomy, the incidence of backache has almost nothing to do with "minor trauma." Furthermore, the incidence of back "injury" has proved refractory to successive waves of ergonomic advice and devices, of clinical and rehabilitative inventiveness, and of regulatory and legal machinations. Back "injury" remains the bane of the workforce despite the fact that the tasks in the modern workplace are far less physically demanding than those of earlier generations. Nonetheless, back "injury" accounts for the majority of the cost of workers' compensation indemnity schemes, and workers' compensation costs consume 2 to 4 percent of the gross earnings of American employers. We've known for decades that we were missing something, but the response was to fine-tune rather than alter our approach.

Fortunately, modern science has probed for and discerned associations with disabling backache that supersede the "injury" paradigm. The result is an entirely different conception of backache. Like the "common cold," backache is an intermittent and remittent predicament of life. If you are a perfectly well, working-age adult, it is abnormal for you to make it one year without at least one important episode of low back pain. For many, backache is memorable; for many more, it resolves and is soon forgotten. Most of those who seek care, including medical care, heal rapidly whether they seek care in the context of work or not. Some, a substantial minority, heal slowly if at all. For these, overcoming the biomechanical challenges imposed by backache colors each day. In the context of work, performance may be so limited that the worker sees no option but to seek a disability award — under workers' compensation if the backache is viewed as an "injury." Common sense dictates that the reasons one is more likely to find backache memorable, worthy of seeking care, or disabling relates to the intensity of the pain, the physical demands of tasks, or the effectiveness of health-care interventions. Common sense is often wrong, and it is particularly wrong in the case of the compensable back "injury." Alexander Magora was the first to understand this over thirty years ago; I was to echo his message not long after. We entered the twenty-first century armed with an extensive and compelling science supporting the premise that there are confounders to coping with backache lurking in the psychosocial context of work that are consistently associated with disabling backache to a far greater degree than the confounders to coping that result from the actual physical demands of work. More recent studies from Manchester, London, Leiden, Helsinki, Copenhagen, and elsewhere bolster this inference. Still, the back "injury" construct is entrenched; it supports and is supported by an enormous ergonomic and "safety" enterprise that is unshaken by study after study impugning its validity.

The convergence of Mixter's inferences and the workers' compensation insurance scheme has transformed backache into a surrogate complaint. If life is bleak, particularly life at work, and we see no alternative, the next backache is likely to seem more than the proverbial "straw"; it is an "injury." No physician, employer, human-resource professional, claims adjuster, or worker is likely to realize that the backache is intolerable and disabling because the job is hateful, unsatisfying, or insecure; the supervisor is insensitive, hostile, or cruel; coworkers are antagonistic; or the worker feels undervalued, underpaid, or overburdened by personal baggage and sees no way out. "I injured my back" is this semiotic.

That's why downsizing and outsourcing is met with a spate of workers' compensation claims whenever such a management decision is impending. A study of the United Parcel Service (UPS) workforce is illustrative. UPS is a private-sector company with hundreds of thousands of employees. About half work in the 1,000 or so "hubs" scattered across the country. Their job, which is physically demanding and nocturnal, is to unload trucks, sort parcels, and load trucks, thereby effecting distribution. The physical demands at the hubs are monitored, quantified, and extraordinarily uniform. So too is the frequency of workers' compensation claims for regional musculoskeletal disorders — with a few hubs exceptionally high. Those high-claims hubs are not faced with more physical demand. Nor was there any indication that jobs were at risk. Rather, they are characterized by inadequacies in shop-level management style.

Does it matter that back "injury" is a sophism, and a workers' compensation claim for a back "injury" is often a surrogate complaint? After all, the backache can be disabling nonetheless — not because of what is lifted but whether or when it is to be lifted. We might countenance such a surrogate if the result of launching a workers' compensation claim was likely to succor the worker who is hurting. However, the consequences of playing out the surrogate complaint as a workers' compensation claimant are unlikely to advantage workers, either individually or as a workforce.

Damnable Disability Determination

The Prussian social legislation created a "welfare monarchy" far more extensive that just workers' compensation insurance. Prodded by Otto von Bismarck's drive to assuage a skittish labor movement, the legislature established three tiers of worthiness for those who claimed work incapacity. The worker who is injured at work is the most worthy and therefore should be compensated for any loss of wage-earning capacity through workers' compensation insurance. If wage-earning capacity is compromised by some disease rather than a work-related injury, that worker is not quite as worthy. When subsistence is challenging, "Invalid Pension" is provided as the remedy (Social Security disability insurance is the U.S. version). However, if the person claims to be fully unable to work and has not worked in the past, the level of worthiness is diminished, as is the pension (supplemental security insurance is the U.S. version). The challenge in administering such a scheme is to quantify whether there is any work left in the person for the lower two tiers and how much work is left in the injured worker. The solution that was offered as rational by the Prussian medical establishment rules today despite its dismal track record. It is this solution that leads to the current spate of complaints regarding disabled veterans. It needs to be understood so that it can be put into perspective and, hopefully, supplanted.

In its day, Prussian medicine was considered exemplary. Prussian doctors taught that all symptoms (the illness) must have a biological cause (the disease or impairment), which must first be identified and then treated with the expectation that the symptoms will regress. This notion is the bedrock of Western scientific medicine. When asked by Bismarck to solve the disability-determination conundrum, however, Prussian doctors confidently offered up the converse: name the disease, the symptoms are predictable. Furthermore, the more disease, the more symptoms are expected, including symptoms of work incapacity. In the context of disability determination, "impairment" is used as the synonym for disease or damage. For workers' compensation, one can base awards on the quantity of impairment without concern for symptoms. For invalid pensions, if the quantity of impairment does not meet a certain threshold, the award can be denied. This is called "impairment-based disability determination."

As mentioned above, in the United States the early decades of the twentieth century brought only state-administered "workmen's compensation insurance." Social Security disability insurance was a political football, finally scoring in the Eisenhower administration. Supplemental security insurance waited for the Carter administration and was tossed back to the states in the Clinton administration. All of these U.S. schemes are wedded to impairment-based disability determination.

In the early days of worker's compensation, impairment-based disability determination took the form of "schedules" stipulating the compensation for the loss of an eye, or a limb, or a life. They were never rational. For example, few workers are disabled by the loss of a fifth finger, unless the worker is a professional pianist. When it became clear that workers could be harmed by more than physical force, such as by mercury and lead exposure or anthrax, new legislation provided a remedy for occupational diseases. Even so, the notion of "injury" was contentious from the outset, as was the inflexibility of the "schedules." Today, schedules are largely supplanted by a convoluted process in all jurisdictions, one that is paralleled in the Veterans Administration and the Social Security Administration. All invoke some medical determination of impairment, often going to great lengths and expense to quantify disease. All consider the estimate of impairment far more determinative than anything the claimant can say about symptoms.

All of these impairment-based disability schemes are efficient when the impairment is readily quantifiable. Amputations, terminal disease, psychosis and dementia, and the like are seldom contentious in disability determination. Overtly traumatic injuries that lead to major damage can be contentious if the particular insurance system is designed to consider more than the biomechanical consequences, aspects such as self-image, pain, or suffering. There is no way to objectively quantify any such consequence; trying to do so is nothing more than a challenge to the veracity of the claimant. Trying to do so will predictably compromise the coping ability of any of us: if you have to prove you're ill, you can't get better. The influence of pain and suffering in rendering a traumatic injury disabling bedevils impairment-based disability determination for veterans injured in battle and many injured in motor-vehicle accidents. Imagine the challenge when there is no overt damage.

Let's take the example of a worker who finds her or his "regional back pain" miserable, and particularly miserable when trying to perform physically demanding tasks at work. A workers' compensation claim for a back "injury" ensues. It is likely that there are factors lurking in the psychosocial context of work that are compromising this worker's ability to cope and thereby driving the claim. Nevertheless, money will be spent to "fix" the "injury." To this day, the United States is first in the "advanced" world in the likelihood of doing surgical violence to the lumbosacral spines of workers with compensable regional back "injuries"; the incidence varies from region to region, with some communities contriving surgical indications ten times more frequently than others. The worker can't readily refuse surgery or anything else that is offered: to do so implies that he or she really doesn't want to get well. That's why most of the people who have undergone multiple procedures are workers' compensation claimants. They are often labeled "failed backs" as if it's their fault that the poorly conceived interventions were unsuccessful.

Once the medical "fix" reaches its iatrogenic ending, and the claimant is labeled "fixed and stable" or "maximum medical improvement," the next level of contest is enjoined. Money will be spent in attempting to teach the disabled worker that the "injury" is not disabling. This is sustenance for all the "pain clinics" and "work hardening programs" but not for the injured worker, who is unlikely to return to work despite all these ministrations. More money will be spent to blame the worker for not returning to work that was unpleasant, even abhorrent in the first place. And when a halt is called, an effort will be made to determine how much work is left in the worker, so that a financial award can be provided that compensates for some approximation of loss of wage-earning capacity. Impairment-based disability determination is no match for this semiotic. Money will be spent in demanding the worker prove that the "injury" is disabling, often requiring litigation to reach a conclusion.

All this largesse is expended to provide the worker with a back "injury" treatment that is tinged by racial bias, ineffective surgery, and invalid, if not fatuous, determinations of residual disability.

Certainly the resource-advantaged world owes its workforce employment that is comfortable when workers are well and accommodating when they are ill, even ill with such predicaments of life as the next episode of disabling backache. Even more important is a workplace that appreciates our humanity — our need to be valued, our need to feel secure, our need for some autonomy, and our need to see a future.

For such a challenge, whether in the context of workers' compensation or Social Security or veterans' benefits insurance, impairment-based disability determination makes matters worse. There are other options, some that have been considered for generations and tested in the past. We need to generate a public debate about such options. We need to stop punishing disability claimants with an approach that has been shown to be harmful.

Ergonomics, Psychophysics, and Metaphysics

The compensable back "injury" has been the rationale for a dramatic shift in the purview of industrial engineering. At mid–twentieth century, ergonomics was the specialty in industrial engineering that analyzed the motion elements of industrial tasks with a view toward maximizing performance. This remains a primary raison d'être. Thanks to the pioneering efforts of Ernest Tischauer and later Stover Snook, maximizing worker comfort without sacrificing effectiveness became another goal. Tischauer incorporated biomechanics into the principles of tool and machine design. Snook's approach, termed psychophysics, was to explore the physical content and context of tasks to optimize worker acceptance. Enter the "injury" construction. Could it be that if a task was not designed according to principles of biomechanics or of psychophysics, it was hazardous? Could it be that ergonomics, and its handmaiden psychophysics, were the Grail in the quest to spare workers the misery of backache (or arm pain)? Given the "injury" social construction, the affirmative answer made sense. Thousands of studies tried to define ergonomic hazards, studies notable for inconsistent outcomes and minor associations. Ergonomic advice flooded the industrial world and spilled beyond. Advice as to task design and safe biomechanics was welcomed and heeded since there was a social construction that rendered such advice sensible. The advice may still seem sensible, but it has never been shown to decrease the incidence of compensable backache. Social constructions die hard. Ergonomics keeps its political currency. An "Ergonomic Standard" was proposed and passed at the end of the Clinton administration, but Congress blocked its implementation. Hopefully, it will not reemerge. All it does is cement the injury construction, thereby diverting attention from the major challenges faced in the modern workforce.

The scientific refutation of the social construction that considers regional backache an "injury" is comprehensive, compelling, and reproducible. It is not incontrovertible. However, I argue that whatever element of physical hazard outside of work or ergonomic hazard in the modern workplace is being missed must be minor and heterogeneous. It is so minor and so heterogeneous as to be irremediable. One need be highly circumspect in postulating any meaningful association between task content and disabling regional musculoskeletal disorders for a wide range of such exposures. Such associations can be detected, albeit inconsistently, in surveys where no alternative association is sought. However, nearly all multivariate, cross-sectional, and longitudinal studies seeking associations between disabling back or arm pain and both the psychosocial context of working and the physical demands of tasks discern the former, generally to the exclusion of the latter. Since regional musculoskeletal disorders are intermittent and remittent predicaments of life, the likely explanation for these observations does not discount the morbidity. Rather, it directs our attention to the psychosocial context in which the morbidity plays out, a context that confounds coping and renders the morbidity more memorable, less tolerable, and often disabling.

Outside the workplace, psychosocial confounders operate to render regional back pain memorable, if not intolerable (chapter 9). Why shouldn't the same pertain to backache at work? The distinction is that the sufferer has the option of seeking care for a back "injury," instead of backache, if all agree the backache arose out of and in the course of working. Such care is indemnified by workers' compensation for as long as it takes to reach maximum medical improvement, during which time income is maintained. Furthermore, if the "injured worker" has persistent work incapacity once at maximum medical improvement and is thereby faced with a loss in wage-earning capacity, she or he will suffer no financial loss. He or she will be compensated by workers' compensation insurance for lost wages.[1] Realize that for the significant minority of American workers who have no health insurance and therefore no coverage

---

1. This assumes the claimant can prove disability. That's a slippery slope beyond our scope here but discussed extensively in my recent monograph (Hadler 2005).

for medical care for a backache, seeking care for a regional back "injury" is the only medical option. For others with health insurance, workers' compensation offers a far more advantaged form of recourse, in that wages are indemnified. Hence, the ergonomic "injury" social construction is a "sacred cow" of all labor advocates, even though the medical recourse and ergonomic interventions have been shown to be effete, useless, or even harmful.

Whenever a worker finds a regional musculoskeletal disorder disabling, the response should pivot on empathy, understanding, and community support. In all likelihood, this is a surrogate complaint indicating adverse aspects of the context of work that may be remedial. Medical recourse is ancillary. As I will emphasize below, when a workforce is struck by an epidemic of disabling regional musculoskeletal disorders, the overwhelming likelihood is that there is an important defect in management style or the architecture of work. Approaching such a circumstance under the "ergonomic injury" banner is likely to lead to a cluster of workers bearing permanent scars from the quest for maximum medical improvement and a workplace dripping ergonomic modifications to no demonstrable avail.

A Psychosocially Adverse Work Context Is Hazardous to Your Health

The frontier for epidemiology is to further define "psychosocial context." That's an exercise that is nearly as daunting as defining the psychosocial correlates of poverty. Some of the common threads emerging from studies in the workplace include aspects of job "stress," "strain," "allostatic load," and motivational "flow." These measures are sampling such complex psychological functions as job satisfaction, perception of psychological demand, job autonomy, motivation, and the like. No wonder that associations with "psychosocial" variables are weak, even inconsistent. There may be much that is idiosyncratic. However, that does not diminish the implications: working in a psychosocial context that is adverse compromises coping with the next episode of a regional musculoskeletal disorder and places longevity at risk. The adverse psychosocial context may be peculiar to a particular worker who then finds back pain disabling. However, there are well-documented examples where the adverse context affects a workforce. As with the UPS example mentioned above, there are many large companies with multiple stereotypical facilities where epidemics of disabling back or arm pain occur in a single facility or a small number of these sites. The physical demands of tasks are uniform across the facilities and therefore not the culprit. Comparing the affected with the unaffected sites proves informative. Usually this is a reproach to management style in the affected facility; it's not easy to work for a fascist, for example. I have suggested to executives in some of these companies that they gather their plant managers together in small groups and ask the managers of the plants with fewer complaints to offer insights as to how they deal with psychosocial challenges. Perhaps they can discuss hypothetical circumstances — the difficult worker or manager, substance abuse, or other problems.

The modern economy is providing us with another example of an adverse context peculiar to work sites, entire corporations, or industries. The specters of downsizing, outsourcing, or bankruptcy engulf the entire workforce in an adverse context rife with job insecurity and contentious personnel issues. The adverse health consequences for these workforces are considerable. There are a number of cohort studies that render this point incontrovertible. All entail "natural" economic experiments in a setting where health outcomes were monitored.

In the early 1990s, the Finnish economy suffered a considerable setback lasting several years. Many workers were dismissed. The effect of impending downsizing on the government employees in one small city was monitored. The rate of absenteeism escalated, most markedly for sick leave ascribed to regional musculoskeletal disorders, particularly among employees over the age of fifty.

The "Whitehall" studies, cohort studies of British civil servants, long ago documented an inverse relationship between civil-service grade and mortality rate, particularly mortality from cardiovascular disease. In recent years it has become clear that the association with grade paled next to the association with psychosocial job "stress," particularly job "control," regardless of grade. Similar relationships pertain to sickness absence from back pain. One nested Whitehall cohort, faced with impending outsourcing, suffered a fate similar to that observed in the Finnish cohort just discussed. Impending downsizing wreaks havoc on the psychosocial context of work inflicting "stress" and "strain" on all, particularly the aging worker. Downsizing exemplifies the noxious, insalubrious, and lethal process we are denoting as an adverse "psychosocial" work context. And it does so without regard for prior station in life.

Even without the inflammatory influences of downsizing, an adverse psychosocial context works its harm. Slowly it will deprive one of favorable "self-rated health" (SRH). Like SES, SRH is a powerful predictor of all-cause mortality. In a cohort of 5,001 Danish workers, adverse "psychosocial" work context was shown to erode SRH over the five years of observation. A similar association has emerged from analysis of the nurses' health study: a perception that psychosocial work conditions were unfavorable predicted declining functional status among some 21,000 nurses followed for four years.

Several years ago, Wal-Mart and investigators from the National Institute for Occupational Safety and Health designed a cohort study to test whether wearing "back belts" prevented disabling back pain. It didn't. This was a large study, following some 6,000 employees in 160 stores for six months. At inception of the cohort, volunteers were interviewed and queried extensively in an attempt to quantify their sense of psychological comfort at work. There was minimal discernible influence of the physical demands of tasks on the incidence of disabling back pain. However, the perception of high job intensity demands and scheduling demands, as well as overall job dissatisfaction, were discernible as associating with the incidence of disabling back pain.

Stress and Well-Being

Stress is a difficult concept to define or grasp, probably because its meaning is so dependent on context. "Stress" is not always bad.

Physical stress in biological systems has the same U-shaped cause-effect curve that we discussed in chapter 3. For example, bone remodels to be stronger with a certain amount of physical stress, but too little leads to fragility and too much to fracture. Furthermore, muscles are more effective, tendons stronger, and cartilage thicker. The ergonomic thrust aimed at banning physical stress from life, including life in the workplace, is a biologically flawed notion.

Psychological stress is not all bad, either, nor can it be avoided. Psychological stress can lead to enhanced performance, which is satisfying, pleasing, and a goal in many aspects of vocational and avocational life. Learning how to overcome or cope with psychological stress is prerequisite to a mature and effective role in family and society. Stress cannot be avoided, at least not for long. Attempting to avoid it is stressful.

In the workplace, safety can be regulated. Violent injuries are unconscionable, and all feasible efforts should be expended in enhancing safety so that accidents are vanishingly rare. Can "stress" be regulated? How do you set up parameters of the context of work so that it is as stress and strain free as possible, so that as many workers as possible feel "good in their skin" often, or usually, or always? The industrial psychologists can define work autonomy in a particular setting, but when they measure the association with job satisfaction, the variability is enormous, reflecting the difference between individuals. That research dilemma is what makes life and people so wonderful. If there is to be any regulation of the psychosocial context of working, it would have to have a very broad tolerance for individual differences. Anything else would smack of Orwell's *1984*.

The humane solution is not in regulations. It resides in informing the body politic of the critical importance of the psychosocial context of work. It resides in valuing workers, particularly workers who have the innate talent to assist coworkers to cope effectively with stresses. Perhaps someday this can be taught. Today, it is best modeled. The modern workplace offers an important opportunity to help those who are lacking in wherewithal to improve their self-esteem, coping skills, and longevity.

Working Well

None of this will come to pass until we displace the social constructions relating to notions of "injury," "in your mind," and "human capital." Today, workers choose to be patients and claimants with regional musculoskeletal disorders because their ability to cope is overwhelmed by the challenges in maintaining employment. The occupational-health establishment must learn that anatomical landmarks do not delineate this illness. Just as we have learned that impediments to coping beleaguer the elderly with knee pain (chapter 9), society must countenance discussions of life in the workplace for the sake of these patients. Doctors may be as powerless as patients to put things right. Or some solution may emerge. The latter becomes more likely if we gain expertise about the dynamics of the workplace and identify resources that can assist us, much as we have done regarding life in the home. Society should bridle whenever "human capital" is held up as expendable.

The Aged Worker

Aged workers are not old. "Aged" has nuance beyond the chronological; there is the ripening of skills, the familiarity of space, and the comfort with station. Americans who came of age in the last half of the twentieth century considered "aged" a goal. Today, it's a tenuous station in life. It is one that tolerates change poorly. And it is one that is far less valued. It is the aged worker that faces the specter of redundancy bent and bowed. It is the aged worker who finds downsizing and outsourcing a knell. Disgruntlement, disillusionment, and resentment are the advantages they realize when their company declares Chapter 11 bankruptcy. The personal price they pay for a loss of security as pensions disappear is incalculable in its morbidity and mortality.

The Retired Worker

I am saddling you, the reader, with quite a burden in terms of your health. Even if my profession approached perfection in the healing art, it would not be enough without your essential contributions. You must be aware of much more than your own socioeconomic status. You must be aware of much more than your own sense of accomplishment at home and at work. The greatest burden I am placing on you is the understanding of the political context that shapes your well-being. If yours is lacking, you will pay a personal price. If too many around you are lacking in this understanding, you will find yourself in a world that is angry, even desperate and possibly violent.

As for the octogenarians, to be well at your age means you have managed to cope with a laundry list of life challenges. To be well, now, means you voyaged through life in a comforting socioeconomic stratum. To be well, now, means you managed to avoid being mired in circumstances that rendered you disaffected or hostile at work or at home. To be well means you were sophisticated enough, or lucky enough in your choice of providers, to have negotiated with health-care professionals so as to enjoy interactions with favorable benefit/risk ratios, to avoid iatrogenesis, and to avoid medicalization. I have written this book to offer guideposts to the generations behind you who aspire to be well octogenarians. However, if you're a well octogenarian, then what? You are of a ripe old age. Can this be an enjoyable and joyful time of life?

Family and community are the precious underpinnings for a joyful last decade. The other prerequisite relates to the entitlement of senior citizens to the best health care money can buy. Senior citizens are a powerful lobby in that regard. However, they have been duped into marching arm-in-arm with the pharmaceutical industry, the hospital industry, and components of the medical industry. Is Plan D of Medicare an advance in health care or in Type II Medical Malpractice? Analysis of Medicare data documents that excess spending and excessive care transfers considerable wealth but does nothing for the well-being or satisfaction of the elderly. All they gain is the hazards of iatrogenicity.

Beware of medical schemes that are offered to prolong your life. For octogenarians, the goals of self-effectualness, independence, interaction, and comfort are primary. Besides, the goal of prolongation of life by medical interventions for anything but acute intercurrent events is even more ephemeral at eighty than it was at sixty.

Beware of the use of pharmaceuticals to serve the primary goals of self-effectualness, independence, interaction, and comfort. The drugs that are available to serve these goals are limited in number and efficacy. They are severely limited in effectiveness. Their therapeutic indices, the tightness of their benefit/risk ratios, are inversely related to your age. That means that side effects are almost as likely as benefits. Don't take any drug for these goals that is not clearly moving you in the right direction. Negotiate with your doctor for trials of agents where the trial has an a priori end point: either you are clearly better or you will stop the drug. Otherwise, you will join the majority of your cohort that is consuming pills; 40 percent consumes five or more different prescription drugs each week, and one out of every eight pill takers suffers a serious side effect each year.

The same sophistication in health-care utilization that will avail those in the generations that follow is as relevant to you who are attempting to enjoy the ripe old age you have attained. I wish you love. I wish you friendship. I wish you well.

chapter thirteen

"Alternative" Therapies Are Not "Complementary"

As you no doubt understand by now, to be well is not the same as to feel well. To be well requires some sense of invincibility. No one is spared symptoms for long. It's abnormal to go one year without upper respiratory symptoms or pain, notably backache. Lurking in our future are heartache and heartburn, shoulder and knee pain, headache, rashes, and skipped heartbeats, not to mention bothersome fatigue, sore muscles, bowel irregularity, insomnia, and so much else to challenge our sense of well-being repeatedly. To be well requires the wherewithal to cope with these predicaments of life until they remit, cope so effectively that they are not long memorable.

If you experience crushing chest pain or excruciating headache, if you have a fever and are coughing up green sputum, if you start vomiting blood — common sense and your caring community demand that you seek the attention of a member of my guild, the guild of physicians and surgeons. No other course is reasonable. These are not ordinary predicaments of life; they are extraordinary. Only my guild can respond in the affirmative if you ask whether you are clearly more likely to be advantaged by our ministrations than not.

But most symptoms are not so extraordinary. We have options to consider. Over the past decade, epidemiologists have ventured into the community to probe the fashion in which we cope with these intermittent and remittent predicaments of life. Most of us, most of the time, cope on our own. "On our own" is not in a vacuum; we are bombarded by advice and marketed ceaselessly to avail ourselves of all kinds of unctions and potions and widgets. Rare is the person who does not succumb; American medicine cabinets bear witness. All this "help" is a cultural phenomenon fostered by legions of purveyors, a cultural phenomenon with roots in antiquity and with inventiveness across time and cultures that boggles the mind. It's a waste of money to participate unless you like the taste (chicken soup, fish, and garlic are examples) or the feel (massage chairs, meditation, and girding your loins are examples) and a waste of breath to decry it. For most of us, most of the time, our symptoms improve no matter what we do. When the particular symptom recurs, we are likely to cope in our precedent fashion, convinced that what we did or what we took or what we avoided was palliative. So be it.

For some of us, some of the time, coping on our own seems inadequate. One of the most important scientific revolutions in our lifetime, ranking with those in genetics and immunology, is unheralded and largely unappreciated. Community epidemiology has provided insight into why coping on our own seems inadequate. In all likelihood, our coping with these predicaments is not overwhelmed by the intensity of the symptoms. Rather, something else in our lives is compromising our ability to cope. Usually the culprit can be found in the psychosocial context upon which the symptom is superimposed: something adverse in our lives at home or at work, something financial or interpersonal that renders the symptom the last straw. If you are tired and have financial worries, you will be more tired. If you have back pain and a hateful job, the back will hurt more (chapter 12). If your marriage is in turmoil, you will have more difficulty ignoring a change in bowel habits than you would when the sailing is smooth (chapter 10). You are not abnormal, or sick, or nuts, or weak to respond in this fashion. You are human. The symptom is not changed; the suffering it engenders is exacerbated by psychosocial confounders in our lives. Will we ever learn this lesson? Are we forever destined to seek out someone who offers to fix or heal or cure the surrogate symptom rather than redress the confounders? In missing the forest for the trees, we risk a Sisyphean quest for well-being regardless of the practitioner in whom we decide to place our trust. The alternative treatments that are available all focus on the symptom rather than the person with the symptom. They are complementary only to the extent that they share this mindset.

Your first stop, usually, is my guild. Seeking our guidance when you find a predicament of life overwhelming can be as sensible as when you find a physical symptom extraordinary. However, we all need to get beyond the traditional complaint "What's wrong with me, doc, that I have this symptom?" and move on to a rational discourse: "Is there any important disease that is causing my symptom? If so, can it be treated? If not, can we discern why I can't cope with this episode?" For nearly all the predicaments of life we're discussing, reassurance regarding underlying important diseases should be rapidly forthcoming, often based on the quality of the symptom and the physical examination, occasionally requiring some testing. If this leads to a "maybe you have," beware. Diagnostic uncertainty in the absence of demonstrable disease is reassuring enough; dwelling on residual uncertainty is a pall that interferes with returning to well-being. And don't leap to swallow "symptomatic treatment." The prescription of such treatment carries with it the notion that pills will help you cope. Since nearly all the drugs you hear about are marginally effective for these predicaments of life, you are setting yourself up for disappointment and desperation. All have adverse effects that may further compromise coping. None of this should surprise you, since treating the physical symptoms is missing the point. There are other warnings regarding the approach taken by my guild. No patient escapes a physician's office unchanged. You will learn a new language, the language of biomedicine. You will acquire new idioms of distress invoking putative pathophysiological insights. You will never forget them.

So much for my "dirty linen"; more is aired in many other chapters.

Many of you will shop among the alternative therapies. All offer the promise of a special insight into the cause of your predicament. Most want to do something to you, apply a "modality" for which application the therapist has acquired some special skill. The modality is never applied without fanfare and intense human interaction. That's the treatment act. These modalities are said to redress the specific defect that the therapist has determined to be the root cause of your predicament. These are theories, beliefs, none of which have survived scientific scrutiny. Nonetheless, you will learn to color your narrative with their idioms: parts that want yanking and those that want soothing, spots that merit probing or sticking and spots that should be spared, chemicals that are unbalanced, missing, or threatening, and the like. You will learn to think of your body in their terminology. And if all they offer and all they say are palatable, comfortable, and sensible, you will enter a long-term relationship that renders questioning the theories anathema and invests power in the therapist. You will share their beliefs. Realize that nearly all "modalities" have been subjected to scientific scrutiny and fare even more poorly than the symptomatic pharmaceutical treatments discussed above. You are choosing an alternative conception of well-being. You will be changed forever. However, your ability to identify the psychosocial confounders that thwarted coping in the first place will be lost in the sectarian jargon, just as it was in biomedical jargon.

I can't blame you if you participate in any or all of these alternative experiences. I am saddened to realize how few of us have access to more effective support when we find our next predicament of life to be more than we can manage on our own. All I can say is don't lose control of the process, regardless of the alternative chosen. Don't lose your ability to say "I am well without you." And don't ask me to share the cost of any alternative that is not devoted to returning you to your prior state of well-being.

I can't blame you, but don't expect my applause. Let me be up front with my prejudices:

1. I am convinced that "complementary and alternative" therapies thrive best whenever my guild, which requires an M.D. for admission, is behaving in an unconscionable manner. We are doing so today.
2. I can countenance no treatment modality or treatment act that has an unfavorable benefit/risk ratio, regardless of the purveyor.
3. I am willing to share the cost for someone to query as to whether the benefit/risk ratio of any therapeutic modality or treatment act is favorable.
4. I am willing to share the cost of the therapeutic modality if the benefit/risk ratio is favorable.
5. As for treatment acts that some find beneficial yet are based on modalities that are neither harmful nor beneficial, I reserve the option of refusing to share the cost.
6. However, I bridle at having to share the cost of underwriting any "therapeutic envelope." I will explain what I mean by "envelope" in detail later in this chapter. Briefly, it is the contract one enters into with any treating professional, a deeply personal contract that forces upon you a privileged vocabulary, alters your self-perceptions, and changes you indelibly. You are entwined in a metaphysical cocoon. That's not what I want for you or for my patients. I want you to leave the treatment act better, not different, to return to being the person you wanted to be before entering the treatment act.

These prejudices are anything but straightforward. Defining them, let alone serving them, takes science to its limits. Even with definitional license, the ramifications are considerable. That will become clear in the following discussions of the history of "complementary and alternative" therapy and the notions of "treatment modality," "treatment act," and "therapeutic envelope."

Before we embark on this odyssey, let me tell you about a study that illustrates the power of belief in the context of alternative therapy. Investigators in Boston recruited nearly 300 young adults with regional musculoskeletal disorders of the arm (chapters 9 and 12) of at least three months duration. They were randomized into one of two randomized controlled trials for two months. In one trial, they were subjected to acupuncture or sham acupuncture: both groups spent time twice weekly with an experienced acupuncturist, who undertook five to ten punctures each session and used a sheathed needle that, for sham acupuncture, looks and feels like it's doing its acupuncture thing but never pierces the skin. In the other randomized controlled trial, subjects were treated with the drug amitriptyline or a placebo pill. Everybody improved in both trials. However, the point of this exercise was not the separate trials but a comparison of the two placebo groups. Those who underwent sham acupuncture improved at a faster rate than those who received the placebo pill. A placebo pill is no match for the acupuncturist's treatment act: the rituals, the beliefs, the body language, the explanations, and whatever else went on even though the needle didn't pierce the skin time after time.

A Brief History of Complementary and Alternative Therapy

The ancient Egyptians prayed to Imhotep. The Romans borrowed the Greek demigod Asclepios. Aesculapius was a son of Apollo who begot two sons, Machaon the surgeon and Podalirios the physician, and two daughters, Hygieia and Panacea. For the ancients, gods and demigods could cause and cure diseases and wounds. Healing gods were enshrined in special temples open to all who were ill and suffering. Physicians were itinerant craftsmen, ministering and operating in the homes of those who could pay their fee. Mythology began to give way to scientific medicine thanks to Hippocrates, who was born on the island of Cos about 460 BCE. On his death at the age of eighty, he left a legacy of shrewd clinical observations and ethical commentaries that have held theological and superstitious clinical theories and practices somewhat at bay ever since. Hippocrates' clinical observations were complemented by the theories of his contemporary Plato to spawn the school of medicine of the "Dogmatists." Health care would never be the same. For the Dogmatists, observation was a poor substitute for reasoning. Their reasoning led to many vitalistic theories and to extreme therapeutic measures, including purging, bleeding, and dehydrating the ill. The history of medicine ever since involves the discarding of vitalistic theories in favor of those that are scientifically tenable and the fashioning of remedies that bridle therapeutic zeal with requirements for evidence of effectiveness. However, the trajectory of progress is anything but linear; there are many false starts and much backtracking. Despite centuries of progress, much of illness remains beyond the reach of tested theories, as does much therapeutic zeal.

The history of the care of the ill and the history of medicine are parallel but not monolithic to this day. Many around the globe who are ill still seek refuge in superstition and theology, some by choice and some by default. Furthermore, today and always there are purveyors of remedies that are beyond the reach of testing, often based on theories that defy contemporary reasoning and therefore earn the scorn of the modern Dogmatists. Others are beyond the reach of testing and so earn the scorn of scientific medicine. Scorned or not, treatments of all varieties flourish. Some predate my guild. Some that are only a century or two old remain active participants in the Western health-care-delivery scene today. In the resource-challenged world, alternatives to my guild often predominate. In fact, it is only in the past century that Western medicine has managed to secure its position on the pinnacle.

A millennium ago, Europe sacrificed its intellectual roots and traditions to superstition and wallowed in the Dark Ages. Meanwhile, science, philosophy, and medicine thrived in the Arab world, with centers of excellence such as Alexandria. Japanese and Chinese medicine and medical education also advanced in rationality and organization. The Western resurgence began with William Harvey's observation on the circulation of blood and made slow progress through the eighteenth century in terms of theory, some progress in terms of surgery, but painfully slow progress in medical therapeusis. It took Louis Pasteur's theory of putrefaction in 1861, followed shortly by Lister's principles of anti-sepsis, for modern therapeutics to gain a foothold and have promise. Nonetheless, purging, bleeding, and other forms of therapeutic violence predominated for generations as the legacy of the Dogmatists.

At the turn of the nineteenth century, Samuel Hahnemann, a German physician, offered an alternative approach to treatment. He had turned to experimental pharmacology, looking for agents with greater benefit/risk ratios than those in common use. He experimented on himself and his family, first with Jesuit's bark (see chapter 9); he termed these experiments "drug provings." He developed his theory of "similia similibus": if a drug produced symptoms in a well person, then very small doses (the "law of infinitesimals") would cure similar symptoms in someone who was ill. He named his system of therapeusis "homeopathy" and termed the standard practice of the mainstream physicians "allopathy." Allopathic physicians, he argued, administered drugs that counter the symptoms of illness (then conceptualized as the disease)—for instance, an antipyretic for fever. He advocated administering tiny doses of a drug that could cause fever in high doses. Sometimes people still label me and my guild "allopathic physicians," but I find that unacceptable since so much that we offer is no longer symptomatic treatment (antibiotics, for example).

Homeopathy proved very successful in recruiting patients, practitioners, and advocates in Europe and in North America. In 1842 Oliver Wendell Holmes, then dean of the Harvard Medical School, delivered two lectures entitled "Homeopathy and Its Kindred Delusions" in which he warned against "fatal credulity" in any of the alternatives then claiming "wonderful powers." Here we have the greatest mind in medicine of his generation casting such aspersions as a spokesman for a profession that was still bleeding and purging. Homeopathy was unfazed. Indeed, homeopathy remained so successful that it challenged the dominance of the traditional medical guild in the American market. President William McKinley was a supporter who, in 1900, dedicated the statue to Hahnemann that still dominates Scott Circle in Washington, D.C. Shortly thereafter, organized medicine capitulated and assimilated the homeopaths and their educational institutions (Hahnemann Medical School in Philadelphia is now part of Drexel University; Flower-Fifth Avenue School in New York City is now the New York Medical College in Valhalla). Homeopathy remains an alternative system of therapeusis in much of the Western world to this day and is having a resurgence in North America.

A contemporary of Hahnemann, Franz Anton Mesmer, became a celebrity because of his theories of "animal magnetism." His Magnetic Institute in Paris was a magnet for the somatizing rich — particularly the young, female somatizing rich — until he and his followers were banished to Switzerland for operating beyond the bounds of moral propriety of the day. Mesmer left two legacies: hypnotic suggestion (hence to "mesmerize") and this notion of magnetism. Therapeutic magnets are enjoying such resurgence that an august medical journal (*JAMA*) recently felt it appropriate and relevant to publish a study that fails to discern therapeutic benefit. Across the channel from Mesmer and Hahnemann, Dr. James Graham was operating his Temple of Health and Hygiene in London. Graham is remembered more for his therapeutic diet, particularly his therapeutic cracker, than for his medicalizing of moral turpitude in a fashion that rivaled Mesmer. While all this is happening, Edward Jenner discovered vaccination.

In the eighteenth century, only the wealthy could afford to partake of the wonders of modern medicine, though these wonders hardly had much to recommend them. The masses made do, or turned to the apothecaries who functioned as the primary-care practitioners of the day (and seek to do so yet again). All sorts of potions were purveyed. The nineteenth century may have witnessed Pasteur and Joseph Lister birthing modern scientific medicine, but the birth was more of theory than practice. For the mainstream practitioners of my guild, the nineteenth century was the century of "heroic medicine." Therapeutic zeal seemed to recognize no iatrogenic boundaries. Bleeding, purging, fever therapies — along with administering heavy metals and toxic botanical potions and unctions — were the order of the day. "Heroic medicine" was a term that grew out of the carnage on the battlefields and in the military hospitals of the Civil War. Not surprisingly, society welcomed old alternatives and invented new ones. Homeopaths claimed recovery rates in the cholera epidemic of 1849 that outstripped the track record of mainstream ministrations. This was a century before epidemiology started to contend with confounders and bias in such observations, so there must be uncertainty about such claims. Perhaps the sicker patients chose mainstream physicians, or perhaps the mainstream ministrations ushered more to their deaths. Regardless, it was sensible to seek alternatives if you or someone dear to you was ill. The nineteenth-century menu of alternatives was extensive. There were schools of hydrotherapists and botanical therapists. North America's answer to Graham's dietary-plus approach to wellness was thriving in Michigan, where Dr. John Harvey Kellogg offered hydrotherapy, colonic irrigation, purging, abdominal surgery, and clitoral stimulation along with his therapeutic corn flakes. In response to "heroic medicine" and all the quackery, the nineteenth century birthed a religious backlash that included Christian Science and the Pentecostal movement. Metaphysics was a match for heroic medicine. By the way, Mary Baker Eddy founded Christian Science, arguing that worry could make one sick and faith could heal. Please believe me that in choosing the title of this book, I mean no obeisance to this bit of history.

Homeopathy and other therapeutic movements that challenge the tenets of mainstream medicine from within or without are termed "sectarian" by the mainstream membership. "Sectarian medicine" is a chauvinistic, if not pejorative, term. In use today, it is not meant to imply that all sectarian practitioners are cultists or even true believers. It is meant to designate the systems of health care that compete with each other and with mainstream medicine. All are capable of taking off their gloves to protect their turf. However, today they all seek licensure as certification of the specialized nature of their knowledge and skills and thereby codify a competitive advantage in that regard. They are perhaps more akin to guilds of old than to present-day unions. All compete for the "health-care dollar." Like other businesses, some flourished, some merged, and many folded. Homeopathy in the United States is one that merged, disappearing into mainstream medicine, though it appears to be rising anew. Naturopathy (which keeps the legacy of the botanists and herbalists) has managed to build schools and attain licensure in some states. Others simply maintain a life of their own. Two made-in-America examples of sectarian medicine are worthy of our attention: osteopathy and the chiropractic.

As a young man, Andrew Taylor Still (1828–1917) was apprenticed to a physician. He became disillusioned with medical practice when he witnessed the heroic measures undertaken by the physicians attending his three children as they succumbed to meningitis in the epidemic of 1864. The son of a Methodist minister, Still believed that imbibing alcohol was sinful. If alcohol is sinful, then aren't other drugs as well? Still was drawn to the theories of Mesmer and the magnetic healers, with their belief that diseases were caused by interruptions in the pathways for magnetic fluids in the body. The magnetic healers employed magnets to redirect that flow. Instead of magnets, Still postulated that the manipulative techniques (long practiced by bonesetters and the like) would work as well as magnets, if not better. He founded his school of osteopathy in Kirksville, Missouri, teaching others how to "realign displacements" — obstructing musculoskeletal segments, usually in the spine. Once realigned, natural healing could proceed without recourse to allopathic drugs. By the turn of the twentieth century, Still had an infirmary in Kirksville, over 700 graduates, and a sizable following. Osteopathic schools opened elsewhere. Patients who were under the care of osteopaths fared better than those treated to "heroic medicine" in the influenza epidemic of 1918–19, harkening back to homeopaths' claims in the 1849 cholera epidemic. Over the objections of Still, then eighty-seven years old, the American Osteopathic Association decided to incorporate the "materia medica" of mainstream medicine into the curriculum in the early twentieth century. By the middle of the century, there were fifteen schools of osteopathic medicine with curricula similar to that of the traditional medical schools. By the 1960s, all states licensed osteopaths with privileges comparable to an M.D. Nonetheless, the American Osteopathic Association maintains control over accreditation of these schools, grants a D.O. degree, and mandates courses in musculoskeletal manipulation, although the vitalistic theories that seduced Still are long gone. Michigan State University houses curricula leading to either the M.D. or D.O. degrees in the same facility, with courses in common.

The chiropractic and mainstream medicine have no such cozy relationship. The chiropractic was founded by a grocer in 1895 in Davenport, Iowa. Daniel

David (D. D.) Palmer (1845 – 1913) was, like Still, into vitalism. He reasoned that excessive "tone" produced "impingement, a pressure on nerves," from which disease resulted. "Adjusting vertebrae, using the spinous and transverse processes as lever" could relieve that "tone." Palmer claimed to have cured a janitor of deafness and to improve heart failure by manipulation of the neck. By the turn of the twentieth century, D. D. Palmer had a school, an infirmary, students, and a moniker for his sectarian therapy. The name "chiropractic" is derived from the Greek *cheir* (hand) and *praxis* (specific use). His son, B. J. Palmer, was one of his first students and later purchased the school and managed to turn it into a successful enterprise. B. J. and his followers were proponents of pure, "straight," unadulterated chiropractic. However, this example of sectarian medicine itself soon turned sectarian. "Mixers" were willing to incorporate the practices of other sects into their own — "napropaths" who treated irritated ligaments instead of impinged nerves, "neuropaths" who felt the impingements were outside the spine, and others, such as "naturopaths" and "physiotherapists." Several (but not all) of these splinter sects have faded away, and several are making a comeback. To this day, a schism persists in the chiropractic between "mixers" and "straights," particularly "straight-straights" who adhere to D. D. Palmer's vitalistic theory.

The bickering within the chiropractic pales next to the open warfare with the medical establishment that played out through much of the twentieth century. By midcentury the American Medical Association held the chiropractic to be quackery and declared interactions with chiropractors on a professional level to be unethical. The chiropractic thrived nonetheless and now number around 60,000, mainly in the United States. Furthermore, the chiropractic took my guild to task in the courts, so that by 1975 the chiropractic was licensed in all states, and in 1979 the formalized prejudice of the AMA was found to be illegal. "Straights" and "mixers" are licensed to perform manipulative therapies and imaging studies but not to prescribe pharmaceuticals. What is less defined, somewhat contentious within the chiropractic, and very contentious for mainstream medicine is the purview of the chiropractic. Is their purview solely the regional musculoskeletal disorders? That is not the stance of many chiropractors and many schools of chiropractic. There are chiropractors who "reduce subluxations" for a range of ailments from headache to asthma. "Subluxations" are the chiropractic diagnosis that implies spinal malalignment. Subluxations are imaginary; there are no such specific skeletal changes that correlate with symptoms. However, chiropractors are skilled at applying brief, high-velocity force to the vertebral column sufficient to create a vacuum phenomenon in the small joints of the spinal column. The vacuum phenomenon snaps back with the cracking sounds and sensations that cause chiropractors to feel accomplished and their patient to feel treated. That anyone can imagine such an event can salve asthma, diabetes, or the like is a testimony to the tenacity of vitalistic theories.

Turning the cracking of backs and necks into a fastidious art form is the triumph of the chiropractic. These maneuvers take their place in the ancient tradition of manual therapy. Therapeutic massage can be traced back through history. Medical luminaries of their day employed and wrote about massage, traction, and manipulation, including Avicenna in the eleventh century, Charef-Ed-Din in the fifteenth century, and Ambroise Paré in the sixteenth century. Manipulation of the skeleton is practiced by the mainstream in osteopathy, where the manipulation traditionally entails the application of shearing force using less acceleration and generally a longer lever arm than the chiropractic. It is central to the system of "orthopedic medicine" formulated by James Cyriax in London thirty years ago and the physiotherapy school of Robert Maigne that is commonly practiced in Europe. Manual therapy is part of the fabric of life today in all cultures, and it always will be.

I am a rheumatologist, a mainstream physician with an M.D. who is schooled in and committed to the care of patients with musculoskeletal disorders. Do I have to learn manual medicine? Should I seek such a salve for my own next predicament of a regional musculoskeletal disorder? Should I refer my patients to such practitioners?

There are corollary issues. Should I encourage or applaud recourse to the morass of putative neutriceuticals, herbal and botanical remedies, dietary supplements, and the like? We are exposed to a barrage of yea saying. There are professionals who claim skills in the purveyance of these remedies, including naturopaths and homeopaths. Does their ministration advantage their patients? As we discussed in chapter 9, mainstream physicians were all herbalists until quite recently. Herbal remedies, botanicals, and other naturally occurring organic and inorganic substances were all that was available until the twentieth century and remained the mainstream physician's stock in trade until the last half of that century. To wit, frankincense and myrrh were expectorants and astringents as well as ecclesiastical accoutrement. The advances of the last half of the twentieth century include the ability to purify and synthesize pharmacologically active compounds, the ability to establish dose-response curves, and the mandate to assess benefit/risk ratios. Do you really think there is something important being overlooked among the folk remedies or the formulations of naturopaths and homeopaths? Maybe you are right in such thinking. Maybe the pharmaceutical industry is so interested in profit margins that substances that cannot be patented lay fallow. Certainly there are botanicals with pharmacological effects yet to be discovered and, more certainly, biologicals with pharmacological effects yet to be purified. But there are none that should circumvent the benefit/risk gauntlet to marketing. Why should we forego the assessment of benefit/risk ratios just because these are naturally occurring substances? Some may be harmful or have tight therapeutic ratios (margin between effect and toxicity). That's true for some of the classic botanicals, such as digitalis and colchicine, which are still in use (though in pure form). Digitalis was isolated from the foxglove and is still used for some cardiac disorders, even though the line between benefit and fatal toxicity is very fine. With colchicine, still used to prevent gouty attacks, the fine line is between benefit and diarrhea.

There are many purveyors of many remedies. Can we infer a favorable benefit/risk ratio for any of these remedies?

Modalities, Treatment Acts, and Therapeutic Envelopes

Modalities are the particulars of what is done for us, to us, or with us by any purveyor of therapy to whom we turn. The treatment act is not so objective; seldom do modalities operate without human interaction with their purveyor. The context in which the modalities are offered and administered is the treatment act. It's the whole process of intervention by the provider on behalf of the patient. The therapeutic envelope speaks to the fashion in which we are changed by the treatment act. The therapeutic envelope is our new being, the sum of our altered self-perceptions and our idioms of distress, and our narratives of illness and our peer affinities, as well as our expectations from our healthfulness in our communities. The therapeutic envelope is the new persona we might take away from treatment acts. Entering into a treatment envelope is entering into another station in life, often never to return regardless of the clinical outcome. The patient or client must become aware of the far-reaching personal impact of accepting treatment prior to initiating the process. I am arguing that the patient/client must tune into the perceptual impact of the process as much as into the effectiveness of the various modalities. No one should enter a therapeutic envelope without awareness of the passage and acceptance of the outcome.

OVER-THE-COUNTER MODALITIES

There are modalities that seem free of a treatment act, let alone a therapeutic envelope, because there is no professional directly involved in their purveyance. That's a false impression. The choice to purchase a putative neutraceutical, botanical, or other dietary supplement is always informed. These substances are darlings of the lay medical press and aggressively marketed to boot. Wherever you make your purchase, you will have access to "informed" and helpful salespeople. There is a community to welcome you, a community of believers, nearly all of whom feel advantaged in some way by participating in this form of sectarian treatment act. You will join their therapeutic envelope, or not. There is no middle ground.

There also is no attempt to provide any assurance of purity, safety, or efficacy. That is a policy decision. The Dietary Supplement and Health Education Act of 1994 permitted the unregulated sale of herbal and other botanical products that were already on the shelf. It was argued that such substances are foodstuffs, not pharmaceuticals. The manufacturer may describe physiological effects and imply benefits but may not promote effectiveness. As for purity, there are many studies demonstrating the enormous variability in the constituents marketed as the same substance by different manufacturers. One study of Asian patent medicines sold in California in 1998 demonstrated that a third of these so-called botanicals were adulterated with undeclared pharmaceuticals or heavy metals that were biologically active and potentially toxic; ephedrine, chlorpheniramine, methyltestosterone, phenacetin, lead, mercury, and arsenic were detected.

And even apart from these undesirable contaminants, herbs themselves, like conventional pharmaceuticals, can have unexpected side effects that are not systematically screened for. Any adverse effects, if they are reported at all, are to be detected in the post-marketing arena. Even with this haphazard surveillance, the FDA has identified toxicities. Table 10 is a partial listing.

Ephedra belongs on the list. Ephedra was in a number of "diet" preparations. It is also called Ma Huang and epitonin. It has well-documented cardiovascular and central-nervous-system effects that have caused adverse events. Its benefit/risk ratio is very small, at best. Various authorities, including Sid Wolfe, who directs the Citizen Health Research Group, assaulted the FDA to ban this agent in order to protect the uninformed and unsuspecting. The agent was pulled from the market despite arguments by its purveyors that too few are harmed to be concerned. I agree that few are harmed, but that's too many given its benefits. Caveat emptor.

There also is a growing list of dietary supplements that can perturb the effectiveness of licensed pharmaceuticals. Some potentiate and others inhibit some conventional drugs' effects. No one should be surprised since foodstuffs,

TABLE 10. Adverse Effects of Herbal Concoctions

Herbal Product	Adverse Effect
Chaparral, comfrey, germander	Liver disease
Slimming tea	Nausea and vomiting; possible death
Jin bu huan	Depressed heart, mind, lung function
Lobelia	Coma and death at high dose
Yohimbe	Kidney disease, seizures, and death

Source: < http://www.cfsan.fda.gov/~dms/ds-ill.html >.

not even dietary supplements, can potentiate and inhibit the effectiveness of licensed pharmaceuticals. Who would have thought that grapefruit or rhubarb would be on the latter list? Physicians and pharmacists are apprised and apprise patients (with uncertain efficiency) as further drug-food interactions are uncovered. That seems a proper function and pressing need in the setting of prescription agents. However, there are enough people in the "dietary supplement" therapeutic envelope that it behooves physicians and pharmacists to consider supplement-drug interactions, particularly in the surgical setting. The Memorial Sloan-Kettering Cancer Center offers a free website (‹http://www.mskcc.org/aboutherbs›) that currently reviews the data as to the upsides and downsides of hundreds of herbal preparations. This is as reliable a resource as is available for any reader who feels the urge to seek benefit from herbal remedies.

Are you waiting for me to tell you which herbal remedies and supplements pass scientific muster in terms of benefit? No surprise, I am not convinced that there is anything in the health-food shelf that has a worthy benefit/risk ratio. Ginkgo is of questionable use for dementia. St. John's wort is a poor excuse for an antidepressant and offers considerable concerns about interactions with licensed drugs. Ginseng and echinacea are useful only as statements that you have disposable income and are unfazed by the clinical trials that fail to discern benefit for either, in particular for ginseng for dementia and echinacea for the common cold. Saw palmetto may do something for you if you have prostatism (chapter 7), but it may not and did not do anything in an impressive randomized controlled trial in San Francisco. Even though there are herbal remedies and dietary supplements that may do something good, they all have downsides. As far as I'm concerned, they are all worthless unless they taste good.

However, that is not the "word on the street," nor the word in advertising. Remember, companies can market herbal remedies and other dietary supplements without approval of the FDA or any other regulatory agency. There are many examples of egregious marketing practices, particularly on the Internet. Even when controlled by the FDA and other agencies, advertisers still often play fast and loose with the truth. The editor of the *New England Journal of Medicine* has felt compelled to decry the license taken by advertisers with science published in his journal. A systematic review of the content of advertisements in leading medical journals performed several years ago documents the plethora of assertions that outside experts find misleading. The uninformed person is at a disadvantage in the marketing arena and will be well served by skepticism when faced with claims about dietary supplements. For that matter, they will also be well served by skepticism when faced with claims about licensed pharmaceuticals in the direct-to-consumer marketing that assaults us every day. I suggest you close your eyes when the next televised advertisement for a prescription drug appears. Listen to the convoluted and obfuscating prose without being distracted by someone on ice skates, or a football coach, or whatever. As for print media, have someone else read the prose to you without your seeing the pictures. These exercises will do wonders for your skepticism.

Then there are the vitamins. Public-health regulations ensure that foods are supplemented with vitamins to assure against deficiency. If you are well, well nourished, and not unusual in your dietary proclivities, you are not vitamin deficient. Nonetheless, it is estimated that half of the U.S. population uses vitamin supplements regularly, surely a testimony to marketing and the preconceived notions of the lay medical press. The people who consume "multivitamins and mineral supplements" tend to be wealthier in order to afford participating in this envelope; they are the segment of the population that is healthier, anyway. Do multivitamin/mineral supplements contribute to their being better off? Is the marketing correct and the lay press prescient? Are well people, or some well people, poorly served by the recommended daily intake upon which basis food is supplemented? Or are vitamin and mineral supplements a waste of billions of dollars?

The answer to the last question is an affirmative with a couple of items of uncertainty. An analysis of the available data was undertaken by the NIH and reached this conclusion. There is no compelling reason, other than your comfort in the vitamin envelope, to take multivitamin/mineral supplements. One unequivocal exception is that the daily recommended intake of folic acid is too little in the first trimester of pregnancy. With further supplementation, the likelihood of neural-tube defects (spina bifida and the like) is reduced significantly. Are there other examples, other subsets of the well and well nourished, that would be advantaged in some clinically meaningful way by vitamin supplements? The lay health press and the industry that purveys vitamin supplements have conspired to render this an urgent matter. In response, large and expensive trials have been undertaken, and more are under way. There is no shortcut to testing whether a vitamin supplement will lead to a subtle advantage or disadvantage than a large and long-term trial. One wonders whether such a subtle health effect is worth so much effort, or whether any subtle effect that is discerned will be convincing, reliable, or even meaningful.

It turns out that some of the most compelling effects to emerge from these trials are negative. Take the carotenoids. There are hundreds of carotenoids, all are antioxidants, and many have pro–vitamin A activity, meaning they are converted in the body to retinol, the active vitamin necessary for normal vision and other functions. It has long been known that you can ingest too much vitamin A, leading to skin and liver disease. However, the doses recommended by those who think the daily recommendation inadequate fall far short of these toxic doses. Antioxidants in general, and carotenoids in particular, are thought by some to have the potential to prevent a variety of degenerative diseases. Carotenoids have been formally studied in cohort and randomized controlled trials to see if they prevent emphysema, coronary artery disease, or prostate cancer. No consistent benefit has been discerned. However, if you abuse tobacco and take carotenoids, your risk of lung cancer is increased. Furthermore, supplements have been shown to increase the risk of fractures, so much so that some are wondering if the recommended daily intake is too much.

Vitamin E is another antioxidant. There are several randomized controlled trials in coronary artery disease. Most discern no effect at all. The "HOPE" trial (the Heart Outcomes Prevention Evaluation Study) randomized almost 10,000 patients at risk for cardiovascular events because they had prior events and a high prevalence of the "Metabolic Syndrome" (chapter 3). Treatment with vitamin E for 4.5 years had no discernible clinical effect on cardiac outcomes; neither was there a discernible effect of vitamin E supplementation for the risk for stroke or respiratory tract infections. In fact, if one looks at all the various trials, the suggestion is that high-dose vitamin E supplementation is worse than a placebo. It may increase all-cause mortality a tiny bit.

If you insist on continuing to spend your money on antioxidants, there are a few suggestions you can hold up as your rationale. Vitamin E supplementation may diminish the likelihood of dementia. The Rotterdam study is a cohort study, not a drug trial. Over 5,000 older people were followed for an average of six years. Careful dietary histories, emphasizing antioxidant consumption, were collected at inception and at intervals. Two hundred developed some cognitive deficiency, of which 150 qualified as Alzheimer's disease. Those with cognitive deficiencies were more likely to have avoided high intake of vitamins E and C. Vitamin E has emerged, barely, as beneficial in decreasing the likelihood of dementia in two other cohort studies. Vitamin C and other antioxidants remain rumors in this regard. However, beta carotene, vitamins C and E, and zinc may slow progression of age-related macular degeneration, the most prevalent cause of irreversible blindness in developed countries. That has emerged from analysis of a number of cohorts, including the Rotterdam study. If I develop this condition, then I, too, would be ingesting antioxidants. But nothing else would compel me.

We should return to folic acid. It has been shown that an elevated plasma-homocysteine level associates with coronary artery disease (so do many other things). It is also known that folic-acid supplementation reduces that level. Folic-acid supplementation of flour has only been practiced in the United States since 1996. Prior to that, uncooked leafy vegetables, whole-grain cereals, and animal products were the richest natural sources. Maybe the new policy (initiated because of the spina bifida experience) is doing much more good beyond pregnancy. Longevity continues to increase, but there are better explanations than folic acid in our bread. Randomized controlled trials of lowering homocysteine with folic acid led to no discernible reduction in vascular events in vascular disease or effect on cognitive performance.

HANDS-ON MODALITIES

According to a recent telephone survey of some 2,000 randomly selected homes, about a third of adult Americans recall back or neck pain last year (see chapter 9 for a discussion of the dynamics of recall). Of these, a third participated only in complementary treatment acts. A third sought care only from a member of my guild. A quarter played it safe and used both. The National Health Interview Survey is a representative, population-based survey of the civilian, noninstitutionalized U.S. population. About two-thirds of us avail ourselves of "complementary and alternative medicine" (CAM), and more if we're diagnosed with "arthritis." We choose from an extensive menu and often sample many items, some repeatedly but seldom exclusively. All CAMs discussed in this chapter are well represented.

Fueled by social constructions and the broadening of coverage by HMOs and other health insurers, the trend to seeing both physician and nonphysician practitioners has escalated in the past decade. It is not clear whether seeing both represents an increase in conjoint service delivery or fragmentation of care. I suspect the latter. It is not clear how often physicians are aware that their patient is being attended simultaneously by a nonphysician clinician. It is also not clear how often a physician coordinates treatment acts with the nonphysician or confronts the cognitive dissonance of the different therapeutic envelopes. I suspect patients fend for themselves in this regard. Table 11 displays relative frequencies of choosing from the menu of alternatives. For the 10 percent of adult Americans who turn to alternative providers instead of or in addition to members of my guild, "physical modalities" have the greatest appeal. In this survey, the three most commonly purchased treatments were chiropractic, massage, and relaxation techniques. The treatments were rated as "very helpful" by 61 percent, 65 percent, and 43 percent, respectively, by the people participating in these treatment acts, whereas only 27 percent of patients attending a member of my guild found their treatment act "very helpful." Before you leap to the conclusion that the increased satisfaction expressed by those treated by nonphysicians is a reflection of the modality, there are "complementary" studies that can disabuse you and which I will discuss shortly.

Another survey of American adults who chose alternative therapies demonstrated that they were predominately white, married, middle-aged, and educated, had less robust self-reported health status, and described the alternative treatment acts as more congruent with their own values, beliefs, and philosophical orientations toward health and life. This was borne out in a survey of chiropractic patients, with the additional insight that their self-reported "mental health" was as worrisome as their self-reported general health status. Taken together, these observations are consonant with those discussed in chapter 9. Life challenges that impair coping are an incentive to seek treatment for physical illness, and the treatment act offered by my guild is unsatisfying compared to that offered by some others. Also, the more satisfying alternatives require, or provoke, agreement between the provider and the recipient as to beliefs in the efficacy of the particular healing system. The 10 percent of Americans identified in the table above are therefore comfortably ensconced in a therapeutic envelope, which requires their sharing the belief system on which the alternative treatment act is grounded. This may be therapeutic, but is it sophistry nonetheless?

There is a wealth of science testing the effectiveness of the physical modalities listed above, and some that are not listed. There have been so many randomized controlled trials of various forms of massage, acupuncture, acupressure, and spinal manipulation for regional back and neck pain that there are not

TABLE 11. Therapies Frequently Used by the 10 Percent of American Adults Turning to Alternative Providers

Modality	Treatment Act	Percentage of People Using
Physical		35
	Chiropractic	20
	Massage	14
	Yoga	2
	Acupuncture	1
	Osteopathy	0.3
Digestives		5
	Homeopathy	3
	Vitamins	2
	Herbs	1
	Naturopathy	0
Cognitive		17
	Relaxation techniques	11
	Imagery	6
	Biofeedback	0.5
	Self-help	0.3
	Hypnosis	0
Other		16
	Spiritual healing	5
	Energy healing	4
	Aromatherapy	3
	Neural therapy	2
	Special diet	1
	Other	2

Source: Adapted from Wolsko et al. (2003).

just systematic reviews and meta-analyses; there are also systematic reviews and meta-analyses of the systematic reviews. These are studies of the modalities, of particular forms of "laying on of hands." With one exception, there is no compelling or even suggestive evidence that any of the physical modalities in the table offer any discernible benefit. A similar conclusion pertains to trials of acupuncture, physical therapy, and massage. There are even randomized controlled trials of "therapeutic touch" and "distant healing" that yield little encouragement, if any.

The one exception relates to spinal manipulation. In 1987 my colleagues and I published a randomized controlled trial we had performed with funding from the Robert Wood Johnson Foundation. We recruited from the community young people who were suffering from acute regional back pain for less than a month, who had never undergone any form of spinal manipulation in the past, and whose predicament was not confounded by issues of work incapacity. All were examined by me and reassured. All underwent a mobilization: they were gently moved from side to side and administered flexion/extension by my colleague and coinvestigator, a professor of family medicine who had been trained by James Cyriax in London in "orthopedic medicine." Half underwent a long-lever arm, high velocity, lateral thrust "back crack" — the bread-and-butter maneuver of osteopathy. All subjects felt better on leaving the office, regardless of the modality. For those who were hurting for two weeks or less at the time of the intervention, all were better two weeks later, and the pace of healing was not influenced by the modality. For those who were hurting for two to four weeks at the time of the intervention, all were better two weeks later, but those who received the single "back crack" healed more rapidly.

The world of spinal manipulation holds this investigation up as a landmark. It has been reproduced many times. However, it does not reproduce in any other subset of the universe of people suffering back pain. Only those who have nonconfounded regional backache for two to four weeks are advantaged by spinal manipulation, and only by a single encounter. Furthermore, the benefit is measured in days of extra relief, not more.

All these studies are an attempt to test the therapeutic modality independent of the treatment act. If the treatment act is allowed to play out, benefit is demonstrated more often than not. The risk of most of these modalities is low. There are anecdotal reports of neurological consequences of manipulating the neck. Otherwise, untoward physical consequences are rare.

The Ethical Conundrum

I am willing to admit that much that is therapeutic in the practice of medicine as purveyed by my guild relates to the treatment act and not just to the modality. I am further willing to admit that many of our therapeutic modalities barely pass scientific muster. Furthermore, I am willing to admit that becoming a medical patient is entering the medical therapeutic envelope more often than not, and clearly too often. This book stands witness to the fact that I am willing to recognize and decry many a medical modality that masquerades as "proven effective." It takes its place in the scientific tradition that Western medicine holds sacrosanct and that is embodied in the philosophy of Karl Popper. The proud history of Western medicine is the history of recognizing, decrying, and discarding all therapeutic modalities found to be lacking in adequate benefit/risk ratios (though not always with blinding alacrity). The process may be inefficient, is sometimes contentious, and currently is denigrated. But it is sacrosanct. Therein lies progress.

Alternative and complementary modalities are widely perceived to work and indeed have a life of their own. They survive in the face of science by relying on such lame defense as the idiosyncrasies of their application or preparation; practitioners argue that they do something differently or purvey something different than whatever proved ineffective in a randomized controlled trial. Circumlocution masquerades as progress. The treatment act, palliative or not, is grounded in such fallacious reasoning, in beliefs that are buffered from refutation. There is no progress, only the self-perpetuation of the treatment acts.

"So what?" you ask. "Who cares if the modalities are fatuous, as long as the treatment act is not harmful and the clinical effect is palliative?"

I do. I care if fellow citizens are being duped into thinking that they are participating in a therapeutic contract that is more than magical. I care that I am being forced to underwrite such magical therapies. And I care if people are unknowingly being drawn into a therapeutic envelope.

Life has many aspects that are beyond reason. Poets conceptualize "love" better than neurobiologists dissect it. Religion has a place, for some a healing place. There are even attempts to study the fashion in which religion might create a therapeutic envelope. Ethnic identities, cultural norms, and social constructions all have their place in the fabric of our lives. We need our beliefs as individuals, and we need their pluralism as a global village. All can provide for beauty, caring, and comfort. All can have excesses and require close scrutiny in this regard. None of these aspects of life is supported by health insurance. Individuals choose to participate in and support these values in their own fashion. They are not aspects of life supported by health insurance. Treatment acts based on modalities whose effectiveness has been scientifically refuted are not treatment acts; they are belief systems. I am aware of no insurance scheme that sets out to indemnify a belief system. Treatment acts based on modalities that have yet to be tested may also be belief systems. Many are indemnified, probably far too many.

Finally, any treatment act that fosters a therapeutic envelope is lacking. For me, such is anathema. This book is a diatribe against medicalization. The proper role for medicine is to collaborate with any patient with the goal that they become a person again. If there is no modality up to that task, then the treatment act must compensate. No one should ever be a "diabetic" when they can be a person coping with diabetes. No one should be a "rheumatoid" when they can be a person coping with rheumatoid arthritis. No one should learn that they have a spinal disorder when their illness is more a consequence of contextual factors that compromise their ability to cope with one of life's inter-mittent and remittent bedevilments. If I am able to craft this diatribe against medicalization, why should I condone chiropractorization, or herbalization, or acupuncturization, or the like?

The supplementary reading for this chapter is a comprehensively annotated bibliography.

chapter

Assuring Health, Insuring Disease

fourteen

Teaching medicine at the bedside is my calling. As I said in the introduction, I know no higher calling. About a decade ago, when my skills as a bedside teacher were finely honed, I found myself faced with one of Robert Frost's forks in the road. I was invited to round as visiting professor around the world, and I did so with pleasure. But whenever I returned to American hospitals, including my own, pleasure in rounding was increasingly contrived. My beliefs as to the reason medicine existed and the directions American institutions of medicine were taking had diverged to such a degree that I felt more and more like an anachronism in my own hospital and the other American hospitals that invited me to perform as a visiting professor. I could have confronted the local system, but the issue was anything but local.

Besides, I knew better. As one wise and wizened patient told me, "Doc, taking on the bureaucracy is like teaching a pig to sing. It's a waste of time and it angers the pig." So, I decided to take on the "institution of medicine" in the tradition of Maximilien Robespierre, maybe Thomas Paine. I'm not a revolutionary and certainly not a politician. I'm a physician who wants to do right by his patients and teach others how to learn to do even better than I know to do. I have paid a great personal price — but not what you might imagine. I sorely miss the twenty-five years that I influenced students and residents at UNC and North Carolina Memorial Hospital. That's what we called the hospital when I arrived there; a large wooden sign stood in the driveway, proclaiming it was "built by and for the people of North Carolina." Now North Carolina Memorial Hospital is UNC Hospitals. It has a large public relations department, a logo some find striking, and an enormous bureaucracy. The sign proclaiming "by and for the people" was trashed long ago.

It became clear to me that there would be a major change in "health care" in the United States because the current system was ethically bankrupt and the current approach financially unsustainable. It became clear to me that the likeliest scenario was a period of chaos, followed by a period of experimentation out of which a Phoenix could rise. However, that scenario would have a human cost far greater than we are paying for the current unconscionable state of health care. So began my ten-year odyssey.

I took advantage of invitations to address Congress and the leadership of such "stakeholders" as industry, insurance, and labor. All understood my message. Some shared my zeal. None were willing to act for reasons ranging from self-interest to fear of being accused of rationing. It became clear to me early on that reform would require a change in the social construction of health. Formulating a reasonable, alternative health-care scheme is straightforward; convincing people that it's reasonable is anything but. That is where *Worried Sick* and other efforts come into play. I have made myself available to the finest of print and broadcast health journalists, and they have learned. I have written a series of commentaries for ABCnews.com, and I am speaking even more widely to even more varied audiences. I am trying. I will not succeed against a status quo that commands some 16 percent of the Gross Domestic Product of the wealthiest nation the world has ever seen. But I am trying.

All prior chapters lead up to this one. Here I will set forth a rational approach to health care. There are alternatives, but we missed the opportunity for those fifty years ago. I will set forth a rational approach that can be superimposed on our history. If you are captured by the arguments in the previous chapters, you will find this approach obvious. If not, I need to start over. And I will.

None of us needs to be told: the health-care delivery system in America is indefensible. About $2 trillion fuels the system, some 16 percent of our national productivity. If we were all covered, that's more than $6,500 per person. Despite such a fortune, about 40 percent of us can't afford the care we are told we need, either because we are inadequately insured or payments out of pocket would bankrupt us. Medical bills broke the back of over 40 percent of us who declare bankruptcy. Even those who feel adequately insured are bedeviled by difficulties accessing care; those inadequately insured are tormented by them. Despite outcries, this sorry state continues to deteriorate. Why? Clearly the cause is not a lack of money. Every other resource-advantaged country indemnifies their entire population with less, usually far less, than half we expend—and with better national health statistics. The problem must reside in the fashion in which the money is spent. Some initiatives at "reform" are concrete: legislated distribution at fixed cost, expunging administrative inefficiency by maintaining a single payer, going "paperless," and so forth. Others in national and state leadership are advocating a more fundamental foray at this inefficiency. I will describe this assault and then explain how the assault is doomed because it, like redistributing care, is missing the mark, the unspeakable mark.

First, we need to understand the basic tenets that underlie health insurance.

Moral Hazards

At the turn of the twentieth century, few westerners were insured for anything. There were burial societies, most modeled after the Friendly Societies in Britain, that offered the advantaged worker the peace of mind that his family, which would probably be left bereft of support by his death, would not be further burdened by his funeral expenses. But insurance was largely unavailable. That was not because it was unheard of. To the contrary, indemnity was a pressing political issue in Victorian times. There was no debate that there are hazards that cannot be wholly avoided and that are catastrophic for any single victim unless the impact is blunted by sharing the fiscal consequences with others at risk. There was no doubt that indemnity schemes could offer a solution to this human predicament. The debate that raged then, and will not be stilled, relates to "moral hazard." If one could afford fire insurance for one's home, then the catastrophe of the house burning down would be blunted and the fiscal burden obviated. That's all to the good. However, if one needs cash, what's to stop one from burning down the house? Therein lies the moral hazard, at least as it was traditionally framed. In terms of property damage, society polices for this moral hazard and is resigned to inflated premiums to compensate for stealth immorality.

Property insurance set the precedent. Personal injury and the rest of social insurance followed in a dialectic that knows no closure. I devoted a good deal of my career as a clinical investigator and much of my monograph *Occupational Musculoskeletal Disorders* to this topic. Its history is grounded in the Prussian "welfare monarchy," which was fathered by Bismarck and rapidly adopted by Lloyd George and the rest of the industrialized world early in the twentieth century. (I touch on some of this in chapters 9 and 12.) When Bismarck was finished, Prussia had a national health-insurance scheme and a stratified disability scheme. The debate regarding the latter, and to a lesser extent the former, was heated, relating to the moral hazard inherent in choosing to be a disability claimant. Even Wilbur Cohen, when he was crafting the Social Security Disability scheme in the United States at midcentury, had to contend with the moral-hazard argument. Would a worker claim disability as a reflection of job dissatisfaction or insecurity rather than work incapacity? How does one police such behavior?

It is traditional to frame moral hazard as a failing of the claimant. It is traditional to seek administrative remedies in light of this moral hazard. Much has been written of this nature, many a finger pointed, and many a tear shed. Chapter 12 touches on the price paid by any claimant who is drawn into the Kafkaesque experience of having to prove illness. But little is said of the other moral hazards that lurk in the personal-injury and disability indemnity schemes and how they pollute the "health"-insurance indemnity schemes, which I term "disease" insurance.

Disease indemnity schemes carry their own constituencies. If they are publicly held, the constituency is comprised of administrators and supportive politicians. If they are private enterprises, the constituency is the administrators and stakeholders. But there is a feature to private insurance that is diabolical and little appreciated. Most is employer based: health insurance is a "benefit" of employment. The larger employers are covering about 60 percent of the American workforce. Nearly all large employers "self-insure." The employer burdens the risk; the insurance company processes claims at a fixed and negotiated overhead. For example, I am an employee of the state of North Carolina. My state employee's health-insurance plan is comprehensive. It is administered by Blue Cross – Blue Shield of North Carolina (BCBSNC), a so-called not-for-profit, which tells the state how much care has been billed for and therefore how much money the state must transfer to BCBSNC to pay the various providers (plus the BCBSNC administrative fees). So if I were to need a heart transplant, BCBSNC might forewarn the state that next month they will need to transfer an additional $500,000 or so. BCBSNC takes no risk administering a self-insured plan. Furthermore, the more "health care" that is consumed, the more money passes through the BCBSNC coffers and the larger the administrative fees. I think moral hazard whenever BCBSNC is offering some cholesterol- or diabetes-screening program (see chapters 3 and 4). The administrative fees are such that seven-figure executive salaries are commonplace in the health-insurance industry. William McGuire, when forced out as the CEO of United Health Care, was realizing annual bonuses greater than $100 million and had accumulated stock options in the billions. United Health Care is a private company and a darling of Wall Street. BCBSNC is a not-for-profit; the CEO salary is a paltry few million and the corporate jet is rented. Pardon my outrage.

If I were somehow forced to relinquish tenure (don't give them any ideas) and left state employ without health-care coverage, I would find myself faced with the challenges that the self-employed and all small employers know all too well. The state of North Carolina employee health benefit costs about $6,000 per year per employee, reflecting the fact that the state is assuming the risk, not BCBSNC. Neither I nor the small employer can assume that degree of risk; that's why we need insurance in the first place. We want BCBSNC to assume the risk and distribute the risk to other policyholders. Indeed, it is willing to do so, but to the other individual policyholders and small employers. Hence, the premium would jump from about $6,000 per year for the state to about $20,000 per year for me to get a comparable policy. No wonder 40 percent of the workforce is uninsured; these are the self-employed or the employees of small companies whose owners probably can't afford health insurance either.

Premiums will diminish if claims are reduced or if their processing is more efficient. In that case, the size of the enterprise and the power of its administrators will diminish as well, usually dragging down their compensation and the profits paid to stockholders. There is a moral hazard in the drive to maintain the size, scope, and profitability of the insurance enterprise. This is a moral hazard that is bounded on one side by the social constructions that relate to coverage needs and how much it should cost, and on the other side by the depth of the pockets of the insured to afford putatively adequate coverage. All forms of "alternatives" to mainstream medicine vie for insurance coverage. The osteopathy has gained full access. The chiropractic has gained full access to workers' compensation indemnity schemes, and some to health insurance schemes. Other alternatives are making inroads. Health-care and workers' compensation premiums escalate as the costs of some sectarian care is added to the sharing of the escalating costs for the interventions covered in the earlier chapters, and much more. Where is the value?

The Cart and the Horse

The guiding principle of all health-care reform in America is the belief that American medicine is the "best" in the world. Reform tackles misdistribution and the inconsistencies in the quality of care. Once these are overcome, all of us will be afforded the "best" to prevent us from getting sick and the "best" to heal us when prevention fails. The savings that would result from a decrease in the national burden of illness would underwrite adequate distribution of care. It follows that the goal of health-care reform is to be certain that American medicine is performed expertly so as to provide optimal "quality" of care.

Serving this agenda are national committees to establish the criteria for expert care for particular diseases, national committees to collect the data on the degree to which care in particular states, hospitals, or practice groups approaches these standards, and national committees to see if it matters. For example, the Hospital Quality Alliance is a public-private collaboration to gather performance information of all acute-care, nonfederal hospitals. Much of this effort has taken heart disease as the target because of the volume of cases, the costliness of treating these diseases, and the consensus as to best care. Many a program has been implemented to move practice up to these standards. In their 2006 report, the National Committee for Quality Assurance (‹http://www.cmwf.org›) assures us "there is hope." To get beyond hope, several payers are developing a stick-and-carrot, "pay-for-performance" approach that bases medical fees on the degree to which practice meets standards.

The "Quality Movement" is enjoying its day in the sun. Legislators and potentates in the hospital and health-insurance industries are beating the drum. Few are questioning the basic premise of the Quality Movement. Does it matter to the patient if practice meets these consensus standards? There is a crying need for such heresy. A recent analysis of the Medicare experience should muffle the drumbeat. The degree to which practice met the accepted standards for Medicare patients admitted for heart disease did not predict who lived. Even for the poster child of the Quality Movement, heart disease, something is amiss.

Why wouldn't performing up to these standards of care for heart disease — to "high performance" — advantage the patient? Maybe the Medicare analysis was not able to detect shortcomings in the fashion in which doctors and hospitals meet standards of care. More likely, the standards of care are far less important than the committees that formulated them claim. If what we do to you doesn't work, or doesn't work much, then it doesn't matter how well we do them. It also doesn't matter how cheaply they are provided; if it doesn't work, it's worthless at any price. The Quality Movement is putting the cart before the horse. The horse is "effectiveness."

The Quality Movement overcame great odds to gain its current influence. Physicians and surgeons, like other professionals, are not reflexively disposed to "outsiders" questioning their competence. Even peer review is a prickly process. I applaud the Quality Movement and admire many of its leaders. However, "quality" is not the goal, it is the process. Efficacy first, then quality promotes effectiveness.

There is an "Effectiveness Movement," bloodied and bent but unbowed. It can muster far more illustrative science than the Quality Movement. *Worried Sick* is exemplar. But the forces that thwart the demand for effectiveness are powerful, wealthy, and predictable. Most of the high-ticket items (procedures and pharmaceuticals) are minimally effective or ineffective. Many of these are considered standards of care. Many are cash cows, touted by vested interests. They may be resistant to a voice such as mine, but I can teach you how to advocate for yourself.

Let's say I have to treat more than fifty people in the hope of doing something important for one. Do you believe that's an effective treatment? Nearly all of us involved in biostatistics will tell you that such an outcome is barely measurable and not likely to reproduce. Here's a partial list of treatments (most the topic of chapters herein) that would not even qualify at this level of effectiveness based on scientific trials designed to test their efficacy:

- Coronary artery bypass grafts, angioplasties, or stents to save lives or improve symptoms
- Arthroscopy for knee pain
- Any surgery for backache
- Statin therapy to reduce cholesterol and thereby save lives
- Newer antidepressants for situational depression
- Drugs for decreased bone density
- PSA screening and radical prostatectomy to save lives
- Screening mammography to save lives
- Many a cancer treatment to save lives

The list of treatments that have been studied and fail at the one-in-fifty level goes on and on, including many of the new drugs touted as "breakthroughs." Many surgical treatments have yet to be studied. From my perspective as a clinician who has cared for patients and taught students for over three decades, if I have to treat more than twenty patients to do something really meaningful for one, I regard the treatment as marginal; I do not prescribe or advocate it and would have no problem if it was not covered by health insurance. Furthermore, designing trials to test whether new or old treatments meet this one-in-twenty level of effectiveness is not difficult, expensive, or time-consuming. We would no longer be marketed to prescribe and consume minimally effective treatments or treatments that offered no important improvement over the tried and true.

If we have effectiveness at the base of our health-care insurance system, adding cost-effectiveness and quality would be rational and straightforward. We could well afford such a rational health-care delivery system, with most of the $2 trillion to spare. We would be more "high performance" than any other country. And our unsung, well-trained, and caring physicians, nurses, and allied health professionals could get back to serving patients instead of the health-care delivery system.

Indemnifying Rational, Not Rationed, Health Care

At the outset of *Worried Sick*, I promised to set forth a "solution" that would promulgate rational health care. I also acknowledged that no such solution was possible until the people, both the well and the ill, were prepared to seek and recognize the sophisms that riddle America's vaunted "health-care delivery system." If I've done my job and you've done your reading, you are prepared, indeed. I will keep my promise. You are also prepared to grasp the substance of the solution I am proposing.

The current approach to health benefits in the United States is uneven, unwieldy, ineffective, and unsustainable. Nearly all attempts at reform target its costliness with the assumption that improvement will translate into an improved benefit/cost ratio. The shibboleth of the current iteration is "quality," a construct weighted heavily toward efficiency (usually in the industrial sense of "throughput"). It is argued that if care was delivered more efficiently, it would be less costly and therefore more cost-effective. This iteration of reform, I predict, will prove as counterproductive as the precedents of recent decades.

Worried Sick is a primer on the fashion in which science calls into question the basic tenet of the "quality improvement" approach. If medicalization and Type II Medical Malpractice are the scourge, then the solution is to first target effectiveness to improve the benefit/cost ratio. Yes, "evidence-based medicine" (EBM) provides the scientific footing, but no more. But the innovation is to harness evidence to the task of informing effectiveness. If any clinical interaction has been studied and cannot be shown to be meaningfully effective, it is worthless at any cost.

Such a simple precept demands definition of "meaningfully effective" in a fashion that vests *all* interests in the well-being of the recipient of the care and caring. The definition must preclude any other motivation. There are very few unequivocally salutary events in medicine or in life. Hence, I am proposing an indemnity plan that institutionalizes this creed. It is conceived as a benefits plan to be provided by larger employers, although it is expected that mechanisms will be developed to offer the plan to smaller employers (through chamber of commerce organizations, for example). In fact, this approach could be state based; each state would fund a plan based on income-tax revenues with provision for those who have no substantial gainful employment. But the modeling we have done, for convenience, is for an employer-based plan.

Financing of the Plan

Employers will contribute a fixed sum — 12 percent of wages. It matters little if these moneys are collected by the state as a form of income tax on all employees (my preference) or contributed by all employers and wage earners individually. The money generated needs to be used to purchase the form of private insurance I will describe. I fear that a federal program will be no match for the pressures of Big Pharma and similar political action committees, a fear that truly saddens me. However, competing private-sector insurance companies constituted as I will describe should live out the "free-market dream," or all is lost. These moneys will be apportioned as follows:

1. Administrative costs for running the indemnity scheme will be fixed at 1 percent of wages.
2. Likewise, 1 percent will be the "profit."
3. There will be multiple codicils attached to the contracts of employees of the indemnity scheme regarding conflicts of interest. Furthermore, no officer will be allowed remuneration greater than five times that of the average wage of those employed by the plan.

That leaves some 10 percent of annual wages, tithed monthly, available for Plans A and B of the indemnity scheme.

Plan A: The Health Plan

As you are aware (since I emphasize it repeatedly in *Worried Sick*), there are important lessons that derive from the work of social epidemiologists. Life-course epidemiology pegs our optimal species longevity near eighty-five. The major confounders to longevity reside in the course of life in a resource-advantaged country such as the United States. When one examines our mortal hazard, some 75 percent of the risk is subsumed by two questions:

1. Are you comfortable in your socioeconomic status?
2. Are you satisfied in your employment?

Based on these realities, monies in Plan A will be available to the worker to underwrite self-improvement activities of her or his choice, which are offered by professionals *licensed* in the state of residence. Examples include English as a second language, skills training, child care, and clinical activities not covered in Plan B, such as the services of licensed complementary and alternative health-care providers. The indemnity scheme will offer an advisory service, informing the worker of the likelihood that particular services will diminish their mortal hazard as discussed above.

Plan A is financed with the moneys not expended in Plan B. Plan A is not a shared-risk pool. Co-pay will be a function of years of service and cost to the plan. Indemnified workers will be educated to realize that moneys poorly spent in Plan B compromise their Plan A resources. Likewise, moneys not poorly spent in Plan B provide more of the advantages inherent in Plan A. Moneys in the employee's Plan A account that are not expended transform into a pension at retirement or are expended to support Plan B premiums when the employee is between jobs. These moneys are conservatively invested and secured from any other expenditure.

Plan B: The Disease Plan

Plan B is the more traditional "health-insurance" component of the indemnity scheme. It follows from the theoretical considerations underlying Plan A that only some 25 percent of our mortal hazard can be ascribed to "proximate-cause epidemiology," or the diagnoses on our death certificates. Underwriting programs designed to improve longevity are limited by this reality. Plan B underwrites this "disease insurance" by indemnifying those interventions that are designed to manage or cure intercurrent disease so that one is afforded the longevity predicted by life-course epidemiology. "Disease insurance" also indemnifies interventions that palliate illnesses consequent to diseases that cannot be cured.

Plan B will be informed by a vast science, the work product of international collaborations of investigators who are quantifying the evidentiary basis of diagnostic and therapeutic options. Several thousand such documents are in the public domain, supplemented by FDA analyses and, to a lesser extent, by similar analyses in journals. It is estimated that some 10,000 systematic reviews will be needed for a comprehensive EBM library. Furthermore, it is estimated that reviews must be updated with some frequency, approaching every four years. This effort will not be duplicated in the indemnity scheme. Rather, a group of individuals trained in this effort will cull the practical essence of the extant EBM library.

Realize that the thrust of the EBM movement is whether there is reliable evidence for or against a particular clinical interface. That question is only the first order for "disease insurance." The reviewing group in the indemnity scheme will be charged to review the EBM literature with the goal of discerning *effectiveness*. If reasoned attempts have failed to discern benefit from a particular intervention, that intervention will be considered useless and therefore not indemnified under Plan B.

Plan B only indemnifies fully when there is evidence that the clinical interface leads to a meaningful outcome for the individual patient:

1. For a "hard outcome" (death, stroke, heart attack, renal failure, etc.), interventions are indemnified if they clearly advantage one in every twenty patients treated (NNT = 20).
2. For a "soft outcome" (feel better, function better, etc.), there must be a clear advantage to one in every five patients treated (NNT = 5).

These cutoffs are set at my level of comfort. They are driven by one's philosophy of life, one's value system. I would argue that a NNT = 50 is ephemeral; it is too small a health effect to measure reliably. I would countenance a debate as to setting the cutoff at greater than NNT = 20 but less than NNT = 50 for hard outcomes. However, the debate must be transparent and public, so that all who are indemnified understand that this indemnity plan is not designed to "save money." Rather it is designed to "save your money," since moneys not expended in Plan B revert to Plan A. All of us have to realize that by setting the cutoff at NNT = 20, we are demanding something approaching a 5 percent absolute likelihood of "hard" benefit. If the plan were to share the cost of interventions with lesser likelihood of benefit, all the indemnified are tithed and each of the indemnified have less Plan A largesse as a consequence.

However, the debate is to NNT cutoff, not co-pay.

To the extent that any clinical interface (diagnostic or therapeutic) falls short of NNT criteria, co-pay will be levied. Furthermore, co-pay is categorical — either 100 percent or nothing. The plan will utilize the federal Medicare-billing scheme with the above co-pay provisions. Many chapters in *Worried Sick* bear witness that nearly all the elective "high-ticket" items (in terms of expense per event or cumulative expense for screening/prevention) will not be covered in Plan B without 100 percent co-pay according to the criteria I am advocating. For example, the co-pay for coronary angioplasty, stenting, and bypass grafting would be 100 percent. If you are convinced you need it, you can use your Plan A moneys, and when they run out, you can pay out of pocket. This is not a "hard-nosed" posture to rationing; Plan B will not pay because the data says these procedures are not worth paying for.

Furthermore, there is data speaking to the effectiveness of all pharmaceuticals licensed by the FDA for thirty years. If an agent does not meet Plan B's effectiveness criteria when compared to an older agent, there will be 100 percent co-pay. Therefore, the co-pay for cholesterol screening as primary prevention would be 100 percent, as would the cost of pharmaceutically altering serum cholesterol levels as primary prevention.

Obviously, this approach will seem counterintuitive in the United States, a country that is medicalized both in terms of personal health and social constructions regarding medical miracles. The introduction of the indemnity scheme will call for a major public education and public-relations effort. The readership of Worried Sick will be recruited to this effort. It is greatly facilitated by the realization that all moneys not expended in Plan B reverts to Plan A. Therefore, the levying of co-payments is designed to spare the insured unnecessary/ineffective medicine and not to "save" money. The patient has the right to draw available funds from her/his Plan A reserve to cover co-pay. However, the insured will be asked to sign a form acknowledging an understanding that the plan is levying co-pay because the value of the particular intervention has proved elusive in systematic studies, and not to "save" money.

Coverage in the absence of quantification of effectiveness. Many aspects of health care that are common practice have not been tested; many are not testable. Most of these are not "high ticket items." However, some provision needs to be made for their indemnification. For example, it is proposed that each insured worker will be afforded a certain number of primary-care hours each year (one or two) and counseling hours (one or two) without co-pay under Plan B. Hours not expended will accumulate. Additional hours incur 100 percent co-pay, which can be funded through Plan A.

Administering the Plan

The entire indemnity scheme will be online. Each provider will have a PIN to access a personal web page, and each insured worker will have a PIN. The provider web interface will be interactive. Based on details of the diagnosis, available options will be listed with co-pay. That is true even if a patient is a candidate for hospitalization or arrives at an emergency department. For pharmaceuticals, the worker will be offered a menu of pharmacies convenient to his/her residence when enrolling. Prescriptions will also be accessed online.

Billing will be electronic at the point of service and at the time of service. Moneys will be transferred instantly to the provider's bank account. Administrative overhead will be minimized for providers and the plan.

Every insured worker will receive a summary of the charges. If the worker has ready access to the Internet, an e-mail will instruct the worker to visit a personal website. Otherwise, summaries will be mailed. The worker will be responsible for monitoring the accuracy of charges. Software exists for nearly all the elements of this process, albeit for other purposes in the current health-care delivery system.

Cost/Effectiveness

Based on the per capita health-care expenditures in other resource-advantaged countries, it is likely that no more than 5 percent of wages is required to insure a worker and family under Plan B. This reflects the value inherent in underwriting only effective interventions and the savings inherent in an online processing scheme. It is hoped that pressure can be brought to bear on the U.S. provider enterprise to reduce the current 50 percent overhead costs by more than 50 percent, bringing them into the range of the national health schemes operating elsewhere. That would lead to a substantial increment in moneys funding Plan A by further reducing the cost of the effective "health benefits" under Plan B.

"Quality"

The indemnity scheme is designed to be intrinsically free of moral hazard by institutionalizing the fiduciary responsibility of its administration. The design also facilitates minimizing moral hazard on the part of providers and patients. Effective care is its raison d'être. Measuring "quality" in terms of efficiency and safety is rational in a scheme that indemnifies effectiveness. It is also highly feasible in a scheme that utilizes the Internet so extensively. Even pharmacovigilance becomes feasible; patients can be monitored for the incidence of adverse drug effects over time.

Up the Republic

For the first twenty-five years of my career, I honed my skills as a medical educator at the bedside of the ill. Much of my self-esteem relates to that effort. Slowly over that period, the "institution" that calls itself the "health-care delivery system" veered from the care of the patient toward self-service. I wrote editorials pointing out the trend and the dialectic. By the mid-1990s, the U.S. health-care delivery system and my sense of what was defensible and ethical had diverged so that I felt an unbearable tension, even in my own institution. That tension was not with my colleagues who toiled at the bedside, nor with our students and patients. It was with the "institution" across the nation. Furthermore, that "institution" was no longer to be led by scholars of the clinical sciences. Rather, the leadership was chosen and valued for putative administrative prowess. Administrators proliferated and vied to accumulate titles that were deemed indicative of their growing power. The infrastructure became the superstructure. The generation of the moneys necessary to support the growing superstructure became the goal. Medical schools and their function vanished into the monster called the "academic health center." By the mid-1990s, the medical "academy" had lost its moral compass, and I had lost my dream.

I knew there was no yield in attempting reform from within. The personality traits that made my colleagues in the "underground clinical departments" so valuable at the bedside rendered them ineffective reformers. Patients already have enough on their plate, and students know no better when they are taught that "managing the case" is the same as caring for the patient. So a decade ago I stepped back from my life at the bedside (not entirely, since I still see many patients) to carry out a productive clinical research program and do many visiting professorships. However, the many months that I had spent each year in the hospital at the bedside growing increasingly frustrated were sacrificed. I felt compelled to become a reformer.

Because of my decades of research regarding workplace health and safety, I was long sought after as a resource for various congressional committees and the like. So, I took off my blinders and began to poke around "the Hill," seeking an ear that could hear that all was not right with the American health-care system, and that costliness was the least of it. I could find many an ear, but none that were not captured by lobbyists for Big Pharma, the big hospitals, the American colleges of whatever, and so forth. Congress was owned.

So, I decided to learn about the advocacy world. I would meet with many a leader and discovered many an appealing thinker. However, the world offers these leaders little security and much resistance. Each has had to find a niche. None were willing to mentor me, even though I required no financial support or physical facilities. I came away more aware and appreciative, and a bit wizened.

So I fell back on the world I have come to know as a clinical investigator, the world of management and labor that has responsibility for the health and safety of the workforce. This is a world reeling from the costliness of "health care." Benefits obligations are sinking some corporations and threatening others, placing pensioners and workers in peril. Furthermore, nearly 40 percent of the workforce is the "uninsured employed" today, including the small employers, and that trend is relentless. I found my audience. I have delivered keynote addresses to the annual meeting of the National Business Group on Health and the Consortium Health Group (the leadership of the major "Blues"). I have spent hours with the executives of United Health Group and Cigna and their major account administrators. And I enjoy the camaraderie and mentoring of important leaders in HR (human resource and benefits administrators) and the union movement. I have no hope for the "health"-insurance industry; much of the leadership is either too dull to understand the error of their ways or would rather sail on in the *Titanic*, enjoying the unconscionable luxury their industry affords them. But tucked into this world are a few individuals whose moral compass matches mine and who understand. I firmly believe that the moral imperative of capitalism is not the accumulation of wealth; it's the provision of sustaining jobs. Several of these individuals lead large corporations, and several are leaders in their industries. They support my efforts, although they offer moral support only. None are able to step out front yet.

The reason relates to the proposed reform that I've just outlined and that I published as an editorial in the *Journal of Occupational and Environmental Medicine* in July 2005. The plan I propose harnesses reason to the benefits of employees. It is ethically sound. However, unless you have digested *Worried Sick*, you are likely to conclude that the proposal calls for rationing rather than rational behavior. I have written this book for the general audience to foment debate and thereby open minds. The science that informs a radical change in the social construction of health and the provision of health care is mature and compelling. Any such radical change must confront social entropy. Without an informed public, the enormous and entrenched enterprise committed to the current approach will be applauded instead of reviled. Until we all see the new clothes for what they are, the emperor will prevail.

Supplementary Readings

Introduction

There are three concepts put forth in the introduction that are crucial to understanding the basis of *Worried Sick*. One relates to the philosophy of science, one to the social components of morbidity, and one to medicalization.

It is easy to paraphrase the central point of Karl Popper's philosophy of science. He described truth as tentative at best. Truth is the hypothesis yet to be disproved. But that's too easy. I would urge the reader to spend time with Popper's *Conjectures and Refutations*, first published in 1963 (Popper 2000). An alternative would be David Miller's *Popper Selections* (Miller 1985), which will introduce the reader to Popper's social philosophy as well as his philosophy of science. There's also the highly engaging and informative biography by Malachi Hacohen (2000).

Popper's refutationist treatment of truth was as discomforting as it was revolutionary. Is there no way to generate more certainty? I think not. However, epistemology since Hume has sought reasonable compromises that might offer some hope of a valid approximate. Inferential reasoning relies on documenting the consistency of observations, the strength and specificity of associations, and the coherence of theories in generating causal inferences. Bayesian philosophy recruits probability theory to approximate truth. This book adheres far more to refutationist principles, explaining how to recognize, quantify, and cope with uncertainty. I will demonstrate repeatedly how inferential reasoning has led us astray. Bayesian approaches are sorely limited because they demand we have a handle on the likelihood of truth up front, a priori, which is a rarity in clinical medicine and in life. I would recommend the elegant and accessible collection of essays *Causal Inference* to the interested reader (Rothman 1988).

Popper's constructions fell into disfavor late in his career. This was in part because his social philosophy was deemed less politically correct in the postwar era than during World War II, when it was written in an attempt to come to grips with the rise of fascism. His refutationist philosophy of science also had to be modified in light of Thomas Kuhn's *The Structure of Scientific Revolutions* (Kuhn 1970). Kuhn brought us the realization of the "paradigm shift" as the fashion in which important hypotheses are rejected.

The image I teach, my philosophy of science if you will, is that there is a vast swamp of ignorance. In this swamp are discrete islands composed of rejected hypotheses. At the high point of each island, scientists are feverishly trying to reject the hypothesis that is the basis of that island. Each island is isolated from the others, not just by the teeming swamp waters but also because the language and perspective of those laboring on each are unique, constructed around the preconceptions and histories of the clustered scientists. The size and scope of the enterprise on each island is determined by society, which looks down on this swamp with proprietary zeal. The hypotheses deemed particularly relevant are socially constructed. When society is convinced that one socially constructed enterprise is more "relevant" or "important," resources are deposited on the shore and scientists young and old immigrate there, adding energy to the testing of the paradigm. My philosophy, so stated, countenances Popper's *Conjectures and Refutations*, Kuhn's paradigm shifts, and the social construction of "science."

As I mentioned, the "illness of work incapacity" is a focus of my scholarship. I refer the reader to the third edition of my monograph *Occupational Musculoskeletal Disorders* (Hadler 2005). The book is an exercise in dissecting the social components of musculoskeletal morbidity, which we will sample in chapters 9–12.

Medicalization is a concept promulgated mainly by medical anthropologists in the last half of the twentieth century, although one can find like observations much earlier. Kaja Finkler defines it as follows: "Medicalization restructures reality by intruding on the world people take for granted, on their tacit understanding of what is normal, by transforming the taken-for-granted state into an abnormal, disconcerting state, separating the individual from the larger whole." You'll find that quote on page 176 of Finkler's elegant *Experiencing the New Genetics* (Finkler 2000). That monograph explains how the genomic revolution is medicalizing the concepts of family and kinship. It is an incisive and insightful analysis of a dramatic new example of medicalization, in the tradition of medicalizing homosexuality, menopause, puberty, orgasm, and the many examples in the later chapters herein. The book could also serve as a primer on medicalization in general. As an aside, the dialectic by which the saving grace of genomics has become a social construction is as pressing as it is scientifically flawed (Hadler and Evans 2001).

Chapter 1

Many of the points made in chapter 1 will be developed in detail in the subsequent chapters. There are several references to the recent literature on social epidemiology that warrant scrutiny. I recommend Richard Wilkinson's classic *Unhealthy Societies: The Afflictions of Inequality* (Wilkinson 1996) for the concept of income gap, discussions that he expands in *The Impact of Inequality: How to Make Sick Societies Healthier* (Wilkinson 2005). I recommend *Social Epidemiology* (Berkman and Kawachi 2000) for a general overview. I like the Lantz paper for support of my assertions that only 25 percent of the hazard to longevity resides in the proximate causes of death (Lantz et al. 1998). As a corollary, Schroeder (2007) argues that lack of "health care" accounts for only 10 percent of our mortal hazard. That the proximate causes of death are increasingly likely to mark our eighty-fifth year is well illustrated by a data set analyzed for the American Cancer Society (Jemal et al. 2005). Many studies have demonstrated the transnational discordance between health-care expenditures and health outcomes (Nolte and McKee 2003), with the United States as the outlier (Bodenheimer 2005).

Some of my own papers explore the concept that proximate causes pale next to SES and job satisfaction in determining our mortal fate (Hadler 2001, 2005a). These articles develop the argument that job satisfaction holds as much of a key to longevity as more traditional measures of SES. An essay by Fitzpatrick offers yet another perspective along the same lines (Fitzpatrick 2001). We will revisit this topic in depth in chapter 12.

The divide between the students of life-course epidemiology and the students of proximate-cause epidemiology is nowhere more striking than in the hallowed halls of British academia. British epidemiology has set the pace in both arenas. Professors M. Marmot and R. Wilkinson are pioneers in the former; Professors W. R. S. Doll, R. Peto, and R. Turner of Oxford are pioneers in the latter. Seldom do their perspectives and analytic techniques converge on the same cohorts. That pertains to the epidemiologists of the respective schools elsewhere. Take the example of the recent studies of the beneficial effects of the "Mediterranean diet." This is a diet that is touted as salutary because of the relative longevity of the citizens of a number of Mediterranean countries, notably Greece (Trichopoulou et al. 2003), where the diet is rich in unsaturated lipids (i.e., olive oil), cheeses, wine, grains, legumes, and fish but lacking in meat. Two large, ten-year prospective studies of samples of the elderly population of many European countries were undertaken to explore this association. Dietary intake and other lifestyle attributes were monitored to see if there was an association with longevity. In both, educational attainment was the only surrogate measure for SES. In both, the more closely the elderly adhered to the diet, the longer they lived (Trichopoulou et al. 2005; Knoops et al. 2004). However, in neither study was the income gap in the various countries, let alone regions of the various countries, considered despite the data from Wilkinson (1996) that this measure will supersede education and diet in accounting for the enhanced longevity in the Mediterranean countries included in these cohort studies. Education, IQ (Batty et al. 2006), even the wherewithal to adhere to medical advice (Simpson et al. 2006) are all important, but they are important as windows to one's position in society.

When there is convergence of the perspectives of proximate-cause and life-course epidemiology, it is telling indeed. Take, for example, the work of Herman A. Tyroler, a colleague of mine at the University of North Carolina at Chapel Hill who passed away in early 2007 at age eighty-three. He had been one of the American pioneers in the study of the proximate-cause epidemiology of coronary artery disease, probing the influence of hypertension, hypercholesterolemia, and the like for decades. Some twenty years ago, the Atherosclerosis Risk in Communities Study cohort was established by sampling adults from the populations of Forsyth County, North Carolina; Jackson, Mississippi; suburbs of Minneapolis; and Washington County, Maryland. The cohort was forty-five to sixty-four years of age at inception. During almost a decade of observation, 615 coronary events occurred in 13,000 participants. The poorest whites were three times more likely to be afflicted than the wealthiest whites; for blacks this hazard ratio was 2.5. These ratios were unaffected after statistically adjusting for established biological risk factors. Most daunting is the observation that the hazard associates with the SES characteristics of the neighborhood more strongly than those of the individual. If you are living your life in a disadvantaged neighborhood, you are marked — regardless of whether your own income or educational achievements outstrip your neighbors' (Diez Roux 2001). We can only guess at this point as to the elements of life in a dismal neighborhood that places such a burden on the biology of the resident. I, for one, would call for improving the quality of neighborhood life rather than expend energy in dissecting its mortal mediators. But even this agenda has caveats. Winkleby et al. (2006) recently published an analysis of mortality rates for 8,000 Californians followed for over seventeen years. The results echo the transnational experience with income gap. People of low SES who resided in wealthier neighborhoods had a higher mortal risk than people of low SES who lived in poor neighborhoods. Proximity to resources and to neighbors who are advantaged does not compensate for a meaner and more meager lifestyle. Rather, it magnifies the toll.

It turns out that social hierarchy influences the health of primates other than humans. In other social species, it can be shown that low ranking in a dominance hierarchy associates with numerous adverse biological outcomes (Sapolsky 2005). The study of rank-health correlations are usually framed in the context of "stress." The corollary construct in humans will occupy us in chapter 12. However, here we are examining the descriptive statistics. Socioeconomic status is tightly aligned with functional capacity (Minkler et al. 2006). SES predicts mortality after heart attacks (Alter et al. 2006; Shishehbor et al. 2006), an easily reproducible observation (Kaplan 2006) that seldom is considered by the epidemiologists committed to the analysis of outcomes from interventional cardiology (see chapter 2). As to the structure of society, SES weighs more heavily on the health status of Americans than of the British (Banks et al. 2006). It all boils down to how we measure SES and what it means; it clearly is an attempt to probe the nature of satisfaction in life (Braveman et al. 2005).

The Virchow quote is taken from E. H. Ackerknecht's biography of Rudolf Virchow (Ackerknecht 1953).

The Cochrane Collaboration resulted when it was realized that the "literature" of medicine had grown so voluminous that no clinician could be expected to grasp even that which was relevant to a particular subspecialty, let alone to a specialty (Levin 2001). Over 6,000 journal articles are published every day, and many more find their way to open sites on the Internet. The solution to making sense of this glut reflects the convergence of the genius of a number of leading academics starting about twenty-five years ago. Archibald Cochrane emerged from medically ministering to his fellow POWs in Germany in World War II burning with the need to define clinical efficacy. He studied epidemiology at the foot of the pioneering Bradford Hill, commenced his academic career in Cardiff, Wales, and in 1972 issued a clarion call for analyzing randomized clinical trials (RCTs) as the most scientific way to inform the practice of medicine. Ian Chalmers, an obstetrician in Cardiff, found the call compelling and set out to assemble the RCTs in his field. The cause was taken up by thought leaders at McMaster (notably Brian Haynes and David Sackett) and Yale (Alvan Feinstein in particular). In 1993 these and some seventy others announced the formation of the Cochrane Collaboration "to prepare, maintain and disseminate systematic reviews of the effects of health care interventions." Today the collaboration is made up of review groups and method groups organized into fifteen centers dispersed across thirteen countries. An elected steering group oversees the entire effort, supported by a secretariat based in Oxford, England. Topics are chosen for review, and the relevant literature is systematically searched out and analyzed as to quality by pre-defined criteria. The format is highly structured and the criteria for the systematic review so rigorous that typically only a few high-quality articles are identified for any given topic. The group then sets to the task of drawing some conclusion as to whether evidence has emerged and to what degree it is compelling. Most of the participants are volunteering their time. The entire undertaking survives on meager contributions from many countries. It is estimated that some 10,000 reviews are necessary to provide a comprehensive "evidence-based medicine" library with periodic updating of all reviews (Mallett and Clarke 2003). There is much work to do, particularly since the available reviews (and probably the available RCTs) do not reflect the global burden of disease (Swingler et al. 2003).

To date, the Cochrane Collaboration has shunned support from pharmaceutical firms and the like, although individual reviewers are not restricted in that regard. There is another body in Britain that is government funded and charged with creating practice guidelines based on evidence (Pearson and Rawlins 2005): the National Institute for Health and Clinical Excellence (NICE). Here, too, some of the experts have industry links, but the institute itself is independent of industry. Although the Cochrane Collaboration and NICE have some conflict-of-interest taint, the degree pales next to common practice. In a survey of more than 200 practice guidelines from around the world, more than a third of the experts on the panels had ties to relevant drug companies, and more than 70 percent of panels were affected (Taylor and Giles 2005). Over a third of the members of "institutional review boards" in American academic institutions have ties to industry (Campbell et al. 2006). These boards, composed of scientists and lay participants, are charged with oversight for the safety of subjects and the ethical conduct of clinical trials. No one on such a board should have any other agenda. No subject of a clinical trial should have to be concerned that members of the oversight board might have priorities that could be in conflict with the ethical conduct of the trial (Nabel 2006). Furthermore, industry-supported systematic reviews, when compared to Cochrane reviews on the same subject, are less transparent, less demanding of methodological quality, and more likely to reach favorable conclusions (Jørgensen et al. 2006). Unfortunately, one cannot rely on the peer review process to assure that published papers meet high methodological standards (Seigel 2003), although such reliance is commonplace among the usual readers and seems more an attribute of those performing systematic reviews that are sponsored by industry. I find all this highly distressing, and so do others, with good reason. Chapter by chapter, I will repeatedly demonstrate the fashion in which conflict-of-interest operates. Health-industry practices are designed to create conflicts of interest (Brennan et al. 2006). Even clinical trials can be viewed as marketing exercises if the prescribing habits of the participating investigators are telling (Psaty and Rennie 2006; Andersen et al. 2006). Fortunately, the Cochrane Collaboration has only minor taint. However, conflict of interest should exclude "experts" from panels and editorial authorships simply because self-interest, subliminal or not, cannot be weighed by those who are to be influenced. This, too, is an argument to which I will return.

It is not clear how efficiently evidence translates into the quality of care in practice. The randomized controlled trials that are the fodder for Cochrane reviews and most similar exercises are seldom designed to seek evidence for clinically relevant effects, only evidence for effects. The systematic reviews are similarly limited (Malmivaara et al. 2006). Today, whatever its impact probably depends more on word of mouth and physician networking than any systemic application (Gabbay and le May 2004), including practice guidelines (Freemantle 2004). No one likes to have their preconceived notions and comfortable practices challenged, not even physicians. I, for one, am uncomfortable delegating all responsibility for "keeping up with" the literature. I have subscribed to some twenty journals for much of my career, reading them all and many others. As an editor of one of the yearbooks, I read hundreds of papers that are sent my way each year and identify the forty in my area that are worth discussing. It is not the burden it seems, or it becomes progressively less of a burden. There is very little that is really new or novel, so that once one builds a foundation it is easy to focus on advances, even minor advances. True, my "search" is not comprehensive, but equally true is the fact that nearly all important advances appear in the primary journals either in the form of the original research or a review that follows. My "search" allows me to consider the meaningfulness of the evidence and not just its existence. I am far more likely to bring information derived from my efforts to the bedside, to peer interactions, and to *Worried Sick* than I am to rely on the latest Cochrane review. As I will discuss in chapter 14, there is a way to systematically apply Cochrane reviews to the advantage of patients, a way that lends itself to rational health insurance.

Chapter 2

A voluminous literature supports nearly all the points I make in this chapter. I will offer a sampling, topic by topic, and try to keep a damper on my editorializing.

The decline in mortality from coronary artery disease is well documented. Representative papers examining the trend before the mid-1980s are Pell and Fayerweather 1985; Gomez-Marin et al. 1987; Goldberg et al. 1986. Similar data pertains to the incidence and severity of strokes (Carandang et al. 2006). Even the vaunted "Framingham Study" investigators were hard-pressed to ascribe the decline in incidence and survival simply to a reduction in risk factors (Sulkowski et al. 1990). An argument has been made for a role of risk-factor reduction in the continuation of the trend into the 1990s (McGovern et al. 1996), but that argument will seem less convincing after you read the next chapter. And I can assure you that any attempt to ascribe this happy trend to the contemporaneous practices of cardiology and cardiovascular surgery must contend with the fact that the trend predates "advances" and a science that rejects the inferences one at a time, from the availability of coronary care units to drugs that treat disorders of cardiac rhythm. That doesn't stop many from wanting to take credit (Rosamond et al. 1998; Levy and Thom 1998). However, it is increasingly clear that any reduction in cardiovascular risk factors does not benefit those in the lower socioeconomic quintiles (Kanjilal et al. 2006); their fate is sealed by their station in society, not their serum cholesterol.

Neither can one ascribe the improvement to the horrifying proliferation of unproven and/or improvable invasive procedures in the 1980s that continues to this day. The three classical studies that could demonstrate no important benefit (except for the 3 percent with Left Main Disease) led to multiple publications (CASS Principal Investigators 1984; Veterans Administration Coronary Artery Bypass Surgery Cooperative Study Group 1984; Varnauskas 1988; and many more). Even Mark Hlatky, a leading cardiologist and cardiovascular epidemiologist on the Stanford faculty writing a "Perspective" article in the vaunted *New England Journal of Medicine*, can be no more charitable than to say, "Despite uncertainty about who benefits from coronary bypass surgery, the procedure has been embraced widely. The growth of surgery has been fueled by anxieties about sudden death from cardiac causes and patients' wishes for a seemingly definitive procedure" (Hlatky 2004). Hlatky and I were "Established Investigators of the American Heart Association" at the same time, a privileged and highly competitive award that supported us for five years when we were junior on neighboring faculties. Given his career path, this editorial is about as outspoken as I can expect him to get. At least he is trying.

If you dig through this literature, you will see how inventive statisticians, driven by the presuppositions they and the cardiovascular community hold as sacred, have eked suggestions of benefit beyond Left Main Disease. The proper term for these statistical exercises is "secondary analysis." When one designs a large randomized controlled trial, it is critical to define the outcome to be tested *before* the trial is undertaken. After all, these are undertakings that recruit patients often by the thousands and make measurements by the hundreds over long periods of time. When all is said and done, these studies generate many thousands of data points. If one starts looking for associations once the data is collected, one will surely find them — often and often statistically impressive. For example, let's take one of these large trial data sets and test 100 associations for statistical significance. Perhaps you are curious whether patients with Right Coronary Disease who have high cholesterol do better with CABG than patients with Right Coronary Disease and normal cholesterol do with medical therapy. Assume you test 100 such reasonable (or even unreasonable) associations for statistical significance. Let's say you are willing to accept that any association that is strong enough so that it would happen by chance less than five times in a hundred (5 percent) is probably meaningful (as you would in an analysis where the associations to be tested were decided in advance). In the secondary or subset analysis of 100 possible associations, five will be found to be statistically significant, but these five are likely to be the five in 100 that reflect chance alone. This pitfall is minimized if you test for a limited number of associations that you established as "primary hypotheses" up front, a priori. Another term for "secondary analysis" is "data torturing," defined by James Mills as: "If you torture your data long enough, they will tell you whatever you want to hear" (Mills 1993). I ignore subgroup analyses, except as an exploratory analysis. It might point the way to the next generation of research protocols, but it does little to enhance my level of confidence in any inference anyone else draws from the data. I am not alone (Legakos 2006).

Data torturing of the randomized CABG trials has served the cardiovascular industry very well and patients very poorly. A secondary analysis of the U.S. multicenter Coronary Artery Surgery Study (CASS) leads to the conclusion that angina patients with plaques in all three major arteries, particularly if their heart muscle was functioning poorly, were a little better off for their CABGs (Passamani et al. 1985). This is the justification for all those multiple bypasses.

This is the fountainhead for that peculiarly American narrative of illness, whereby survivors of CABGs and their families boast of the number of grafts they received as if these were notches on the handle of a pistol. It's a sophism — and it's not their fault.

Whose fault is it?

Mine is not the only lonely voice long decrying the discordance between the zeal for cardiovascular invasiveness and the science demonstrating any benefit for patients. I have been railing in the literature and on rounds for over twenty years. Others have also written scholarly discussions to or toward this end dating back nearly as long (Friedman 1990; Schoenbaum 1993; Herman 1993), to no avail. If these procedures were pharmaceuticals, I can't imagine the FDA of that day permitting their sale (I'll have more to say about the FDA of today in other chapters). But the regulation of procedures is far less stringent than the regulation of pharmaceuticals. And the cardiovascular industry was in full control, though not yet in full flower. Realize that by 1987, cardiovascular disease was the largest source of health-care spending in the United States. Inpatient hospital costs accounted for the majority of medical spending, and cardiovascular disease accounted for 15 percent of those costs (*Mortality Morbidity Weekly Report* 1994). Realize, also, that conflicts of interest abounded (we will return to this as well), with many cardiologists and cardiovascular surgeons having financial ties to providers and purveyors of this technological and pharmaceutical boom. Arnold Relman, then the editor of the *New England Journal of Medicine*, decried the "growing entrepreneurship among clinical investigators" (Relman 1989). One pride of such investigators went so far as to write "conflict-of-interest guidelines" (Healy 1989) for interventional cardiology research. Those efforts did not stem the tide. They were buried by the proclamations of cardiology potentates who saw the CABG data through rose-colored lenses, proclaiming the promise of a new age where patients will be carefully categorized so that they can be afforded the benefits of particular forms of CABG or angioplasty. Thus spoke Eugene Braunwald, then the Hersey Professor of Physic at Harvard (Braunwald 1983), whose career is tainted by the Darsee scandal (his subordinate who was caught falsifying data) and the Genentec affair (where the experts hired to monitor the thrombolysis trials had vested financial interest in their outcome).

Speaking of entrepreneurship, the CABG and the angioplasty enterprises are in competition. The former is the turf of the cardiovascular surgeon; the latter is the turf of the invasive cardiologist. There are many comparative trials and comparisons failing to show one in a decidedly and consistently more favorable light. For example, if you were one of the 37,212 residents of New York State who were afforded a CABG for multivessel disease between 1997 and 2000, you were more likely to survive three years than the 22,102 patients with multivessel disease who underwent angioplasty with a stent (Hannan et al. 2005). Of course, one has no way of knowing from a study such as this if you would have been still better off on medical therapy, or if the patients were stented because they were too sick for CABG (despite the attempts of statisticians to account for such bias). It is not unusual for patients to be afforded the largesse of both industries. After all, failure to get better coincident with angioplasty is generally considered an indication for CABG, if the coronary anatomy seems ripe. There is one study comparing angioplasty with "medical therapy" for angina that is particularly illustrative, if one doubts my assertion that neither angioplasty nor CABG is worthwhile (RITA-2 trial participants 1997). Of 70,000 patients who underwent cardiac catheterization for coronary artery disease at twenty centers in the United Kingdom and Ireland, about 3,000 were considered eligible for enrollment in this trial. The eligibility criteria are difficult to understand, somewhat subjective, and certainly won't generalize. Nonetheless, 1,000 of the eligible were randomized to either angioplasty or medical therapy. Results were first reported after three years. During follow-up, thirty-two angioplasty patients (6.3 percent) but only seventeen medical patients (3.3 percent) died. That absolute difference was statistically significant and it exceeds my 2 percent clinical credibility level. These patients were better off if their coronary arteries were not invaded! There was also no important difference in the incidence of myocardial infarction. There was a trivial difference in whether the medical patients were deemed worthy of a CABG or an angioplasty during follow-up; the authors and the cardiology world hold up this difference in order to gloss over the strikingly disappointing result of this study. The RITA-2 patients were followed for another four years (Henderson et al. 2003) with still no disadvantage for those initially randomized to noninvasive treatment.

The Swiss published a randomized trial of optimized medical therapy versus early invasive therapy with either angioplasty ± stent or CABG (Pfisterer et al. 2003) and followed up at four years (Pfisterer 2004) in patients with angina who were less than seventy-five years old. It's no surprise that there was no advantage of the early invasive strategy in terms of death or myocardial infarction. The early invasive strategy was followed by fewer rehospitalizations for all reasons, but notably for invasive treatments. Of course, the need for such is in the eyes of the beholders, eyes that peer through glasses fogged by preconceived notions. These authors attempted to assess the quality of the lives of the patients following randomization. Maybe the patients who were afforded early invasive therapy were more likely to be spared later invasive therapy. But none of this did anything for their quality of life.

"Progress" of this sort continues apace despite a growing awareness that trials with multiple treatments and composite end points are inherently fraught with uncertainties (Ferreira-González et al. 2007) that are ripe for abuse by any investigator or sponsor with presuppositions (Freemantle et al. 2003; Lauer and Topol 2003). Based on a meta-analysis (a statistical technique about which I will have much more to say in the next chapter) of seven trials, a gaggle of leading cardiologists and cardiac epidemiologists (Mehta et al. 2005) are advocating "routine" invasive strategies for anyone who presents with an acute coronary syndrome, selectivity be damned. These investigators reached that conclusion despite the fact that the benefits of routine invasive strategies were inconsistent and marginal, whereas the increase in mortality that results is more consistent. Furthermore, they managed to avoid including the RITA-2 trial discussed above, as well as large trials conducted in the Netherlands (de Winter et al. 2005) and Brazil (Hueb et al. 2004) that also demonstrate an increased mortality with routine invasive strategies. If you live in a region of the United States that is relatively devoid of the wherewithal to invade your coronary arteries, do not despair. You're no worse off should you have a heart attack (Popescu et al. 2006). No patient should agree to angioplasty without the clear understanding that the procedure will not offer a survival advantage over medical therapy. That pertains to CABG as well, unless one can justify ferreting out the occasional patient with Left Main Disease.

However, interventional cardiologists and cardiovascular surgeons and the industry they underpin are all quick on their feet. They are wont to proclaim, "We don't do it that way any more." And indeed they don't. Furthermore, the barriers to these technological innovations are not nearly as stringent as those for pharmaceuticals (Hlatky 2004); hubris trumps the need for scientific testing. So today the interventional cardiologists are no longer content blowing up a balloon inside the occluding plaque. They are wont to leave a "stent," a little piece of tubing, behind it the hope of maintaining the patency of the vessel. Of course, the blood-clotting system does not look favorably on a foreign object in midstream. Stents clot. So the biotechnology industry was recruited, thanks to venture capitalists, to thwart the clotting with costly pharmaceuticals. The triumph is for the stents, not for the patients who are not advantaged whether the stents are patent or not (Mahoney et al. 2002; King 2003). Nonetheless, with stentorian bellow a recent *JAMA* editorial carried the title "To Cath or Not to

Cath: That Is No Longer the Question" because the author (Bhatt 2005) was enamored of the latest bit of hardware. It is true that these drug-eluting stents stay patent longer (Van de Werf 2006). It is true that they are rapidly dominating the annual stent market, much to the joy of the management and stockholders of Johnson & Johnson and Boston Scientific. It is also true that the notion that they are better for patients than stockholders is on increasingly shaky ground (Mitka 2006). The COURAGE Trial discussed in the principal chapter is particularly damning; no one should be told that angioplasty, with or without stenting, prevents a heart attack or stroke or prolongs life (Boden et al. 2007) in patients with stable coronary artery disease. Rather, these patients should be forewarned (Hochman and Steg 2007). The suggestion that patients are poorly served by this technology in the long term (Bavry 2006) is gaining in influence. A multi-center trial, funded by the NIH (Hochman et al. 2006), recruited 2,000 patients within a month of their heart attack because they had persistent blockage of the relevant coronary artery and heart damage. All received optimal medical care; half were randomized to also undergo angioplasty and stent placement. Over the next four years, there was no difference between the two groups in terms of recurrent heart attack, death, or heart failure. After four years, those with the stents fared less well. Not only do drug-eluting stents seem to be plagued with thrombosis long after they are placed (Stone et al. 2007; Lagerqvist et al. 2007) and thereby create major challenges to management (Mishkel et al. 2007), they also may interfere with the development of collateral blood vessels, thereby jeopardizing heart-muscle repair (Beier et al. 2007).

Drug-eluting stents may well be more harmful than plain stents, and plain stents are useless at best. Because of this, the Circulatory System Device Panel of the Food and Drug Administration held an open meeting on 7 and 8 December 2006. There was much hemming and hawing and defending of preconceived notions and vested interests (Shuchman 2007), with little of substance resulting. The believers point to the fact that the randomized controlled trials that led to FDA licensing of Cordis's sirolimus-eluting Cypher stent and Boston Scientific's paclitaxel-eluting Taxus stent, albeit mainly industry sponsored (Spaulding et al. 2007; Mauri et al. 2007), suggested a "breakthrough technology" (Maisel 2007). Many cardiologists are declaring these trials valid and ascribing the late thrombosis to the poor judgment of cardiologists who are responsible for placing several million stents in nonideal, "off-label" patients. The American colleges that house the stentors are coming out with statements that the indications for stenting are exquisitely defined and that patients with drug-eluting stents should be treated with aspirin and colpidigel for many months. They are certain that the latter will prevent more late stent clots than it will cause more bleeds. They ignore the precedent that published industry-sponsored trials are biased toward the positive. I am not one to advocate litigation as the best way to ensure that patients' interests are primary in such a debate. However, I suspect that it will take the plaintiff's bar and the banner of product liability to bring reason and science to the forefront of the debate. If there is no other way, then so be it.

So the cardiovascular industry has flowered. In 2001 more than 300,000 patients underwent a CABG in the United States at a cost of over $6 billion, and twice that number of angioplasties/stents were performed. Entrepreneurs, many with academic titles, hold sway. The ramifications are considerable, as will become clear in subsequent chapters. For now, realize that the medical community is countenancing conflicts-of-interest of this nature as long as they are openly admitted. The current editor of the *New England Journal of Medicine* has so declared yet again. Of course, Dr. Jeffrey Drazen's career is notable for his relationships with pharmaceutical firms in the conducting of drug trials. There is no way the pen is a match for an enterprise of this size and power. The cardiovascular trade controls both academic and community hospitals, not because of the benefits to the people who have cardiovascular illness but because it is still the largest cash cow. In institutions such as mine, there are fixed protocols awaiting anyone who presents with chest pain — protocols that involve the urgent administration of drugs, the urgent definition of coronary anatomy by cardiac catheterization, and some form of violence to the plaques that are likely to be found. Panels of experts abound to define indications for procedures and to denounce the fact that there are people with chest pain escaping the interventional cardiology net. The panels are always dominated by powerful people with forceful beliefs and often-declared vested interests in the interventional cardiology enterprise. The panels torture the inconsistent results of the many trials to generate indications by consensus (Hemingway et al. 2001). These are the same inconsistent trials that I interpret as indicating an absence of compelling data for benefit. Certainly there is no hint of a degree of benefit that justifies the risk of postoperative horrors and prolonged cognitive deficits from CABGs (Newman et al. 2001; Mark and Newman 2002; van Dijk et al. 2007). I find the argument that angioplasty is "as effective" but gentler than CABGs sophistic.

There are many precedents throughout history of medicine losing its way under the banner of hubris. The twentieth century witnessed epidemics of tonsillectomies, hysterectomies, laminectomies, and the like. Seldom can sci-

ence confront such hubris directly and overcome it. Even refutationist s
leaves room for doubt. Hubris, particularly hubris that commands weal?
take advantage of those doubts. Science can inform the debate, and thereby the
public.

The only solution today is to forewarn those who are still well. If you have
a heart attack or think you might have a heart attack, go to a hospital that
doesn't have a cardiac catheterization facility and refuse to be transferred to a
hospital with such. You'll be better off in the short and long run (Van de Werf
et al. 2005). And if you find yourself in a hospital where you are offered cardiac
catheterization, ask to what end. If it is to see whether angioplasty is feasible,
demur. You're likely to do as well (or better) in the long run with an exercise
program (Hambrecht et al. 2004) or a little aspirin (Ridker et al. 2005; Patrono
et al. 2005).

And let's all hope that research in cardiovascular diseases does not remain
mired with the technocrats. The challenge is not in the plumbing; the challenge
is in vascular biology. Maybe we can learn how to identify those of us who
are disadvantaged when it comes to making new collateral vessels and thereby
compensate for those that have hardened. Such is on the horizon (Rosenzweig
2005).

I will not trouble you with a reiteration of all these arguments as they pertain
to interventional neurology, neuroradiology, and neurosurgery in their attempt
to get their day in the high-tech sun. The oft-misquoted trial purporting to
show a benefit of carotid endarterectomy is the North American Symptomatic
Carotid Endarterectomy Trial (1991), which I interpret to demonstrate a benefit
for the carotid artery and not for the patient. The trial of carotid stenting that
convinced the FDA to license the widgets for symptomatic patients who were
too sick for endarterectomy was published by Yadav et al. (2004). One must
marvel at the technical inventiveness. Angioplasty pulverizes plaques wherever, running the risk of releasing debris that floats downstream, occluding
the vessel. So, the widgets employed include all kinds of inventiveness to trap
the debris before it can wreak havoc. Inventive or not, the French stopped a
trial comparing endarterectomy with stenting early, after recruiting only 527
patients, because stenting was the more evil intervention (Mas et al. 2006).
Furlan (2006), who heads the section for stroke and neurological intensive care
at the Cleveland Clinic, argues that this "cannot be considered the final word
on carotid stenting." Furlan bolstered this opinion with prose that is even more
inventive, unconvincing, and self-serving than that displayed by the interventional cardiologists in his institution, about whom we'll have more to say in

later chapters. Remember, stenting is an attempt to avoid the complications of carotid endarterectomy — which doesn't really work.

Chapter 3

Cholesterol. The literature I am citing in this chapter is a fraction of the thousands of relevant papers. But I am citing the papers that represent the gauntlets for all papers that are taken to support the inference that primary prevention of cardiovascular disease is well served by the pharmacological perturbation of blood lipids. The West of Scotland pravastatin study is published by Shepherd et al. (1995). The Air Force experience with lovastatin was published by Downs et al. (1998). The ALLHAT-LLT (2002) pravastatin trial was published with an accompanying editorial by a cardiologist who lists affiliations with no fewer that eight pharmaceutical firms, including the manufacturer of pravastatin, and who ascribes the lack of efficacy to "clinical inertia" in response to the uneven compliance of patients who were to take pravastatin (Pasternak 2002). Dr. Pasternak has many peers, some of whom were involved in writing the U.S. guidelines for cholesterol screening and treatment (NCEP-ATP III 2002) and an update that calls not just for treating but for treating aggressively with statins (Grundy et al. 2004). The CDC has bought into this in its "Healthy People 2010" agenda that sets a goal of screening 80 percent of the adult population.

The principal underlying these guidelines is the supposition that the risk imparted by cholesterol is linear; the benefit of lowering cholesterol should be colinear. It matters little that benefit has proved elusive except in the high-risk groups, mainly those who already have heart disease (Hayward et al. 2006; Manuel et al. 2006; Abramson and Wright 2007). Rather, all the data from primary and secondary prevention trials on 90,056 subjects were massaged to support the contention that statins can benefit all with any risk (Cholesterol Treatment Trialists Collaborators 2005), including women of any age and elderly men about whom data is scant. In a clinical discussion in *JAMA*, Mittleman (2006) argued for treating a thirty-nine-year-old woman who was worried but otherwise well with statins because she had an estimated 1 to 2 percent risk of developing coronary heart disease in the next decade. This line of reasoning was not lost on the marketing departments of the manufacturers of statins. After all, nearly all of the experts conducting the trials and sitting on the panels had formal, lucrative consultative arrangements with the manufacturers of the statins (Steinbrook 2007). Mittleman (2006) disclosed that he served as a consultant to Pfizer and five other pharmaceutical firms. The number of

Americans for whom statins are recommended escalated from 13 million to 36 million in the past five years. There is a muffled cry of outrage from various hallowed halls of institutional medicine, but little else. It may take the plaintiff's bar to drive remedial action. A class-action complaint was filed in the U.S. District Court in Massachusetts on 28 September 2005 on behalf of Teamsters Local No. 35 Health Plans and various others against Pfizer, the manufacturer of the industry-leading statin Lipitor, which had worldwide sales of $10 billion in 2004. The suit alleges "violation of State unfair and deceptive trade practice laws . . . arising from the marketing of the brand-name drug Lipitor" for indications for which there is no scientific support.

This will not be the first time that the plaintiff's bar has used the mechanism of a class-action suit to hold the pharmaceutical industry more accountable (Kesselheim and Avorn 2007). We will discuss below the fates of cerivastatin (Baycol), another statin, and troglitazone (Rezulin), an oral hypoglycemic, both of which bit the dust when it came to light that the published studies minimized their risks. In chapter 9, I'll explore the canard that enveloped the coxibs Vioxx and Bextra. In these instances, along with Redux, Paxil, Propulsid, Zyprexa, and others, we owe the plaintiff's bar a debt of gratitude for forcing the FDA toward regulatory remedies. Before you assume that I applaud the plaintiff's bar indiscriminately, I can assure you that I am well aware of and wont to condemn its excesses.

The reference that discusses the negative psychological effects of labeling a well person as hypercholesterolemic is by Brett (1991). That the FDA has either withdrawn 10 percent of approved pharmaceuticals or appended a "black-box" warning to the package inserts was demonstrated by Lasser et al. (2002). This is all the more remarkable since post-marketing surveillance is not systematic; it relies on hit-and-miss reporting. An analysis comparing the benefits of aspirin, statins, or both for the primary prevention of heart disease in men (Pignone et al. 2006) reached a conclusion similar to mine: if you must, take a baby aspirin, but don't chastise yourself if you don't.

Caro et al. (1997) published the pharmacoeconomic analysis of pravastatin. If you want to read an appraisal of such pharmacoeconomics that is as cautionary as mine, I'd suggest Rennie and Luft (2000). So much of the analysis hinges on the validity of the calculation of the NNT for one year to accomplish something — spare a heart attack, save a life from a heart attack, or the like. This is a very tenuous statistic for any particular statin study and across studies (Kumana et al. 1999). In the case of statins for primary prevention, any cost/benefit analysis is fatuous.

It is now argued that the pharmacoeconomic analysis of pravastatin greatly underestimates the value of the drug. The argument is based on the long-term follow-up of the West of Scotland cohort (Ford et al. 2007). Nearly all of the participants were followed for another decade after the RCT was completed and they had returned to the routine care of their physicians. The differences in outcomes for the men who had been treated with pravastatin during the trial and those treated with placebo persisted for another decade. Namely, there was no meaningful difference in all-cause mortality, in mortality ascribed to cardiovascular causes, or in any other dramatic disease process. The authors also assert that the small difference in nonfatal heart attacks also persisted.

I am even less convinced about that than I was by the results of the RCT itself. The follow-up study has none of the elegance of the RCT. For one thing, the outcomes are based on the use of records held by the National Health Service for Scotland. Administrative data sets such as these are convenient but far less accurate than the laborious review of records that was part of the original RCT. Even for a national scheme such as Britain's, important inaccuracies are readily measurable (Singleton 2007). I am less concerned about the data regarding all-cause mortality. I have some concerns about the accuracy of ascribing death to cardiovascular disease because so many patients have cardiovascular disease as comorbidity at the time of death regardless of the cause, and weighting the proximate cause can be quite subjective. But I have great concerns about the validity of myocardial infarction in administrative data sets, as many a cause of chest pain other than coronary artery disease can be so labeled at the time of discharge. In an editorial that accompanied the presentation of the West of Scotland follow-up, Domanski (2007) asserts, "There should no longer be any doubt that the reduction of LDL cholesterol levels has a role in the prevention . . . of coronary heart disease." I beg to differ. Primary prevention with a statin doesn't save a life. It arguably spares one man in fifty a heart attack if they take the agent for five years. The argument that a well man should take it forever is contrived. Interestingly, little is made in the follow-up regarding the use of statins after the RCT closed. About a third of those who had been on placebo were started on pravastatin, and about a third who had been on pravastatin remained on the agent. This was not a random assignation; we have no idea why the agent was used in either group and for what interval. It is likely that the result is contaminated by some element of secondary prevention, but we do not know if that element biased the small difference in heart attacks that is purported.

I have qualms about structured reviews and greater qualms about meta-analyses. These are statistical exercises, semiquantitative and quantitative, respectively, that attempt to pool all the data from all trials on a single topic and derive a unitary inference in spite of the cacophony of varying methodologies and varying results. I have qualms because these exercises require that the authors of the analysis sit in judgment of the papers as to their quality and then weight the papers accordingly. That's so subjective an exercise that I am not willing to delegate it when the issue is crucial for my patients. I have further qualms about such exercises because we know that most negative studies (particularly those sponsored by pharmaceutical companies) are not published. To remedy this, it was agreed that all trials are to be registered and all results made available, even if the trial is never published. It is not clear that this mechanism has arrived at a state that brings negative trials to the attention of those who do systematic reviews and meta-analyses. Since the existing literature is skewed toward the more positive trials, so too will be the meta-analysis of all these marginal papers. Not only is there bias because negative trials are not published; there also is bias that relates to the influence of funding on the outcome of trials in many disciplines, including cardiovascular clinical trials (Ridker and Torres 2006). It is easy to show that published studies that were sponsored and/or executed by people and business entities with a vested financial interest in the result are more likely to favor the experimental intervention than studies of the same intervention sponsored/executed by people and organizations with no vested financial interest. The implicit reproach is inescapable. But the observation is on firm grounding. In addition to the analysis by Ridker and Torres (2006), who had no conflicts of interest to report, there is a complementary analysis by two Danish scientists who were supported by the government-sponsored Cochrane Collaboration (Kjaergard and B. Als-Nielsen 2002), as well as papers by Lexchin et al. (2003) and Melender et al. (2003).

Speaking of qualms, I am not alone in decrying the hype of "relative risk" and the abuse of NNT. Relative risk seldom is as informative as absolute risk; if your five-year survival is improved from 96 percent to 98 percent by some intervention, does the assertion of a 50 percent reduction in mortality ring as true as 2 percent improvement in survival? As for NNT, if the result of the trial is marginal, say a 1 percent improvement in survival in one year, why should I be offered the supposition that I will save one life for every 100 people I treat for a year? A review of 359 studies of new treatments published in major medical journals found that the majority expressed and emphasized their results as "relative risk" reduction (Nuovo 2002). Furthermore, it is commonplace to find the least informative statistics — those most likely to mislead — standing alone in the "abstract" of papers (Gøetzsche 2006). The abstract is the most read and readily accessible summary of the paper, which is too often a shortcut to "reading" utilized by all. Since the "peer review" mechanism is not up to policing this abuse of statistics, the consumer must be skeptical and learn to ask the telling questions. It's an issue that we will return to repeatedly in the chapters that follow.

The observations of Phillips et al. (2002) fuel my concerns about the potential for long-term insidious muscle damage from statin exposure. They observed symptoms and demonstrated muscle pathology in patients whose serum CK levels were normal. An elevated CK can indicate muscle damage and was the hallmark of the catastrophic muscle inflammation that led to the withdrawal of cerivastatin (Baycol) (Farmer 2001). Even without the elevated CK, there is cause for concern (Thompson et al. 2003). But the pharmaceutical industry is indefatigable in its pursuit of a lower cholesterol level, and its fellow travelers in the FDA, the drug-trial enterprise, the American Heart Association, and the academy are all too willing to support the effort. There are billions of dollars in play. So now rosuvastatin (Crestor) is enjoying the fruits of a seemingly omnipresent direct-to-consumer advertising campaign coupled with an aggressive campaign to win over all who might prescribe statins. This is occurring in the face of disquieting data (Alsheikh-Ali et al. 2005) that Sidney Wolf and Public Citizen have been using to taunt the FDA into action. There are new drugs on the way to market, novel congeners of the statins, that target the putatively more harmful of the lipids or increase lipids that associate with better outcomes. The zeal based on mechanisms far outstrips the science that supports a meaningful outcome for whichever consumer is unaware that marketing is driving the research agenda (Avorn 2005).

By the way, if the specter of muscle disease doesn't make one sufficiently concerned, add the possibility that statins have been associated with the development of osteoarthritis of the hip in elderly woman (Beattie et al. 2005) and perhaps with the risk for Parkinson's disease (Huang et al. 2006).

Metabolic Syndrome. The literature that relates to the "Metabolic Syndrome" is even more voluminous than the literature that relates to cholesterol metabolism. In fact, it largely subsumes that literature to move on across many fields of investigative endeavor. It is remarkable how frequently each component of the Metabolic Syndrome is studied, as if the investigators were barely cognizant of the related research. It's as if those who focus on the details of carbohydrate metabolism are uncomfortable collaborating with those who focus on lipid metabolism. However, biochemists and clinical investigators are not alone in suffering intellectual myopia; epidemiologists do as well. The epidemiologists who focus on proximate-cause epidemiology tend to collaborate with the clinical investigators who study particular proximate causes. In that fashion, we learn of the individual "risk factors." Hence, there are numerous studies of the epidemiology of obesity, dyslipidemias, and various forms of hypertension and type 2 diabetes but far fewer studies of the epidemiology of combinations. The development of the concept of a Metabolic Syndrome is the response to this lack. Recently, the American Diabetes Association and the European Association for the Study of Diabetes have issued a joint statement that asserts that the combining of risk factors into a syndrome is premature (Kahn et al. 2005). The American Heart Association offers the counterargument (Mitka 2005), bolstered by demonstrations that people with Metabolic Syndrome are at increased risk (Gami et al. 2007) and that lifestyle modification, particularly lowering cholesterol — the cardiology shibboleth (Kohli and Greenland 2006) — is the primary recourse.

Proximate-cause epidemiology, which has enjoyed much recognition and generous research support, provides the raison d'être for much that is lucrative for the contemporary pharmaceutical industry. Perhaps that, directly and indirectly, explains why proximate-cause epidemiology has been coddled. However, life-course epidemiology receives little recognition from the proximate-cause epidemiologists in their writings and in the design of their studies. Furthermore, life-course epidemiology deals with the structure of society and therefore offers the pharmaceutical industry and its fellow travelers little hope of a profitable intervention. The greatest gap in the literature on the Metabolic Syndrome is the dearth of input from life-course epidemiology. The greatest challenge for the student of this literature is to read the methods and data analyses and have to wonder how the inferences would change if the design incorporated measures of SES and the like. Yes, American men, children, and adolescents weigh more than ever before; 32 percent are labeled obese (Ogden et al. 2006). Furthermore, it is clear that obesity in midlife is a mortal risk regardless of SES: it results in a shift toward the upward slope of the U-shaped curve (Adams et al. 2006), but often slight. However, the increased prevalence of diabetes or obesity is in ethnic minorities (McTigue et al. 2002; Brancati et al. 2000), particularly the adolescent poor (Miech et al. 2006). SES and its covariates (such as self-reported health status, education, and job satisfaction) explain most associations of this nature, if SES is measured (Beckles and Thompson-Reid 2002; Wardle et al. 2006). It is easy to show that chronic stress at work predisposes to the Metabolic Syndrome (Chandola et al. 2006).

The National Cholesterol Education Program (NCEP) "criteria" for the Metabolic Syndrome (National Cholesterol Education Program 2001) are flawed beyond the fact that they do not take SES into account. These criteria leave me incredulous as to their validity and the mind-set of the panel who constructed them. Realize how many of the panel were (some still are) consultants to pharmaceutical and biotechnology firms. By the way, such arrangements are legal and condoned by their peers (National Institutes of Health 2001). My reservations are borne out by the publication that demonstrated that a quarter of Americans qualify for the label "Metabolic Syndrome" whether they are white or African American females or white males, but only 15 percent of African American males qualify. Furthermore, nearly half of Americans from sixty to sixty-nine years old qualify. Yet they are in their sixties already, and reaching eighty is a reality for most of their cohort, particularly the women (Ford et al. 2002). Most of these people with putative Metabolic Syndrome are normal. A recent analysis of the cardiovascular risk from Metabolic Syndrome in middle-aged Finnish men shows little consistent risk in the 14 percent who qualify by NCEP criteria, whereas there is a three-fold risk for men in the highest quartile by criteria that are more stringent (Lakka et al. 2002). The Metabolic Syndrome grows out of another U-shaped curve. We have little justification in establishing cutoffs before the degree of risk starts escalating. Two groups of investigators from the CDC have analyzed data from a number of cross-sectional national surveys undertaken periodically between 1960 and 2000. It is clear that all cardiovascular disease risk factors (with the possible exception of diabetes) have declined considerably over the past forty years in all BMI groups (Gregg et al. 2005) to such an extent that obesity (BMI between 25 and 30) is no longer a risk factor (Flegal et al. 2005). We need to rethink the public-health imperative regarding weight loss (Mark 2005) and the validity of the notion that because we weigh more today than in the past (Hedley et al. 2004) we will die sooner.

Despite the backpedaling by the experts speaking on behalf of the American Diabetes Association and the European Association for the Study of Diabetes mentioned above (Kahn et al. 2005), it is likely that the various components of the Metabolic Syndrome exhibit synergy; the syndrome is a greater health hazard than the sum of its parts. For example, obesity is a more powerful risk factor when it is accompanied by insulin resistance, or type 2 diabetes (Reaven 2003). Therefore, public-health policy that focuses exclusively on one feature is myopic. That may explain, in part, why the National Task Force on the Prevention and Treatment of Obesity (1994) could discern little hazard in "yo-yo weight loss." Perhaps actual loss of weight is no more likely to lower all-cause mortality then just attempting to lose weight (Gregg et al. 2003). Or maybe it is because lack of "physical fitness" is more of a risk than BMI (Wessel et al. 2004). There are many mysteries to the Metabolic Syndrome, some of which may overlap with the mysteries as to why SES is so crucial. That mystery is not solved by pharmacologic therapy to promote weight loss (Li et al. 2005) or bariatric surgery (Maggard et al. 2005).

Adult onset (type 2) diabetes. For an overview of the contemporary conundrum that is the diagnosis of type 2 diabetes, I'd suggest a paper by Barr et al. (2002).

Although predictable from earlier surveys, Tirosh et al. (2005) demonstrated that young men with fasting blood glucose levels in the higher range of normal are more likely to reach criteria for type 2 diabetes as they age, and this likelihood increases if they have higher BMIs or blood lipids. The accompanying editorial finds this alarming and advocates measuring blood glucose with the goal of advising fitness (Arky 2005). This is the notion of "pre-diabetes," when glucose metabolism crosses a threshold such that consensus considers it to be impaired but not sufficiently impaired to warrant the diabetes label. In 1997 the "Expert Committee of the Diagnosis and Classification of Diabetes Mellitus" of the American Diabetes Association revised the criteria for the diagnosis of type 2 diabetes. One criterion was a fasting blood glucose level of 126 mg/dl. The NIH panel that formulated the criteria for the Metabolic Syndrome listed in the chapter established the cutoff at 110 mg/dl. These panels and others have access to survey data that looks at the prevalence of the clinical manifestations of type 2 diabetes as a function of various measures of blood sugar. Most of these surveys rely on surrogate measures that speak to diabetes-specific microvascular damage, such as subtle changes in the eyes (diabetic retinopathy), rather than less frequent, delayed serious consequences such as blindness, renal failure, heart attacks, or death. There is an experimental literature exploring the molecular mechanisms by which bathing tissue in fluids high in glucose leads to damage (Sheetz and King 2002). The existence of this literature supports the hypothesis — but does not test the hypothesis — that controlling blood-sugar levels will prevent microcirculatory damage. Surrogate measures are convenient for testing the hypothesis *only* if one assumes that they are indeed important measures of long-term risks.

Surrogate measures, such as blood pressure or serum lipid levels, are frequently employed in intervention studies designed to abrogate biological risk factors for macrovascular and microvascular disease and relied heavily upon by the FDA. Caveat emptor, redux. Surrogate and intermediate end points are not reliable in many of these settings (Psaty et al. 1999; Temple 1999). However, surrogate measures are seductive because they tend to be more sensitive to change, both temporally and quantitatively. "Hard outcomes," such as death or stroke, unfold at a pace that demands much more patience and a larger cohort, both of which can tax the resources of any investigative team. Hence, we will always be stuck with surrogate end points — but they need not fool us.

Pardon the digression. In the Pima Indians, a long-studied population with a very high incidence of diabetic complications, there is no increase in the prevalence of retinopathy until the fasting blood sugar rises above 125 mg/dl or so. The general U.S. population starts to climb out of the valley of the U-shaped curve for retinopathy above 110 mg/dl. The relationship between blood sugar and retinopathy is predictable. However, the relationship between blood sugar and other diabetes-associated outcomes is not that predictable. In particular, the risk of macrovascular complications, such as coronary artery or peripheral vascular disease, and blood sugar have less clear cutoffs. Here, the relationship is more monotonic (straight line) than U-shaped, with some risk still apparent in the population with normal blood sugar (no matter how "normal" is defined). That's because type 2 diabetes is only one of the relevant risk factors in the Metabolic Syndrome. So the expert panels are forced to examine the epidemiology of surrogate outcomes and come to a consensus. The consensus cutoff is seldom age dependent, even though insulin resistance is a fact of normal aging. Hence, the "epidemic" of type 2 diabetes may prove a contrived reflection of changing the definition so that more people qualify for the label. According to the CDC, we are already labeling another 1.5 million Americans as diabetic each year (‹http://www.cdc.gov/diabetes/statistics›).

The study of intensive treatment of type 1 diabetes was published by the Diabetes Control and Complications Trial (DCCT) Research Group (1993). The most recent paper describes cardiovascular outcomes seventeen years after the trial commenced (DCCT/Epidemiology of Diabetes Interventions and Complications [EDIC] 2005). The classic study contrasting diet, insulin therapy, and a first-generation oral hypoglycemic in the management of type 2 diabetes was published by the University Group Diabetes Program (UGDP) (1976). This was a study where the oral hypoglycemic was associated with more deaths than the alternatives. The vaunted UK Prospective Diabetes Study (UKPDS) Group paper was published in *Lancet* (1998). Stratton et al. (2000) published the secondary analysis, observing a relationship between exposure to hyperglycemia and important clinical outcomes. This was the result of the meta-analysis when glycosylated hemoglobin, hemoglobin A1c, was the measure of persistence of hyperglycemia (Selvin et al. 2004) and triggered the editorial by Gerstein (2004).

I should mention the Diabetes Prevention Program (DPP) trial, which randomized over 3,000 people with subtle type 2 diabetes to placebo, lifestyle intervention, or a particular oral hypoglycemic (metformin). After nearly three years, the glucose intolerance was less subtle in the placebo than in the other two groups. Based on considerations like cost, lifestyle intervention is the most sensible approach to modifying this surrogate measure (Herman et al. 2005). The lifestyle intervention had a goal of at least a 7 percent weight loss and over two hours of elective physical activity per week. There have been over twenty trials like this, comparing the effectiveness of pharmacological and lifestyle interventions on progression in type 2 diabetes and reaching similar conclusions (Gilles et al. 2007). However, lifestyle modifications are quite variable, both in terms of adherence and outcome (Davey Smith et al. 2005). I suspect we are faced with some of the issues we noted in chapter 1 relating to confounders in elements of SES (Tuomilehto 2005). The impressive downward trend in cardiovascular complications discussed in chapter 2 also advantages diabetics (Fox et al. 2004) and renders their macrovascular hazard less pressing. Hence, the "lifestyle" that needs intervention is a highly relative notion. Does two hours of additional exercise make as much of a difference for a field hand as for a sedentary worker?

Type 2 diabetes is part of the Metabolic Syndrome. It is difficult to define because the hazard it alone imparts escalates very slowly unless the blood sugar is extraordinarily high. And treatment with first-, second-, or third-generation oral hypoglycemic agents drops the hemoglobin A1c but has nothing more to offer than simply suggesting the patient lose weight and exercise. If this is the state of the science, grave questions must be addressed as to the state of the art.

What drives the American Diabetes Association (2006) to recommend screening of all adults after age forty-five? What drove the Ambulatory Care Quality Alliance to propose hemoglobin A1c monitoring as an indicator of the quality of care in April 2006 (‹http://www.ambulatory-qualityalliance.org›), and the Centers for Medicare and Medicaid Services to endorse it a month later? And how can the American College of Physicians come out with a continuing-education document (Laine 2007) detailing a screening program and an intervention program that echoes this party line? When I confront those who formed the committees that produced these documents, they are true believers who feel the surrogate measures are not to be ignored despite the UKPDS trial. One leading investigator went so far as to say that the ravages of type 2 diabetes "are likely to become the major cause of preventable disease and premature death in this millennium" (Nathan 2006). I'd take issue with the notion of "preventable death" and the notion of "premature death," as you know from chapter 1. At least I can find like-minded individuals on the U.S. Preventive Services Task Force (2003), which found "insufficient evidence to recommend for or against routine screening."

The quest for the effective oral hypoglycemic is yet another Grail of the pharmaceutical industry. After all, we are defining an ever-expanding population of diabetics, an epidemic if you will, which represents an ever-expanding market to be captured. The quest is stymied because not only is benefit difficult to document, but many classes of these agents also cause weight gain and do so rapidly. That's not a happy trade-off for reducing a surrogate measure such as hemoglobin A1c. Some are advocating that patients in clinics and studies be "risk adjusted," so that if the A1c drops further in a patient with a higher A1c, we should consider the drug more likely to be beneficial in the long run (Pogach et al. 2007). No one is proposing another UKPDS; neither the investigative community nor the governmental and industry communities leap to mobilize the patience or moneys for such an undertaking. So the mantra of essentially all papers, research and educational, is something like, "The attainment and maintenance of near-normal glycemia reduces the risk of long-term complications of diabetes," referencing the DCCT and UKPDS trials. This is the introduction to the ADOPT trial (Kahn et al. 2007), which compared the effectiveness over four years in 4,600 diabetic patients of three classes of oral hypoglycemics, each with its own mechanism: the biguanide metformin, the sulfonurea glyburide, and the thiazolidinedione rosiglitazone. Each class lowered hemogloblin A1c in the majority of patients. The effectiveness of rosiglitazone was slightly better than the other two at the price of more weight gain and edema, but with less gastrointestinal events and fewer hypoglycemic episodes. A secondary analysis suggests that maybe there were more cardiovascular events on metformin than the other two, but the incidence of any cardiovascular event was quite small; fatal heart attacks occurred in 0.1 percent for example, and absolute difference between the agents for any cardiovascular event was trivial, around 1 percent. More disturbing is that long after the ADOPT trial was published in the *New England Journal of Medicine*, and therefore long after the initial data analysis, the safety data were reviewed only to discover that women on rosiglitazone experienced more fractures, mainly of the arm and foot. Yet the standard of care demands treating the hemoglobin A1c. For example, in "Clinician's Corner," *JAMA* published the discussion of an "expert" related to a particular case. Abrahmson (2007) held forth on the treatment of a thin, otherwise well seventy-four-year-old woman who was found to be "hyperglycemic" incidentally and whose hemoglobin A1c was 7.4 percent despite simultaneously taking maximum doses of all three oral hypoglycemics studied in the ADOPT trial for six years. Dr. Abrahmson waxed eloquent as to what should be done next, including switching her to insulin. He was determined to reach the "ideal" hemoglobin A1c at all cost and at all risk. Talk about treating a test and not a patient. Talk about missing the forest for the trees.

I doubt the enthusiasm would be tempered by the brouhaha that now surrounds rosiglitazone, which is manufactured by GlaxoSmithKline (GSK) and marketed as Avandia. Steven Nissen is a cardiologist on the staff of the Cleveland Clinic who assumed the role of director of the clinic's contracted drug trials enterprise from Eric Topol after the latter became embroiled in the Vioxx controversy about which we have much to say in later chapters. Nissen and Wolski (2007) undertook a meta-analysis of forty-two treatment trials and concluded that rosiglitazone increased the risk of myocardial infarction. At the end of the paper, Nissen declares receiving research support from no fewer than seven pharmaceutical firms, absent GSK. There has followed a heated debate with innuendos of culpability and suppression of data reminiscent of the brouhaha over stents discussed in chapter 2. Experts have weighed in, generally backpedaling on recommending rosiglitazone (Nathan 2007; Psaty and Furberg 2007). It has also provoked reconvening of the relevant FDA Advisory Committee with much chest beating as a result (Rosen 2007).

For me, there is little to debate. Since I am not convinced there's any benefit to be gained from rosiglitazone, I will not prescribe the agent in the first place and am disappointed that the FDA was willing to license the agent because of its effect on surrogate markers. If there is no meaningful benefit, no risk is tolerable.

High blood pressure. There is an elegant demonstration of the J-shaped relationship between blood pressure and mortality published by Boutitie et al. (2002). The JNC 7 report was published by Chobanian et al. (2003). Fortunately, in recent decades there has been a downward trend in the blood pressure of most populations that cannot be attributed to medical interventions (Tunstall-Pedoe 2006). This parallels the downward trend in cardiovascular disease and in all-cause mortality. But it is no match for the escalating zeal of the interventionalists.

The MR FIT trial of step therapy for hypertension was published by the Multiple Risk Factor Intervention Trial Research Group (1982). For a discussion of the fashion in which diuretic therapy may have predisposed to sudden death in that trial, and why the risk of sudden death may be outweighed by the benefits of therapy, I suggest the papers by Bigger (1994) and Heos et al. (1995). A recent analysis of the MR FIT cohort after sixteen years of monitoring for cardiovascular and all-cause mortality and morbidity demonstrates that SES overwhelms all the many other risk factors that were measured. SES is more powerful than "race" (Davey Smith et al. 1998).

The classical trial demonstrating an advantage for the elderly from treating their systolic hypertension is the SHEP trial. The most recent analysis of this cohort experience reemphasizes the effectiveness in terms of a decreased incidence of all kinds of strokes (Perry et al. 2000). However, trial after trial supports the use of nothing fancier than a gentle diuretic in the elderly patient with systolic hypertension, or, for that matter, as first-line therapy in all patients with hypertension (Wassertheil-Smoller et al. 2004; Kostis et al. 2005).

Stelfax et al. (1998) discuss the calcium channel blocker stain on medical ethics. The trial by Tuomilehto et al. (1999) is an example using calcium channel blockers to the advantage of older patients with diabetes and systolic hypertension. Adler et al. (2000) published the observational data from the UKPDS cohort demonstrating the synergy of hazards when type 2 diabetic patients are hypertensive. The demonstration that tight blood-pressure control benefits the UKPDS diabetic patients was a secondary analysis (UK Prospective Diabetes Study Group 1998b). The demonstration that treating the systolic hypertension of elderly diabetic patients is also effective derives from the SHEP study (Curb et al. 1996). The fact that these elderly diabetic and hypertensive patients are so easily and effectively treated argues that they are different from many in the UKPDS cohort. I suspect that the type 2 diabetes in the UKPDS cohort is a reflection of the Metabolic Syndrome, whereas in the elderly the type 2 diabetes label is a medicalization of the relative insulin resistance of normal aging. I am concerned about the trade-offs in treating hypertensive-diabetic patients with multiple agents. I am less concerned about treating the elderly with isolated systolic hypertension. The regimen is gentle and there is data that it will not compromise the quality of their lives (Applegate et al. 1994). ALLHAT (an acronym for the Antihypertensive and Lipid-Lowering Treatment to Prevent Heart Attack Trial) is a testimony to the current fashion of naming trials so that their acronyms are pronounceable. The major thrust of the trial was the comparison of antihypertensive agents (2002), which demonstrated that an inexpensive off-patent thiazide diuretic outperformed an expensive ACE inhibitor and an expensive calcium channel blocker. A third class of agents, an alpha blocker, was also studied, but that alternative was eliminated early because of untoward events. This result of the ALLHAT trial is consistent with the literature in general, according to two recent meta-analyses of trials that, in the aggregate, randomized 56,000 people (Law et al. 2003) and 192,478 people (Psaty et al. 2003) with hypertension to a large assortment of interventions.

The TROPHY trial (Julius et al. 2006) should give pause to the zeal to treat more and more of us with any drug, let alone newer and more expensive pharmacologic agents. At best it's unconvincing (Schunkert 2006); at worst, it's another example of data torturing (Persell and Baker 2006). And it may very well belong in the category of another recent example of vested interests clouding science (Psaty et al. 2006).

The TONE study renders nonpharmacological options a reasonable alternative in the elderly (Whelton et al. 1998). This study is a randomized controlled trial in a targeted population — the elderly, whether they are hefty or not. The PRE-MIER trial was also randomized, with a similar outcome in a younger cohort (Premier Collaborative Research Group 2003).

Chapter 4

Most of the literature on the effects of "lifestyle" on longevity is observational. The most influential studies are longitudinal: cohorts are assembled, characterized, and followed over time to see if particular aspects will associate with all-cause and disease-specific mortality rates. This is another voluminous literature that is remarkably varied in quality. The paper I was picking on from the Nurses' Health Study is by Hu et al. (2002). The analysis at twenty years that discerned no important cardiac hazard from a dietary history that tended toward low carbohydrate, high protein, and fat was published by Halton et al. (2006) to add the voice of the Nurses' Health Study to the carbohydrate-fat nutritional debate. The analysis that dredged out the tiny relative risk of trans fat from the Nurses' Health Study data set was by Oh et al. (2005). However, these are only two examples of the fashion in which these investigators are willing to mine their data beyond the realm of the credible. Realize that they have a parallel male data set, the Health Professionals Follow-up Study, which began in 1986 by recruiting 51,529 male health professionals age forty to seventy-five. The following analyses of these two observational cohort studies, to my way of thinking, cross the methodological boundary to the fatuous. Realize that this observational cohort approach, as is true for case-control, cross-sectional designs, is more powerful at refuting associations than making them. The former is limited by the statistical power of the study design: the ability to claim a negative result is likely to be real rather than reflect the missing of a positive result (a calculation that is based on the efficiency of the measurement of the health effect and usually defines the size of the study population). Positive results are very susceptible to confounding; they may reflect unmeasured influences.

1. The Health Professionals Follow-up Study could find no difference in benefit comparing men who claimed one to two servings of fish per week and those claiming five to six servings in the likelihood of suffering from coronary artery disease. For this disappointing negative result the researchers offer "confounding by unmeasured factors" as explanation (Ascherio et al. 1995).

2. Not to worry. Coffee consumption is safe in this and other studies (Willett et al. 1996). It may even prevent you from being labeled as diabetic (van Dam and Hu 2005). It has been very difficult to pin any blame on coffee or other caffeinated beverages in multiple studies. Even in the Nurses' Health Study, there is no discernible association between habitual caffeine intake and coronary heart disease (Winklemayer et al. 2005).

3. Fiber is good for men's hearts, we are told. But this study massages the data to the same extent as the fish study above to come up with significant reductions in relative risk. Absolute risk reduction is trivial (Rimm et al. 1996).

4. Fiber is good for women's hearts, we are told. The study (Wolk et al. 1999) is as unconvincing as the study on men.

5. Eggs are exonerated! At least, one egg per day won't hurt you. Many eggs may hurt you if you're a diabetic (Hu et al. 1999). Give me a break.

6. An unpublished analysis of the Health Professionals Follow-up Study is alluded to in a review paper and said to result in a relative risk of trans fats similar to that discussed above (Mozaffarian et al. 2006). This review describes a secondary analysis of a large Finnish cohort resulting in an even less compelling relative risk that was not statistically significant.

And so butter is now politically correct. It joins seafood and the constituent omega-3 fatty acids as the smart thing to eat. The supporting literature is as voluminous as it is low in quality. For an analysis of the risk/benefit ratio of fish intake, I'd suggest the review by Mozaffarian and Rimm (2006). My assertion that neither fish nor omega-3 fatty acid itself will spare you cancer is supported by another systematic review of the literature (MacLean et al. 2006). Brouwer et al. (2006) performed an interesting randomized controlled trial of omega-3 fatty acids in patients with implantable cardioverter-defibrillators for life-threatening arrhythmias. There was no effect on recurrences of arrhythmias.

The observational study of survival benefit of adhering to the Mediterranean Diet in Greece was by Trichopoulou et al. (2003). The experimental short-term randomized controlled trial of adding olive oil and nuts to a low-fat diet demonstrated a change in lipid profile that suggested a reduction in risk (Estruch et al. 2006).

Examples of observational cohort studies that demonstrate an inverse relationship between leisure-time physical activity and all-cause and cardiac mortality are the studies by Lakka et al. (1994) and Anderson et al. (2000). These studies are representative of all the observational cohort studies seeking risk factors that are under way around the advanced world. Now you understand why the scare one week may be red meat and next week a study may purport to show that a stake in beef is good for the public health or suggest that pork is a "white meat" and therefore good for your longevity. Epidemiology is not able to discern such subtle health effects in observational studies in a reliable and valid fashion. That's why observational studies suggest antioxidant vitamins are good for your heart but experimental studies find no benefit (Jha et al. 1995).

The four randomized controlled trials of lifestyle interventions I discussed are by Appel et al. (1997), Tuomilehto et al. (2001), the Diabetes Prevention Program Research Group (2002), and the PREMIER trial at eighteen months (Elmer et al. 2006). The first, using the DASH diet, has been expanded to demonstrate that in the setting of a healthful diet, lowering the carbohydrates may be beneficial, though the benefit was tenuous indeed (Appel et al. 2006; M. H. Weinberger 2006). The results from the Women's Health Initiative are more compelling, since the women were not restricted as to baseline diet. However, restricting dietary fats led to modest weight loss (Dansinger and Schaefer 2006) but spared none from invasive breast cancer (Prentice et al. 2006), colorectal cancer (Beresford et al. 2006), or cardiovascular disease (Howard et al. 2006). Many are not willing to give up their true belief (Anderson and Appel 2006).

It's time to admit limitations and call a halt to pseudoscience. In a recent editorial, Davey-Smith and Ebrahim (2002) warn that data dredging, bias, and confounding are tarnishing the credibility of modern epidemiology. Data dredging is the exercise of reworking data analyses until the result fits a preconceived notion. Bias is a systematic error that creeps into the fashion in which the study is conducted. For example, allocating sicker patients to a control group will make the drug being tested seem more effective. Confounding, as we've already discussed, is the influence of unmeasured or immeasurable variables. Data dredging is condemnable; the analysis to be performed must be decided and honed before the study commences. Bias is excusable only if every effort has been made to avoid it. And confounders are, by definition, always lurking. For that reason, only robust results should raise our eyebrows; statistically significant absolute differences greater than 2 or even 3 percent are best published so that they can be ignored. Trumpeting such results in the scientific literature, let alone the lay press, is unacceptable.

If data dredging were not concern enough, the "science" of the benefits and risks of dietary content is not spared being influenced by vested interests. It has been shown that industry-sponsored studies of the benefits of various non-alcoholic beverages are eight times more likely to have favorable results than non-industry-sponsored studies (Lesser et al. 2007).

Chapter 5

The paper that ushered in the scientific era for colorectal cancer screening, the Minnesota Colon Cancer Control Study, was published in 1993 (Mandel et al. 1993) after the cohort had been followed for thirteen years. A second paper was published after eighteen years of observation (Mandel et al. 2000). The result at eighteen years was no different from what I discussed after thirteen years. Both papers speak only of reducing disease-specific mortality, as do all papers in this field. This is missing the forest for the trees, as I discuss in the text. There are other papers examining FOBT as the primary screening modality, nicely reviewed by the Cochrane Collaboration (Towler et al. 1998) and the Canadian Task Force on Preventive Health Care (McLeod et al. 2001). Both miss the forest for the same trees. There's also an entertaining debate on FOBT screening between Jerome B. Simon of Queen's University in Ontario and Robert Fletcher, formerly a colleague of mine at UNC (Simon 1998). Dr. Simon examines the literature with a skepticism that approaches mine; Bob gets it wrong. If one remains wedded to FOBT, realize that a single specimen is not adequate (J. F. Collins et al. 2005) but attention to the details of the method is important (Nadel et al. 2005).

A paper by Lieberman et al. (2001) is an example of a study demonstrating the limited screening efficiency if flexible sigmoidoscopy is the gold standard. Certainly tumors beyond the reach of the flexible sigmoidoscope are elusive. There is a recent study suggesting that one invasive cancer and nine adenomas with high-grade dysplasia would be missed if 1,500 women (half between fifty and sixty years old and the other half older) were screened with flexible sigmoidoscopy rather than colonoscopy (Schoenfeld et al. 2005). The more recent literature has moved the debate to issues of screening colonoscopy rather than flexible sigmoidoscopy. The paper demonstrating futility in individuals younger than fifty is by Imperiale et al. (2002). A paper demonstrating the relative futility of expunging the risk of death from colon cancer in Medicare-age patients was by Gross et al. (2006). The older the patient and the more the comorbidities, the less likely colorectal cancer will play a clinical role in their lives. It is nearly useless in patients over age eighty (Lin et al. 2006) despite their increased prevalence of colorectal cancer. The paper demonstrating that colonoscopists are human and miss lesions was by Rex et al. (1997); they are particularly prone to mistakes if they are in a rush (Barclay et al. 2006). Nonetheless, several studies led to the zeal for colonoscopic screening, particularly the study published in the *New England Journal of Medicine* by Lieberman et al. (2000) with an accompanying editorial by Podolsky (2000).

A cross-sectional analysis of the experience from a large national colonoscopy-based screening program in Poland is illustrative of what can be accomplished (Regula et al. 2006). Some 43,000 individuals between the ages of fifty and sixty-six underwent colonoscopy. This was a voluntary screening program and the volunteers were biased toward a family history of colon cancer, elicited in 13 percent. The authors restrained their analysis to the detection of "advanced neoplasia," or a cancer of adenoma that was at least 1 centimeter in diameter, had high-grade dysplasia, or had a histological architecture that was otherwise abnormal. They detected such neoplasia in the men more than the women. However, they had to screen seventeen men between the ages of fifty and fifty-four to discern one such neoplasm, twelve between the ages of fifty-five and fifty-nine, and ten between the ages of sixty and sixty-six. I don't think you can find an experience demonstrating greater efficiency of screening. Now you have to decide if the screening led to something more important than detection and biopsy. Did it spare anyone from death by colon cancer, or a miserable end of life from colon cancer? No doubt many, many more Americans of Medicare age are now screened, since Medicare decided to reimburse for the procedure, and many more polyps and other neoplasias are discovered (Gross et al. 2006), but there is much doubt as to whether this will advantage these patients (Morris 2006).

In the Polish screening program, the rate of complications was 0.1 percent and no one died. The experience of the Northern California Kaiser Permanente HMO allows a closer examination of this aspect of colonoscopy (Levin et al. 2006). Their experience is based on some 16,000 patients. There were five serious complications per 1,000 colonoscopies (0.5 percent). These complications, mainly perforations and postbiopsy snare bleeding, were most likely to occur with attempts at polypectomy or biopsy, which is why I would have wanted my long-stemmed polyps left alone. There was one death at Kaiser attributed to colonoscopy.

Screening colonoscopy only accounts for the majority of the more than 4 million studies performed in the United States annually. A minority, but a growing minority, is for surveillance, or repeat colonoscopy after polypectomy looking for recurrence. The American Society of Gastrointestinal Endoscopy formulated guidelines that suggest repeating colonoscopy three years after finding a large adenoma and three to five years after a small adenoma; surveillance is not recommended for a hyperplastic polyp. A survey of endoscopists suggests that surveillance is "inappropriately performed and in excess of guidelines." (Mysliwiec et al. 2004). The risk of developing colorectal cancer remains low for more than ten years following a negative colonoscopy (Singh et al. 2006). Nonetheless, Americans tolerate being scheduled for repeat colon checks for no good reason. Maybe now that the $1,000 bill in the cecum is seriously deflated, volume of procedures is compensating.

For further discussions of the risk/benefits of colonoscopic screening, see the comprehensive papers by Ransohoff and Sandler (2002) and the U.S. Preventive Services Task Force (2002). There are several recent attempts at cost-effectiveness analyses. The papers by Frazier et al. (2000), Pignone et al. (2002), and Sonnenberg (2000) are as good as they get, given the need for approximations, suppositions, and guesses. The upshot is that even Ransohoff is wondering if colonoscopy is oversold (2005).

The recommendation of the U.S. Preventive Services Task Force to eschew aspirin (Dubé et al. 2007) and other NSAIDs (Rostom et al. 2007) as a preventative for colon cancer was published in 2007. An analysis of the risk/benefit ratio of low-dose aspirin for primary prevention of coronary heart disease and stroke in men and women over seventy was recently published. Any benefits are offset by the risks (Nelson et al. 2005). In younger women, the offset is slightly more tenuous, though both the benefit (maybe for stroke) and risks are exceedingly small (Mulrow and Pignone 2005). The old saw that fiber intake reduces the risk of colorectal cancer is now debunked (Park et al. 2005). There is a suggestion that statins reduce the risk of colorectal cancer (Poynter et al. 2005), but barely a suggestion. The possibility that "virtual colonoscopy" will diminish the endoscopists' workload is discussed by Lieberman (2004). Given the fact that a goodly number of colonoscopies are "incomplete" because the endoscopists could not visualize the entire colon, it is possible that imaging will prove more sensitive. However, if you see something, you still need colonoscopy for the biopsy.

The New Age has been ushered in with assays for tumor DNA in stool samples and immunochemical testing of stools from neoplastic epitopes (Fraser et al. 2006). Tests of this nature are still too fraught with false negatives to be ready for prime time (Imperiale et al. 2004). Furthermore, the methodological prerequisites for finding the specific needle in the haystack (Ransohoff 2005a) are so demanding as to make one wonder if they will ever be surmounted. Methodological biases were the reason the celebrated proteomics blood assay for ovarian cancer proved spurious (Ransohoff 2005b).

Chapter 6

The twenty-five-year follow-up of the Malmö mammography trial was published by Zackrisson et al. (2006). The discussion of overdiagnosis based on that trial was published by Møller and Davies (2006). We will return to this trial later in the supplementary readings.

For a discussion of medical heuristics, the elegant essay by McDonald (1996) is a good start. As for Oliver Cope, I'd suggest his brief commentary on the education of the physician, "Man, Mind & Medicine" (1968), published near the end of his career. Oliver Cope was one of many innovative surgeons in his generation. But he was a great man because he understood the human context in which he labored. No other surgeon had seen fit to question whether more and more radical surgery served the woman, or just her breast cancer. Few remember Oliver Cope. Many more remember Theodor Billroth, an innovative surgeon of the generation before Cope when medicine in Berlin dominated the world, as did medicine in Boston in Cope's day. Billroth devised surgical procedures for treating peptic ulcers that are largely replaced by advances in pharmacology. So too has time replaced Billroth's advice for educating the physician as to the plight of the patient: "If the whole of Social Medicine must needs be part of the curriculum of the medical student, it must not take more than two hours per semester" (Billroth 1924). Yet Billroth is a name that rolls off the tongue of surgeons around the world. Cope can rest assured.

Bernard Fisher is another celebrated name, still alive and active at the University of Pittsburgh. Shortly after Cope raised the red flag, Fisher put together the National Surgical Adjuvant Breast and Bowel Project. Between 1971 and 1974, Fisher and his collaborators around the country and in Canada recruited 1,765 women with "primary operable breast cancer" to participate in a randomized controlled trial. These were women with a palpable breast mass, a "lump," but no palpable lymph nodes and no metastatic disease detected on chest radiographs or suggested by chemical laboratory studies. The results of this trial were published at ten years (Fisher et al. 1985) and twenty-five years (Fisher et al. 2002a). There were very few relapses after ten years, yet there are very few survivors at twenty-five years. Half of the node-negative patients are "cured" of breast cancer, only to live long enough to die of something else. Seventy percent of the node-positive patients are "cured," likewise to go on to die of something else. The "something" else is termed comorbidities. If you have enough comorbidity, the other diseases will overwhelm breast cancer as a hazard to longevity regardless of the stage of the breast cancer (Satariano and Ragland 1994). The life table analysis of Phillips et al. (1999) places the fearsome malignancy construct into the context of life-course epidemiology.

Fisher et al. followed the mastectomy trial with a trial of lumpectomy versus simple mastectomy. The twenty-year follow-up has been published (Fisher et al. 2002b). Lumpectomy, with or without radiation therapy, is as effective as mastectomy in terms of the impact the disease will have on the longevity of the woman. If the treatment is lumpectomy without radiation therapy, the likelihood of local recurrence is doubled (from about 15 percent in the woman subjected to mastectomy or lumpectomy with radiation). Nonetheless, her likelihood of dying from breast cancer is the same. That is similar to the experience in Italy comparing simple mastectomy with removal of the quadrant of the breast with the tumor followed by radiation therapy (Veronesi et al. 2002).

Of course, all patients with recurrences, and many with positive margins or nodes, were treated to the heuristic of the day: "adjuvant" (jargon for additional therapies that are thought to add to the initial therapy) chemotherapy. If the "adjuvant" of the day was effective, the effectiveness was not contingent on the initial approach to therapy. After all, the likelihood of overall survival is the same as the likelihood of distant disease-free survival at ten years (it's about 70 percent) and at twenty years (50 percent) regardless of the initial treatment. The definition of a "positive" axillary node has evolved since the cohorts were assembled some thirty years ago. By the 1990s, pathologists were applying far more sensitive techniques and finding that 10 to 30 percent of women whose nodes are considered to be negative on the basis of conventional analysis will be found to be node positive (B. L. Smith 2000). Enter the Will Rogers Phenomenon (J. C. Bialar and H. L. Gornik 1997), now applied to staging and its therapeutic implications. Over the course of the past decades, women have become increasingly likely to be treated to adjuvant treatment because tumor cells are detected in their axillary lymph nodes, particularly the so-called sentinel nodes.

The literature on adjuvant medical interventions is extensive. There are multiple trials. Some are designed to recruit thousands of patients for randomization. Whenever I see a trial with thousands of subjects, I bridle. Large trials are deemed necessary if there is great variability in the natural history, or if a small effect is sought. If there is such variability, we need science to teach us how to identify the subsets at most risk and target them in trials. As for the "small but statistically significant" outcome, that's a will-o'-the-wisp. As I discussed in earlier chapters, randomization errors and confounders are too likely for me to buy into the preconceptions of the authors. I also find the trend to more and more toxic interventions disturbing. Metastatic breast cancer is awful and often lethal. However, it is a chronic disease, waxing and waning over years. There is room in the natural history to do more important harm than important good. Furthermore, the heuristic of "killing" the cancer with drugs appears as flawed as the notion of "cutting it out." These malignant cells can resist the onslaught of chemotherapy so toxic as to be lethal were it not for stem-cell transplants to support the patient (Stadtmauer et al. 2000). Even the standard adjuvant chemotherapy is effete in premenopausal women, with a modest 10 percent increase in relapse-free survival at twenty years in premenopausal women (Bonadonna et al. 1995), which translates into a similar improvement in all-cause mortality at thirty years. Unfortunately, postmenopausal women are barely advantaged if at all (Bonadonna et al. 2005). That reflects, in large part, the increased toxicity of chemotherapy in the elderly (Muss et al. 2005) and the prognostic importance of comorbidity (Piccirillo et al. 2004). Considerations of the risk/benefit ratio of adjuvant chemotherapy in the older woman is a demanding exercise that leaves very few candidates for any but the most gentle of regimens, and few for even that (Gradishar and Kaklamani 2005). It is not clear that even radiotherapy adds anything to tamoxifen after lumpectomy (Smith and Ross 2004). Fortunately, the therapeutic horizon for adjuvant chemotherapy has moved away from "killing" cancers to rendering their biology less malignant. The heuristic is lagging.

There have been recent reviews of the spectrum of benign breast disorders (Santen and Mansel 2005; Arpino et al. 2005). There are many changes that occur in the normal breast with aging that have no significance but to confound all attempts to find the early malignancy. There is a suggestion that any lesion manifesting increased cell division, albeit short of the degree of cellular abnormality or degree of invasiveness that would signify malignant change, marks the breast as having malignant potential somewhere (Hartmann et al. 2005). However, this malignant potential is so small, if it is real, that communicating the level of risk to the patient approaches the surreal (Elmore and Gigerenzer 2005). Women in general tend to overestimate the risk of breast cancer, thanks to medicalization, well-intentioned or not. Explaining risk calculations leaves women feeling relieved and more likely to avoid further screening (Fagerlin et al. 2005). One risk that is seldom discussed is the psychological consequence of learning one has early breast cancer. A year of anxiety and/or depression is likely to follow (Burgess et al. 2005). That's all the more reason to be certain that the diagnosis leads to interventions that are beneficial.

It turns out that the public-awareness programs for cancer screening have been far more effective in provoking enthusiasm than reason. Americans are willing to undergo screening without regard to efficiency of the tests or the likelihood that they will lead to unnecessary treatment (Schwartz et al. 2004). America is ripe for any half-baked scheme and ready to either pay or demand indemnity. Witness the epidemic of skin biopsies. The public-health agenda has made Americans aware that sun exposure is leading to an "epidemic" of skin cancers. In fact, the incidence of melanoma of the skin is said to be rising faster than any other major cancer. People are monitoring their skin for the unfamiliar. Physicians are collaborating and dermatologists are accommodating by performing a biopsy whenever there is any doubt. Dermatopathologists can be shown to be less reliable the earlier and more subtle the lesion. The result is that there is an epidemic of the diagnosis of melanoma but not of disease-specific mortality. The inescapable conclusion is that the disease is being vastly overdiagnosed (Welch et al. 2005).

The study of the interobserver reliability of mammography was by J. G. Elmore et al. (1994), as was the study of false positive rates (J. G. Elmore et al. 1998). When the mammography establishment decided to compare digital versus film mammography (Pisano et al. 2005), they spared no expense. Over 40,000 women underwent both studies at thirty-three participating sites. The outcome was determined 455 days later, allowing the various clinical algorithms to play out in terms of repeat studies and biopsies. The experience is an object lesson. The finding of cancer was concordant for the two techniques for about 200 women; nearly 2,000 were found to be "positive" by only one technique, split evenly between the alternatives. Of the 200 women deemed positive by both, eighty-five were diagnosed with an invasive cancer and thirty-six with DCIS by 455 days following the study. Of the 1,000 positive only by film mammography, thirty-five had invasive carcinoma and seventeen DCIS. Of the 1,000 positive only by digital mammography, thirty-eight had invasive carcinoma and twenty-five DCIS. And of those negative by both techniques (nearly 40,000), seventy-three were found to have an invasive carcinoma and twenty-five DCIS. These are the "raw" data. Try as they did, the research statisticians could not demonstrate that digitizing the image improved detection for the group as a whole or the women over age fifty. Of course for every cancer detected, many women had negative biopsies. Many cancers went undetected, even a number that made their presence known in the next year or so. And, as we'll see, many of the "cancers" that were detected bode little of importance, particularly for the older women. There were about 10,000 premenopausal women in the study. Of course, they had far fewer positive studies and developed far fewer cancers. This underlies the differential in predictive value that allowed the authors to suggest that digital mammography was an advance for screening young women. It is, but it's trivial.

The comparison in recall and biopsy rates between the United States and the United Kingdom was by Smith-Bindman et al. (2003). The study probing the psychological price paid by these screened women was earlier (C. Lerman et al. 1991). There are more recent papers (Sharp et al. 2003) documenting the discomfort, even pain, associated with mammography as well as the long-term adverse effects of a false-positive reading (Brewer et al. 2007). A false-positive result increases anxiety, increases self-examining, and tends to render another mammogram less appealing. Thurfjell (2002) provides a brief discussion of the influence of breast density on mammographic accuracy. Similar conclusions resulted from an analysis of the Million Women Study (Banks et al. 2004). The paper by Boyd et al. (2002) demonstrates that breast density is a familial trait.

The literature on DCIS is somewhat muddled by the preconceptions and beliefs of the various authors. Finding DCIS and resecting DCIS and irradiating DCIS are enormous industries in the United States. Furthermore, the mandate to have adequate margins may lead to offers of mastectomy with breast reconstruction on cosmetic grounds. The emotionality of the prose seems to vary if the authors are surgeons or pathologists or oncologists. Here's a sampling that substantiates all my assertions, if you are willing to read with an open mind: Morrow and Schnitt (2000), Page and Simpson (1999), Lerner (1998), Fonseca et al. (1997), and Page and Jensen (1996). Burstein et al. (2004) offer an uninspired "standard of care" update.

The results of the Canadian National Breast Screening Study for the stratum that was forty to forty-nine years old at inception of the cohort were published after a mean follow-up of 8.5 years (Miller et al. 1992a) and after eleven to sixteen years of follow-up (Miller et al. 2002). The results for the fifty to fifty-nine stratum were published after 8.3 years (Miller et al. 1992b) and thirteen years (Miller et al. 2000). No trial of this size and duration can be perfectly executed. There will always be dropouts, patients who miss screenings, lost data points, and the like. However the Canadian study is as close to perfect as such a trial can be (Baines 1994).

The commentary by Woolf and Lawrence (1997) on the politics that swirled around the 1997 NIH "consensus conference" offers more than an insight into the advocacy for screening mammography in the United States; it offers an accessible analysis of the fashion in which political debate can distort scientific debate. Schwartz and Woloshin (2002) performed the analysis of the response of the news media to the controversy. None of the relevant science escaped the deliberations of the U.S. Preventive Services Task Force (Humphrey et al. 2002), particularly since Woolf was one of the principal participants. Nonetheless, the best the U.S. Preventive Services Task Force could manage in 2002 was a compromise posture, based on "fair evidence" for mammographic screening "every 1 to 2 years for women aged 40 and older." To conclude that the evidence was "fair" required accepting the results of lesser studies to temper the inferences derived from the randomized controlled trials. The American College of Physicians has revisited these and more recent studies (Armstrong et al. 2007; Qaseem et al. 2007) to reach a much more definitive conclusion. The risk/benefit ratio favors informed consent before screening in this age group. Schwartz and Woloshin (2007) revisited this analysis and extended it to reach a similar conclusion for older women.

The Nordic Cochrane review of the literature on screening mammography (Gøetzsche and Olsen 2000; Olsen and Gøetzsche 2001) found, as I do, that the Canadian and Malmö randomized controlled trials are by far the most telling of the available science on methodological grounds. Unlike the U.S. Preventive Services Task Force, the Nordic Cochrane analysis was based only on the Canadian and Malmö trials. Unlike the task force, the Nordic Cochrane review concludes that screening mammography offers women of any age little but an increased likelihood of more aggressive treatment.

The randomized controlled trial is the best way we have for testing whether any given exposure (for example, screening mammography) is not associated with any given health effect (such as less deaths from breast cancer). If there is an association, one can only hope it is real. If there is no association, one can hope that the study design was powerful enough so that an important association was not missed. As I've said repeatedly in earlier chapters, I am always skeptical when the trial is designed so that thousands of subjects were randomized and followed for great periods of time. The only justification for such a large trial is that the health effect is so infrequent and/or variable that a smaller, briefer trial would detect too few outcomes to allow meaningful inferences. True. However, that does not mean that the differences detected (or not) in the larger, longer trial can be assumed to reflect only the exposure. A small discrepancy in the allocation of subjects (for example, more in one group have metastasizing tumors by happenstance) can fool you into thinking the exposure was the explanation. That's called randomization error. It can only be avoided if all the important variables can be measured and considered in the allocation or the analysis. In small trials probing a robust health effect, randomization errors from "minor" influences are less important. However, in large trials seeking tiny effects, randomization errors can never be avoided. The very fact that the Canadian and Swedish investigators felt compelled to design trials with tens of thousands of subjects followed for decades says to me that the health effect they target is too small to measure and too small to be meaningful. I don't think such trials should ever be done. They are not necessary.

However, that's heresy. Most leading epidemiologists and statisticians revel in these large randomized controlled trials. They do not think they are inherently flawed, as I do. But they are aware that they are subject to confounding, to the influence of variables they did not think to measure or could not measure that can mollify the exposure on one group more than another.

Enter Olli Miettinen. Miettinen has no quarrel with the undertaking of the large and lengthy randomized controlled trials of screening mammography. He also has no quarrel with the interpretation of the Nordic Cochrane collaborators who accepted the data analysis offered by the investigators. His quarrel is with that analysis. He makes his point, using the Malmö study data set, in a series of papers (Miettinen et al. 2002a, 2002b, 2002c). He argues that the analysis by the investigators obscured an important and meaningful advantage accrued to older women thanks to screening mammography. Miettinen reasons that the supposition underlying screening for early disease detection is that the treatment of disease detected earlier is more likely to cure the disease than treatment started later in unscreened patients. Based on that precept, he reanalyzed the Malmö data to compare deaths in screened and unscreened women over age fifty-five by year since entry to the trial. He can demonstrate no decrease in the likelihood of death from breast cancer until two decades had passed. Then there is a statistically significant 50 percent decrease in deaths in the women who were screened two decades earlier compared to the women who were never screened.

Interesting? Yes, interesting, but not as clinically meaningful to my eye as to Miettinen's. The Malmö study recruited 42,000 women between 1976 and 1978, allocating half to biannual screening and offering screening to the controls after fourteen years. Over the course of follow-up, there were sixty-three deaths ascribed to breast cancer in the screened group and sixty-six in the control. Miettinen's secondary analysis is based on the women who were fifty-five at inception and spared comorbidities, so they were still at risk for a "breast cancer death" twenty years later. If the Canadian life table (see chapter text) generalizes to Sweden, Miettinen's data would suggest the following. Let's assume that half the Malmö cohort was fifty-five or older at inception. Of these, about 4,000 would be alive in the screened cohort and 4,000 would be alive in the control cohort twenty years after inception, and all would be seventy-five or older. About 2,000 deaths will occur in the next ten years in each the control and screened cohorts. However, more of the sixty-six breast cancer deaths that were the fate of women in the control group would have already occurred, whereas more of the sixty-three deaths that were to carry away women in the screened group have yet to occur.

If I am generous, and I grant Miettinen all the assumptions he has taken, I am still left with the impression that this is an outcome that hardly justifies all the screening, let alone all the unnecessary aggressive treatment. We need to relegate mammography as practiced to the archives. Clearly it offers too little; on that point there is little debate (Sox 2002; Goodman 2002; Fletcher and Elmore 2003).

To be charitable and complete, I have raised the issue of efficacy versus effectiveness. The efficacy of screening mammography is marginal at best. However, maybe in practice it is more effective. Maybe there are features of the way it is used that have yet to be defined but are important. Hence, I mentioned the modeling of the BreastScreen Australia data (Barrat et al. 2005; Taylor 2005), which said the benefit/risk ratio of screening mammography was too close to call. There are other ecological experiences. Epidemiologists in Denmark, Norway, and Sweden have examined the effectiveness of the introduction of screening mammography into the public-health agendas of their countries or portions of their countries.

Mammography was introduced for ages fifty to sixty-nine in Norway in 1996 and Sweden in 1986 (Zahl et al. 2004). In Norway and Sweden there was an increase in the diagnosis of breast cancer by some 50 percent in women aged fifty to sixty-nine, but no corresponding decline in incidence after age sixty-nine. The inescapable conclusion is that without screening, one-third of all invasive breast cancers in this age group would have been missed in their lifetime, and it wouldn't have mattered. That's called overdiagnosis. In Denmark, screening was introduced by region. It arrived in Copenhagen and two other administrative regions in 1991 (Olsen et al. 2005). Prior to screening, Copenhagen had higher breast cancer mortality than the rest of the countries for reasons that are not clear. However, that incidence did not increase with screening; to the contrary it was reduced by 25 percent. Furthermore, "owing to a deliberately conservative attitude towards supposedly benign microcalcifications," the incidence of DCIS was only 11 percent of detected cases. The Danes have avoided some of the pitfalls. However, there was little impact on all-cause mortality.

The controversy speaks to the fact that if there is benefit to screening mammography, it is minimal. The U.S. Preventive Services Task Force (Mandelblatt et al. 2003) thinks that the cost of screening justifies the program in women after age sixty-five. They have been looking at the same data we have been pondering. So have the British. The spokesperson for the consultant breast surgeons thinks it's worthwhile (Dixon 2006). British epidemiologists (Irwig et al. 2006), echoing the Nordic Cochrane Centre investigators (Jørgensen et al. 2006), think it's so marginal that women need to be forewarned and required to offer informed consent.

I think it's time to move on.

Chapter 7

The survey of physicians as to whether they had submitted to PSA screening was published by Chan et al. (2005). I am aware of no similar physician survey regarding cholesterol or other screening programs, but I suspect that compliance would be comparable. The Veterans Administration case-control study was published by Concato et al. (2006) and the Canadian case-control study by Kopec et al. (2005).

Eastham et al. (2003) have evaluated the fluctuations in PSA that contribute to its lack of specificity as a screening tool. The transient elevations can reflect inflammation, trauma, and other biological variables. Many men needed a negative biopsy to be certain the elevated PSA was "false." They are relieved, no doubt, but not totally relieved, as they pay a price in persistent worry (McNaughton-Collins et al. 2004). False positives aside, the data speaks to a continuum of PSA levels that correlates with tumor burden. One would predict that there are many men with prostate cancer in situ yet a normal PSA. The Prostate Cancer Prevention Trial enrolled nearly 20,000 men age sixty-two to ninety-one in a randomized controlled trial of a drug that is used for prostatism. Of the half on placebo, nearly 3,000 never had a PSA greater than 4 ng/ml and still underwent prostate biopsy seven years into the trial. Prostate cancer was diagnosed in 15 percent (Thompson et al. 2004). Given the sampling error involved in needle biopsy, the true prevalence of prostate cancer was much, much higher in men. However, given the implications of a normal PSA regarding tumor load and even tumor aggressiveness, neither I nor Carter (2004) can countenance seeking prostate cancer in men with normal or near normal PSAs, regardless of their age. There is data to suggest that the rate of rise of PSA reflects the risk of fatal disease (D'Amico et al. 2004). So if one is faced with an elevated PSA in a young man where there is some suggestion that radical prostatectomy might be lifesaving, repeat PSA levels over time might offer some insight as to which patient might be the more appropriate surgical candidate.

The Scandinavian randomized controlled trial was first published as companion papers in the fall of 2002 (Holmberg et al. 2002; Steineck et al. 2002); the results at ten years followed (Bill-Axelson et al. 2005). Sox (2005) offers an interesting take on this trial. The cohort studies defining the natural history of early prostate cancer were from Connecticut (Albertson et al. 2005) and Sweden (Johansson et al. 2004). When both cohorts were assembled, there were no PSA screening programs. Disease was detected at the time of surgery for prostatism or if a nodule was palpated and then biopsied. That was largely true of the Scandinavian randomized trial. Today, the screening programs are ensnaring many more perfectly well men, many of them younger. The "natural history" of watchful waiting will be perturbed in cohorts defined so differently. This is termed "lead-time bias." It almost certainly will render the PSA even less predictive of an untoward outcome.

The ecological study of the Seattle and Connecticut Medicare cohorts was by Lu-Yao et al. (2002). An editorial by Patrick Walsh accompanied the Scandinavian experiment (Walsh 2002). Walsh, a urologist on the Johns Hopkins faculty, pioneered a "nerve-sparing" prostatectomy that reduced the dismal complication rate of earlier approaches and drove the procedure to the forefront of options. His quarrel with the Scandinavian trial is that "nerve-sparing" was not routine, and that patients older than sixty-five are the most likely to have complications. However, the incidence of complications in the Scandinavian study is well within the range of the recent published experience with the "nerve-sparing" approach. An analysis of a population-based cohort of American men diagnosed with clinically localized prostate cancer at age seventy-five to eighty-four who underwent radical prostatectomy reiterates the Scandinavian result: the absolute risk of dying from prostate cancer was minimally reduced if at all (Hoffman et al. 2006).

Walsh's argument for screening younger men for nonpalpable PSA-positive disease seems shallow. All he is advocating is watchful waiting. In that case, the screening is meddlesome. The other pioneering prostate surgeon, William Catalona, argues for screening at age forty so that young men with rapidly escalating PSA levels would be identified (Catalona et al. 2006). However, such individuals are exceedingly rare, whereas false positives are a great deal more common. Such an approach will turn many healthy men into patients with no demonstrable yield. That was the conclusion of the British survey of the attitudes of men with positive screening tests (Chapple et al. 2002) and of an editorial that accompanied that survey (Thornton and Dixon-Woods 2002) calling for "stronger and braver governance . . . to ensure that responsible decisions about risk management emerge for areas such as screening, which have such potentially enormous individual and societal consequences." It is a perspective that is argued eloquently in an essay by Ransohoff, Collins, and Fowler (2002), calling for informing the public to such an extent that the common sense is to approach recommendations with a critical eye.

That's no mean task. The literature relating to screening for prostate cancer is voluminous, contentious, and difficult. Many an august body has taken on the task of basing recommendations on its analysis. The recommendations are a cacophony (Vastag 2002): the American Academy of Family Physicians recommends counseling men over fifty, the American Cancer Society recommends annual PSA testing for men over fifty, the American College of Physicians recommends individualized decision making, the AMA calls mass screening "premature," the Canadian Task Force on Preventive Health Care found "fair evidence" for screening, and Medicare includes annual screening as a standard benefit. In 2002 the U.S. Preventive Services Task Force waffled on its 1996 recommendation against screening, stating that "the net benefit of screening cannot be determined" (Harris and Lohr 2002). Fortunately, others are willing to join me in decrying screening in the elderly or in men with multiple co-morbidities (Hoffman 2006; Litwin and Miller 2006; Albertsen 2006). Maybe the Veterans Administration will climb on board instead of repeating their screening practices of the 1990s, when half the elderly vets had PSAs (Walter et al. 2006).

The upshot is that no one should have a PSA screen without a discussion as to how a "positive" result will affect clinical decisions. If the trade-off between the benefits and the risks are unappealing a priori, why do the test? Unfortunately, there is no substitute for an interchange with a wise counselor, usually a physician. The publicly available patient-education material regarding early-stage prostate cancer was recently surveyed and found to be woefully lacking about the risks and benefits of treatment (Fagerlin et al. 2004).

Chapter 8

I highly recommend Gadamer's *The Enigma of Health: The Art of Healing in a Scientific Age* (Gadamer 1996). These essays are Gadamer's only foray into the topic that occupies us. I have often wished he had turned his extraordinary intellect in this direction again and again. He might have done so much more than knock at the door. Then again, he would have given short shrift to so many other areas of thought that benefited from his enlightenment. The lengthy quote is from page 107 of *The Enigma of Health.*

In 1979 and again early in this decade (Smith 2002), the *British Medical Journal (BMJ)* undertook a quasi-scientific poll as to the "top 10 non-diseases" from a lengthy listing. In 1979 all those polled thought of malaria and tuberculosis as diseases, but physicians were far more likely to consider senility, a skull fracture, heatstroke, tennis elbow, malnutrition, or drug overdose a disease than nonphysicians, including high school students. All were split fifty-fifty on whether hypertension, acne, or gall stones were diseases. For the second poll, the editors offered up a list of 300 labels that they considered nondiseases and asked the readership to vote for the labels that designated the most "non-diseaseness." The editors also categorized the labels: some were considered misattribution, such as anxiety about size, flat feet, and multiple chemical sensitivities; some were universal changes, such as aging, loneliness, and menopause; some were usual responses, such as borborygmi, stretch marks, bereavement, and pregnancy; and some were variants of normal, such as big ears, baldness, conduct disorders in childhood, and ear wax. Of all these, the top ten were aging, work, boredom, bags under eyes, ignorance, baldness, freckles, big ears, gray hair, and ugliness. More interesting than the list was the heated debate about entries and omissions. Gadamer was correct: if the condition doesn't objectify itself, one is hard pressed to consider it a disease and is likely to do the patient a disservice by labeling it so (Meador 1965). But aging is acquired and objectifies itself in many ways, from graying to weakened bones. Are aging, graying, and weakened bones disease states? Chapter 11 is devoted to this query.

I have long taught medical students that one of the most dangerous acts a physician undertakes is to take a history from a patient. We have no choice but to do so. After all, seldom can we consider a diagnosis, let alone a diagnosis-appropriate treatment, until we discern the "chief complaint" in the patient's narrative of illness. Much of the art of medicine is in the listening to the response to our serial queries. The structure and direction of the dialogue is determined by the physician's interpretation of each response. It is a complex interaction that assumes that the physician and the patient have semantics in common and that demands recognition of preconceived notions on the part of both participants. It is an exercise in semiotics. Both parties are changed by the experience — the physician in the context of the particular patient and the patient forever. The fact that the patient will be changed forever places a heavy responsibility on the physician to assure that the change advantages the patient in the long run. It will not in the short run. The questions probe for clues by forcing the patient to view personal experiences as potential symptoms of disease. All patients have had morbid experiences, often repeatedly, for which they had not thought to seek medical attention and for which medical attention was not necessary. The "history" taking will highlight these experiences to render them more telling and probably more memorable. I teach that we must take a history, but we must learn to "un-take it" by pointing out which symptoms are of no concern. Otherwise, we will surely medicalize the patient.

Medicalization is an important concept. Predictably, it has been overused and misused and become hackneyed. Such is the fate of several of the sentinel ideas discussed in this volume; "paradigm shift" and "evidence-based medicine" are examples of the hackneyed, and "refutationist" is a candidate. The concepts remain important nonetheless. Medicalization is useful, despite its negative connotation, to denote the crossing of boundaries that society had considered or still considers the purview of medicine. It is useful in critiquing pharmaceutical marketing practice, particularly direct-to-consumer marketing, for example (Metzl 2007). The fact that medicine, more than ever, has become part of the fabric of day-to-day living renders medicalization a fact of daily life with political and philosophical implications beyond those that are clinical (Tomes 2007).

The concept of medicalization is part of the legacy of Ivan Illich. Illich was born in Vienna in 1926 and died in Bremen in 2002. His father was Croatian and Roman Catholic; his mother was a Sephardic Jew. He had a secular education in Florence and went on to the Pontifical Gregorian University in the Vatican to be ordained as a priest. There followed a twenty-year career as polyglot cleric, educator, and social activist in Mexico, Puerto Rico (vice rector of the Catholic University of Puerto Rico), and with the immigrant Puerto Rican community in New York City. By the mid-1960s, Illich had evolved into an outspoken reactionary whose philosophy ran so counter to the Church that he left the priesthood in 1968 and spent the remainder of his career as a peripatetic intellectual and academic. He came to believe that all institutions of the industrial hegemony, communist or capitalist, had destructive potential. He saw much of value in a preindustrial society and launched into a career making that argument about organized religion, institutionalized education, and medicine. His influence peaked in the 1970s with the publication of *Deschooling Society* (1971) and *Medical Nemesis: The Expropriation of Health* (1975). Both remain interesting reading today, somewhat prescient, though neither is without serious flaws. In *Medical Nemesis*, Illich argues that the medical enterprise is often more harmful to humanity than helpful, often imperialistic, and given to promulgating unrealistic expectations — that is, medicalization. "The medical establishment has become a major threat to health," he states. Beyond many flaws as a philosopher and some as a man, Illich was a fascinating and erudite scholar. I'd recommend the collection of interviews Cayley (1992) did for Canadian Broadcasting's Ideas Program for an appreciation of Illich's scope, along with *Medical Nemesis* itself (Illich 1976). Illich spent his last decade avoiding medical treatment for a disfiguring facial neoplasm, opting for folk remedies and opium.

I obviously have some degree of ambivalence about Illich and his legacy. I have none about Lynn Payer or her legacy. Lynn was a brilliant medical journalist. We became pen pals about the time she published *Medicine & Culture: Varieties of Treatment in the United States, England, West Germany, and France* (Payer 1988). This little monograph is a classic and a gem. It is an analysis of the fashion in which several particular diseases are conceptualized differently by patients and doctors in the United States, England, West Germany, and France. This was a time in my career when I was busy dissecting the fashion in which legal tenets influence clinical judgment in these countries and many more (using disability as my focus and the World Health Organization for my funding). Our transnational interests obviously overlapped, but our philosophical bent overlapped even more. Both of us were interested in what it means to be a well person and the influence of sociopolitical context on this station in life.

Lynn pursued this as only a brilliant journalist can, finding the wheat in the chaff of opinions. She coined the term "Disease Mongers" for the title of the book that resulted (Payer 1992). I was privileged to review drafts for her and provide lengthy discussions of my research that was relevant to her thesis. Lynn Payer died at age fifty-six of breast cancer in 2001. We are all deprived of a truly remarkable and precious person. "Disease mongers" is part of her legacy — the rubric and the book that tackled such issues as unnecessary surgery, excessive testing, and the "Lyme hysteria," as well as the excesses of the drug companies and why medicine's approach to saving women from breast cancer was an unconscionable overreach.. I highly recommend *Disease Mongers* as a template for print and media medical journalists. Shannon Brownlee needed no such template. Her *Overtreated: Why Too Much Medicine Is Making Us Sicker and Poorer* (2007) picks up where Payer left off and does so brilliantly.

Lynn left me with memories and lessons, lessons that relate to the difficult task faced by journalists attempting to make sense of "health care" in the United States. They all face enormous constraints. Some relate to the social construction of health (about which we will have much more to say in chapter 13). Some reflect the soft underbelly of our capitalistic society. As I discuss in chapter 9 and elsewhere, direct-to-consumer advertising transfers billions of dollars of pharmaceutical profits to print and broadcast media companies. There is an inherent conflict of interest in this arrangement. Without imputing malfeasance, it behooves the media companies to look askance, or choose other topics of interest, or practice circumlocution when it comes to being critical of the products of their advertisers. I believe that this is a subliminal dialectic most of the time. However, it need not be so subliminal. For example, a number of years ago I was honored by an invitation to sit on the editorial board of the *Annals of Internal Medicine*, the journal of the American College of Physicians, which is distributed twice monthly to more than 100,000 subscribers and is the premier journal in internal medicine. We received a paper that we sent out for peer review; it passed muster and was published (Wilkes et al. 1992). It was a simple study in which the authors took an inventory of the pharmaceutical advertisements from several of the premier journals. All these journals are cash cows because they are primary conduits for medical marketing, pharmaceutical marketing in particular. None do much screening of advertisements, particularly if the advertisements are for licensed drugs, since that content is constrained by FDA regulations. In the paper, the advertisements were sorted by topic (infectious-disease drugs, arthritis drugs, etc.) and "thought leaders" were asked to score the validity of the selling points. The advertisements proved disappointing in that regard. The consequences of this publication were considerable, not the least of which was the fact that pharmaceutical revenues of the *Annals of Internal Medicine* dipped dramatically and the editors-in-chief found reason to seek alternative employment.

Given that such forces operate at some level in the print and broadcast media, it is no wonder that many successful investigative reporters shy away from biting the hands that feed them. But some are willing to learn and test these waters. I've been privileged to interact with a number of journalists over the past decade and to watch the gentle evolution of their approach to issues in medicalization and disease mongering. Lynn Payer set the precedent. The likes of Gina Kolata of the *New York Times*, John Carey of *BusinessWeek*, and freelancers such as Susan Dominus, Betsy Agnvall, and Paula Dranov are all notable for their willingness to see, to learn, and to speak out. Reporters at National Public Radio are also at this forefront; individuals such as Gail Harris and Frank Stasio are blessed by fewer constraints on their choice of topics.

In my introduction to this chapter, I offered a litany of experiences that are all too often medicalized, including heartburn and heartache. It is not my style to tackle a topic of clinical importance in a fashion that is less than comprehensive. I will ask for an indulgence regarding the following disorders, which are begging the treatment I am wielding in each chapter. These are affective disorders that are not predicaments of everyday life — mood disorders that afflict without reason, often afflict multiple members of families, and are amenable to pharmaceutical interventions. The last assertion is bolstered by randomized controlled trials, most double blind, which convince the FDA for licensing and the clinical community for prescribing. Fortunately, there are relatively few people who are the victims of these primary affective disorders, and fortunately, as well, the pharmaceutical industry has been inventive on their behalf. However, these afflicted individuals are not the "market." All of us will suffer transient depressive moods, usually for good reason (grief, loss, disappointments, and the like). "All of us" is the market that drives pharmaceutical profitability. However, it is all too clear that these drugs offer more likelihood of toxicity than of benefit for secondary depressions (Lucire 2005). Furthermore, the existence and marketing of antidepressants serves to medicalize these unpleasant, challenging, but unavoidable predicaments to the extent that "mental illness" in America has become nearly epidemic (Whitaker 2005). I could cite many other authors on this topic. Lucire and Whitaker are among my favorites. I recommend also their monographs (Lucire 2003; Whitaker 2002).

Chapter 9

As I mentioned in the text, the supporting literature is particularly rich, voluminous, and compelling. There is a reason. The regional musculoskeletal disorders are the rubric under which much of the expense in workers' compensation and other disability indemnity is cost accounted. In most industrialized countries other than the United States, workers' compensation insurance is a federal benefit, often funded from general tax revenues. In the United States, there are fifty-eight jurisdictions that regulate workers' compensation indemnity schemes, most of which mandate that employers provide insurance themselves or purchase it from private-sector purveyors. The number of claims and the cost incurred has been an issue since the middle of the twentieth century in the United States and elsewhere, escalating dramatically since the 1980s largely because of disabling regional low back pain and other regional musculoskeletal disorders. Furthermore, the claims were escalating in spite of the institution of interventions, notably the ergonomic interventions that were touted by ergonomists to be useful.

In 1983 the Quebec Task Force on Spinal Disorders was constituted by the Quebec Workers' Health and Safety Commission to examine this trend. For example, the commission wanted the task force to explain why the trend was not blunted in spite of the continual increase in physiotherapy treatments in Quebec, which had risen to 641,197 by 1982. Dr. Walter O. Spitzer, chairman of the Department of Clinical Epidemiology at McGill University, chaired the task force. Dr. Spitzer assembled representatives from many of the relevant clinical disciplines, many of whom stayed on board for what was to be a pioneering, though politically truculent, exercise. Dr. Spitzer charged the group with performing one of the first systematic reviews of the scientific literature relevant to the diagnosis and treatment of neck and low back regional disorders. The exercise requires assembling the world's literature and sorting it by quality. Well-done randomized controlled trials were considered most persuasive. Uncontrolled but structured descriptive studies and literature reviews were given little weight, and anecdotal reports were not considered. Of some 4,000 studies considered, 469 were rated as informative. The analysis was published as the first supplement to *Spine* (Spitzer et al. 1987). Its message resounded around the industrialized world. Almost nothing in the diagnostic and therapeutic armamentarium was on firm scientific footing. Several procedures and interventions had been shown to be useless or harmful. The document stood as a reproach to the professions and a clarion call for science of higher quality and reform of the approach to medical indemnity.

The document stands, to this day, as a template for similar exercises in other fields, as well as for similar exercises and updated exercises for the regional musculoskeletal disorders. The most influential of the updates was initiated by the U.S. Department of Health and Human Services nearly a decade later, when Congress funded the Agency for Health Care Policy and Research (AHCPR) to examine the effectiveness and cost-effectiveness of health care delivered under the Medicare program, a national health insurance scheme for retired and disabled workers. A panel was constituted, chaired by Dr. Stanley Bigos and charged with developing an evidence-based "Clinical Practice Guideline" for "Acute Low Back Problems in Adults." Another 4,000 articles, published after the Quebec review, were considered and about 10 percent deemed informative. After a couple of years of effort (I served as consultant to this panel), the guideline was published (Bigos et al. 1994). It reached conclusions very similar to those of the Quebec Task Force a decade earlier.

The fate of the AHCPR Back Pain Guideline and the AHCPR guideline program speaks volumes about the result of speaking the truth to controlling powers in the clinical context. The North American Spine Society (NASS) has a membership comprised largely of practicing spine surgeons. NASS had contracted epidemiologists to perform an assessment of the literature in parallel to the AHCPR exercise, which arrived at contrary conclusions. Armed with their document, the leadership of NASS approached Congress, with the result that the AHCPR guidelines program was rendered defunct along with the AHCPR. It was to be reborn as the Agency for Healthcare Research and Quality (AHRQ), funding studies of the quality and distribution of services but less of their effectiveness and nothing about practice guidelines.

Since then, nearly every industrial country has chimed in with their version, many the product of a task force assembled by a professional organization. Notable is New Zealand's, first appearing in 1999 (‹http://www.rcgp.org.uk›), which specifically addressed diagnostic and therapeutic issues that relate to the psychosocial confounders to coping. Today there is an academic industry generating systematic reviews and promulgating evidence-based clinical guidelines. The Cochrane Library (‹http://www.updateusa.com/cochrane.htm›) is spearheading the international effort to produce and update systematic reviews; nearly fifty collaborative review panels have been recruited to the effort, including a back pain panel. I applaud the exercise, though it is not without serious drawbacks. The documents that relate to the regional musculoskeletal disorders illustrate both the benefits of consigning the reading of literature to someone else—a committee no less—and the drawbacks. They are remarkably consistent, though not entirely so. But the consistency probably reflects common denominators in the evaluative process that predispose to particular conclusions. First, the approach to measuring the quality of trials is not uniform and, more importantly, may not be uniformly valid (Berlin and Rennie 1999). For example, there is little evidence that the results of well-done observational studies and well-done randomized controlled trials differ much in measuring treatment effects (Benson and Hartz 2000), yet whenever they do, most quality scales will favor the randomized controlled trial. Some of the scales have subscales; for example, one measures the quality of the randomized controlled trials based on details of their design and data analysis. Assumptions about and misinterpretations of the published methodologies can result in invalid scores and invalid weightings. And then there are all the value judgments that play out in these panels and task forces as to the interpretation of treatment effects or lack thereof. In many of the earlier chapters, I explained why I am skeptical of and unconvinced by tiny (less than 2 percent) effects, even if they are discerned in elegant randomized controlled trials (I return to this argument at length in chapter 14). Yet, tiny effects are the rule in these exercises. *If there were major consistent effects, there would be no need for systematic reviews or meta-analyses!* Statistically significant tiny effects discerned in elegant trials tend to sway the methodologists who populate review panels much more than they sway me—or most clinicians who much prefer maintaining the autonomy of their clinical judgments (Nolan 1994; Sox 1994). Finally, guidelines are more effective in informing as to the existence of debate than in swaying the preferences of patients (Hlatky 1995; Katz 2001).

Having said all this, I am going to take advantage of recent systematic reviews in referencing chapter 9. Each provides a plethora of references should the reader choose to undertake their own review. And each offers conclusions that are fully consonant with my assertions in the text. Furthermore, the third edition of my monograph *Occupational Musculoskeletal Disorders* (Hadler 2005) offers any reader a wealth of information relevant to this chapter and to chapter 12. To start, there is precious little evidence that there is anything we can do to prevent our next regional backache or predicament of neck pain (Linton and van Tulder 2001). However, there is a wealth of evidence that psychosocial factors confound our ability to cope with the predicament (Hoogendoorn et al. 2000; Linton 2000) or to heal should we choose to be a patient (Pincus et al. 2002). Recent studies from Manchester (Harkness et al. 2003), London (Head et al. 2006), Leiden (Lötters et al. 2006), Helsinki (Kaila-Kangas et al. 2004), and Copenhagen (Nielsen et al. 2006) bolster this inference. This has long been my teaching (Hadler 1994) and is now that of others (Main and Williams 2002; Hagen et al. 2006). Psychosocial confounders are also a leading reason people with the predicaments of regional shoulder (Babcock et al. 2002; Diepenmaat et al. 2006), neck (Bot et al. 2005), or knee (Hadler 1992; Brandt et al. 2000; Mitchell et al. 2006) pain seek assistance with their predicaments. The challenge for the future is to understand the therapeutic ramifications of this insight; current approaches are disappointing (Jellema et al. 2005). Maybe it will require a media campaign (Buchbinder et al. 2005) to assault the semiotic of back pain (Hadler 2004) before reason can drive the patient-physician dialogue.

There are many systematic reviews of interventions for the regional musculoskeletal disorders. Hoving et al. (2001) document the dearth of informative studies for the conservative treatment of regional neck pain. But there is no dearth of informative studies for the treatment of backache and no dearth of systematic reviews. Some reviews attempt to encompass the entire menu of interventions (van Tulder et al. 1997) for acute and chronic regional low back pain. Others take on particular modalities: injection therapy (Nelemans et al. 2001), transcutaneous electrical nerve stimulation (Brosseau et al. 2002), specific exercise therapy (van Tulder et al. 2000), massage (Furlan et al. 2002), and the advice to stay active in spite of the backache (Hagen 2002). There is a systematic review that supports my contention that no newer nonsteroidal anti-inflammatory drug is more effective than aspirin for low back pain (van Tulder et al. 2000b) and another that found surgery perhaps helpful for sciatica but not for low back pain (Gibson et al. 1999). Even for chronic low back pain, rehabilitation trumps surgical stabilization (Rivero-Arias et al. 2005). Spinal fusion surgery has only modest, if any, effects over the natural history (Koes 2005), even for sciatica (Weinstein et al. 2006a). The explanation for the everescalating performance of fusion surgery in the United States (Weinstein et al. 2006b) cannot be clinical indications or outcomes (Deyo et al. 2005). The explanation for the latest in inventive technology, the so-called artificial disc, is our unconscionable regulatory climate for "devices." As I've made clear, the safety bar at the FDA is vastly lower for devices than for pharmaceuticals. There are trials that suggest that these bizarre pieces of hardware are as ineffective as fusion despite serving the latest theory; preserving "motion" of spinal segments is better for you in the long run than eliminating motion by fusing (Zeller 2006). The artificial disc is difficult to put in, more difficult to remove, and very profitable. The licensing of the artificial disc (two manufacturers are vying for this market) is yet another reproach to the fashion in which the FDA safeguards us. It's reminiscent of the saga of the coronary artery stents (chapter 2).

There are precious few systematic reviews of interventions for regional disorders of the knee, in part because quality literature is sparse (van Dijk et al. 2006). However, there are some recent telling randomized controlled trials. The trial from the VA Medical Center in Houston (Moseley et al. 2002) should dampen anyone's enthusiasm for arthroscopic remediation of knee pain in the setting of osteoarthritis of the knee. And read about the Swedish experience (Roos et al. 1998) if you think that meniscectomy is sensible because it spares the knee from long-term ravages. Non-weight-bearing exercising makes far more sense and is supported by a systematic review (Fransen et al. 2002) and notable randomized controlled trials (Baker et al. 2001). Certainly this makes more sense than contributing to the dismal track record of my surgical colleagues. They seem to carry on in spite of the fact that their traditional and reflexive physical exam is invalid (Scholten et al. 2001) and radiological features poorly predict clinical outcomes in knee osteoarthritis (Bruyere et al. 2002). I would argue that the arthroscope is yet another good idea that went nowhere and now belongs in the archives next to coronary stents. As for knee arthroplasty—the so-called total knee replacement—beware of all the hype. Patients are far less pleased with the outcomes than are their surgeons, although they seldom fess up to their surgeons. It takes a more objective observer to gain this insight (Woolhead et al. 2005).

The literature for regional musculoskeletal disorders other than those above is scant, sadly. There is a trial comparing corticosteroid injection of the lateral elbow for lateral elbow pain ("tennis elbow" or "lateral epicondylitis") with physiotherapy or "wait-and-see" therapy. The latter was the better option (Smidt et al. 2002). But little else is worthy of mention, and much else is awaited with great anticipation.

For a discussion of the reason for skepticism regarding the neutriceuticals chondroitin and glucosamine, I'd suggest the editorial by Felson and McAlindon (2000), three meta-analyses (Leeb et al. 2000; McAlindon et al. 2000; Reichenbach et al. 2007), and the NIH-sponsored randomized controlled trial (D. O. Clegg et al. 2006). From my perspective, these compounds are a waste of money. At least copper bracelets can be attractive.

Regarding the NSAID wars, I would recommend two books for further discussions of, and references for, the history of the development of NSAIDs: Chapters 4 and 5 of the second edition of *Occupational Musculoskeletal Diseases* (Hadler 1999) and *The Aspirin Wars* by Mann and Plummer (1991). The former discusses the FDA and the historiography of anti-inflammatory pharmacology and introduces the COXIB debacle. It was in the second edition that I first decried the dialectic that led to the FDA's licensing COXIBS. *The Aspirin Wars* details the colorful politics of the industry in the twentieth century up until the 1980s.

The CLASS trial (Silverstein et al. 2000) purported to demonstrate that Celebrex was safer than ibuprofen. The VIGOR trial (Bombardier et al. 2000) purported to demonstrate that Vioxx was safer than naproxen. The former was published even though Pharmacia (and probably some of the authors) were aware of data that contradicted the published conclusions (Jüni et al. 2002). The VIGOR trial may have demonstrated some advantage to Vioxx in terms of gastropathy but may also have demonstrated a hazard in terms of cardiovascular disease (Mukherjee et al. 2001) — a hazard that was obscured by the fashion in which the data was presented in the original publication of the VIGOR trial, which lead to "expressions of concern" by the editors of the *New England Journal of Medicine* (Curfman et al. 2005 and 2006). Not surprisingly, theoreticians have leaped to explain the putative COXIB-induced thrombophilia, the tendency toward clotting (Marcus et al. 2002; Baigent and Patrone 2003), with zeal that outstrips the certainty regarding the effect. Not surprisingly, academic physicians who are highly visible as consultants to the pharmaceutical industry and as industry-sponsored "thought leaders" rushed to press (Strand and Hochberg 2002) asserting a favorable risk/benefit ratio for COXIBS, an argument they base on a contrived attempt to assert safety and downplay cardiovascular toxicity. Other Merck consultants (Ray et al. 2002) argue that Vioxx is safe at low doses. I am unimpressed by the data that supports an assertion that COXIBS (or any particular COXIB) have less gastrointestinal toxicity than traditional NSAIDS, and I'm not alone (Hippisley-Cox et al. 2005). As for cardiotoxicity, there is a suggestion that Vioxx may have some small risk associated with its use, but it's barely a suggestion that has to be teased out of the observational (Graham et al. 2005; Solomon et al. 2006) and controlled data (McGettigan and Henry 2006; Kearney et al. 2006) at a time when the teasing is eagerly absorbed into the product-liability arena. My response is to eschew these drugs because they offer my patients nothing new except unknown and undefined long-term toxicities. There is no consistently discernible cardiac risk from use of the old standbys (Salpeter et al. 2006). Furthermore, the COXIBS are unconscionably costly (Marra et al. 2000): a COXIB pill costs over $2 in the United States, compared to pennies for an aspirin. My patients with painful regional musculoskeletal disorders usually find acetaminophen as useful as any NSAID (Brandt and Bradley 2001). If that is not effective, I try an over-the-counter NSAID. If that offers little, I explain that pharmaceuticals are not helpful and offer exercises, warm baths, empathy, and time as the alternative. Americans seem wedded to their medicalization, consuming enormous quantities of over-the-counter and prescription analgesics (Turk 2002).

My therapeutic posture is consonant with the recommendations of a European task force (Pendleton et al. 2000). As I discussed in the text, a "subcommittee" constituted by the American College of Rheumatology recommended COXIBS (American College of Rheumatology Subcommittee on Osteoarthritis Guidelines 2000) as did the "International COX-2 Study Group," composed of multiple consultants to the industry and supported by "unrestricted educational grants" from Searle, Pfizer, Merck, and Johnson & Johnson (Lipsky et al. 2000). The lead author of this paper went on to a stint as a senior administrator in charge of extramural research programs for arthritis at the National Institutes of Health. It is not unusual for members of all kinds of "guideline" panels to have financial links to the drug companies that purvey products relevant to the particular guideline. The journal *Nature* undertook to survey panels for such entanglements (Taylor and Giles 2005). About half the panels did not require disclosures. Of the other half, some 685 disclosures, about 50 percent of the panelists, reflected industry ties.

The data I used to illustrate the cardiotoxicity of Celebrex was from a clinical trial of colorectal adenoma prevention (Solomon et al. 2005). Hazards of similar magnitude were discerned after cardiac surgery (Nussmeier et al. 2005) and in general practice (Hippisley-Cox and Coupland 2005; Lévesque et al. 2005). Opie (2005) chronicled the machinations of the FDA advisory panel and Congressman Henry Waxman (2005) of the Government Reform Committee of the U.S. House of Representatives. Steinbrook (2005) offers a critical appraisal of the fashion in which conflict of interest is allowed to sully the advisory function of the FDA's advisory panels. Lurie et al. (2006) surveyed FDA advisory panels for declared conflicts of interest. Realize that FDA regulations do not take exception to such ties to industry as long as they're declared. Of some 3,000 advisory committee members and voting consultants, 28 percent disclosed a conflict. Most were consulting arrangements, contracts/grants, and investments, often for sizable sums. An analysis of the influence of these arrangements on voting patterns suggests that advisors with conflicts are predisposed to voting against the interests of competitor products, although the influence is weak and not discernibly determinative.

The issue of conflict of interest has been receiving increasing attention in lay and medical literature. This is not a trivial issue. We are witness to the corruption of clinical investigation. Authors' conclusions are significantly more positive toward the experimental intervention in pharmaceutical (Kjaergard and Als-Nielson 2002) and device (Shah et al. 2005) trials funded by for-profit organizations compared with trials free of such vested interests. There are many viable explanations for this bias. One is the tendency of industry-sponsored analyses to choose unfairly matched control groups, or to squelch the publication of negative results (Djulbegovic et al. 2000). A recent analysis of randomized trials that compared protocols to the published articles detected, with alarming frequency, incomplete and biased reporting, which carried over into review articles that included these results (Chan et al. 2004).

The CLASS trial saga is an example of a form of data massaging harkening to our discussions in chapters 2 and 3. Large multicenter trials rely on the "coordinating center" for organization, data collection, and analysis; enter the CRO and the issues of vested interest. It is human nature for a decision maker in a contracting company to look more favorably next time on a petition from a CRO that generated a happy result last time. Since nearly all these trials are seeking small effects at most, inaccurate data, slight biases, and nuances in analyses are critical. There are well-documented instances of abuses in all such areas. However, there is precious little call for reforms to cleanse the drug-testing process such as those I offer in the text of this chapter and formulated in a long-ignored paper (Hadler and Gillings 1983). Rather, there is much chest pounding to identify and label potential conflicts of interest in publications (Fontanarosa et al. 2005) and educational exercises so that the readers, students, and consumers are forewarned. Forewarning has an impact on the reader (Schroter et al. 2004), but seemingly little impact on the investigators. There is much chest pounding to define the appropriateness of relationships between academicians, their institutions, and the pharmaceutical industry. There is much chest pounding regarding the perturbation of the treatment act by the trial, regardless of the setting. There is much chest pounding about the ethics of pharmaceutical marketing. Some of this chest pounding is so illustrative as to be worth our attention.

The editors of medical journals have been debating the handling of financial associations of authors for years. As I mentioned in the text, the comfortable solution was to ask authors to declare all associations that may represent a conflict of interest related to the content of the research and leave the interpretation to the readership. That was the solution promulgated by A. S. Relman twenty years ago (Relman 1984) when, as editor of the *New England Journal of Medicine*, he became aware that authors of an article on the effectiveness of TPA (the thrombolytic biotechnology product that did far more for Genentech's stock than for patients with myocardial infarctions) were also monitoring the trial and held stock in Genentech. However, declaration was hardly a solution, as it assumed that authors could identify conflicts and that readers could interpret them. There is nothing straightforward about this. Conflicts of interest are part of life, inside and outside the academy (Korn 2000). We all have dual commitments, competing interests, and competing loyalties. Which need declaring? How can we know which bias our judgment or have biased the judgment of someone else? The challenge is all the more confounded for multicenter randomized controlled trials, even more so when there is a "coordinating center" and a cro involved.

The response of the leading medical journals was to promulgate and publish as a consensus document a detailed guideline for the declaring of potential conflicts of interest and the specifying of the role of each author in the conduct of the trial (for example, *Ann Intern Med* 135 (2001): 453–56). As a frequent author, I can tell you that this is a confusing exercise. For example, if in a future publication I reference *Worried Sick*, am I to declare a conflict of interest since this monograph is a source of royalty income? I have searched my soul, and I can identify no personal conflict of interest in the writing of *Worried Sick*. First Relman (A. S. Relman 1990) and then his successor as editor of the *New England Journal of Medicine*, J. Kassirer (Kassirer and Angell 1993), declared that for review articles and editorials, the declaration of a potential conflict of interest was not sufficient. The "*Journal* expects that authors of such articles will not have any financial interest in a company (or its competitor) that makes the product discussed in the article." Recently, the current editor modified that restriction to "any significant financial interest" (Drazen and Curfman 2002). Drazen had been involved in industry-sponsored drug trials prior to accepting the editorship. He claimed that almost all with appropriate expertise to write such articles were disqualified by the former restriction. He even goes on to define "significant financial interest" as excluding mutual funds and the like but not "major research support" and set an "upper limit on the annual sum that a person may receive before a relationship is automatically considered significant," currently at $10,000. Relman, speaking from retirement (Relman 2002), decried the policy change: "Editors are on safer ground when they prohibit such conflicts of interest altogether rather than attempt to manage them by establishing flexible guidelines and negotiating with authors." Bravo.

However, maybe Drazen's bending the ethic is a reflection of these times. Drazen (Drazen and Curfman 2002b) argues that a zero-tolerance policy "would exclude from the *Journal* the views of some of our top researchers and would instead favor authors who are not actively working in the field." I would argue that not all "top researchers" are excluded by the zero-tolerance posture, and the fresh eyes of scientists from other fields can inform us all. But Drazen is correct in saying that many a "leading scientist" would be excluded. The financial arrangements between pharmaceutical firms and the academy have become institutionalized. Many a medical school has been subsumed by an "academic health center" whose allegiances, alliances, and goals barely encompass the education of the next generation of physicians. Several have developed in-house CROs. Financial arrangements between basic and clinical investigators in academic health centers and private-sector pharmaceutical and biotechnology industries are now commonplace. In 2000, one-fourth of the authors of papers presenting original, quantitative studies had specific industry affiliations, and approximately two-thirds of academic institutions hold equity in start-up companies that sponsor research performed at the same institution (Bekelman et al. 2003). The money involved is substantial. The potential for the shading of ethical constraints, if not for abuse and fraud, is real (Angell 2000; Bodenheimer 2000). The many legal issues (Kalb and Koehler 2002) are not well addressed by many of the contractual agreements between the institutions and industry sponsors (Schulman et al. 2002). Is it possible to live up to commitments as an inventor/entrepreneur and as a clinician/educator simultaneously? Probably not (Kelch 2002; Moses et al. 2002). Just look at the Cleveland Clinic Foundation and Topol's new clothes (Diamond 2006). Or, contemplate whether a physician who is paid (directly or indirectly) to recruit and enroll patients into a drug trial is compromised to serve as their treating (advising) physician (Morin et al. 2002; Miller et al. 1998).

Palumbo and Mullins (2002) detail the history of prescription-drug advertising. Total spending on pharmaceutical promotion grew from $11.4 billion in 1996 to $29.9 billion in 2005. DTC spending increased over threefold in that time but only represents 14 percent of the total (Donohue et al. 2007). There is reason to suggest that DTC marketing has a higher yield than all the money spent advertising to physicians in the media, over meals, in the office, and elsewhere. Critics are calling for another moratorium. However, proponents argue that direct-to-consumer advertising, if done well, would be a form of health promotion (Hollon 2005) rather than an exercise in medicalization. It has been argued that treating physicians must assist their patients in interpreting the barrage of direct-to-consumer pharmaceutical marketing (Rosenthal et al. 2002). Sidney Wolfe (2002) has further argued, "The education of patients — or physicians — is too important to be left to the pharmaceutical industry, with its pseudoeducational campaigns designed, first and foremost, to promote drugs." Relman (2003) echoes this plea. However, the campaigns are pervasive and now part of the fabric of American medicine. The pharmaceutical industry has spawned subsidiary industries in addition to CROs. There are SMOs (site management organizations), contracted to recruit physicians and physician groups to do the trials. There are MECCs (medical education and communication companies), contracted to put together educational programs for physicians. A contracted company, rather than the pharmaceutical firm, often employs the representatives paid to "detail" physicians. All this contractual delegating compounds the vesting of interest (Angell 2000b). The challenge is not just to thwart the pharmaceutical marketing initiative (Relman 2001); it also is to undo its impact. There is compelling evidence that the extent of physician-industry interactions (such as gifts, meals, and so-called continuing education events) directly affects prescribing, beginning in medical school (Wazana 2000). Furthermore, such interactions strongly and specifically associate with requests by physicians that drugs be added to hospital formularies (Chren and Landefeld 1994). I'm not suggesting malfeasance. If not quite malfeasance, these behaviors are a reproach to peer review and to the ethical fabric of my profession. Some are calling for the promulgation and enforcement of standards of behavior for the pharmaceutical industry and the medical profession. I am calling for reform of the fashion in which new drugs are licensed.

The data that supports my contention that NSAID gastropathy is much ado about nothing (with the exceptions I list in the text) has been available for many years (Hadler 1990) and ignored for as many in the zeal to market "purple pills" and prove that the latest NSAID spares the stomach's lining.

Chapter 10

Stone et al. published the study of the "number needed to offend" in 2002. Foucault's *Birth of the Clinic* was first translated into English in 1973, and Payer's *Medicine & Culture* was published in 1988. I use the Kuhnsian term "paradigm shift" advisedly in regard to the illness-disease construction. Nearly all of the many "paradigm shifts," which are commonly announced, turn out to be ephemeral (Atkin 2002). I would recommend the engaging little monograph by Wootton (2006) for an exposition on the harm wreaked by medical heuristics since Hippocrates.

Pain has been something of a will-o'-the-wisp for epidemiology. It is part of life. At least half of us will experience a week of pain, usually musculoskeletal pain, every six weeks. Most of us cope; we ignore, we rationalize, we deny, we complain, but rarely do we feel unwell and rarely do we seek professional help. In all advanced countries, and throughout the developing world, if we feel the need to seek help there are multiple options and multiple providers purveying them (Hadler 1999). Traditional Western medicine is but one option. So when the World Health Organization (Gureje et al. 1998) surveys primary-care practices around the world and discovers that 22 percent (ranging from 5.5 to 33 percent) of patients report persistent pain, one wonders how many people with persistent pain are not attending primary-care practices; they are going elsewhere or simply suffering in silence. Those who attend primary care are four times more likely to suffer anxiety or depression than patients without persistent pain and even more likely to manifest unfavorable health perceptions than patients seeking care for other reasons.

Epidemiology has come slowly to appreciate and explore the issue of persistent widespread pain. Until recently, the focus was on the prevalence and persistence of anatomy-specific pain. Household surveys abound about the prevalence of knee pain, or back pain, or headache, or abdominal pain. Hidden in all of these surveys are the people who answer in the affirmative to many such questions (Natvig et al. 2001). These people are more likely to be found in lower socioeconomic strata (Urwin et al. 1998) and more likely to seek medical care frequently for pain (Rekola et al. 1997) and other somatic complaints (Kadam et al. 2005), independent of medical and psychiatric comorbidity (Barsky et al. 2005). Furthermore, this high level of utilization long precedes a diagnosis such as fibromyalgia and is not perturbed by the diagnosis (Hughes et al. 2006). Only recently has this population been recognized and their plight probed. Some of the most informative epidemiology has been generated on the population of Manchester in the United Kingdom. There, investigators are using a stringent definition of chronic widespread pain that requires persistent pain for at least three months in the axial skeleton and in at least two sections of two contra-lateral limbs. Almost 5 percent of the adult population satisfies these criteria (Hunt et al. 1999). These people feel neither well nor happy. They are twice as likely as others to manifest psychological disturbance, to manifest limitations in function, and to report other somatic symptoms. They tend to have hypochondriacal beliefs and a preoccupation with bodily symptoms.

What is the fate of these people? First, they are no more likely to develop any systemic disease, including any systemic rheumatologic disease, than their age-matched cohort without widespread pain. The prevalence of symptoms in the community is stable, with considerable individual variability (Bergman et al.

2002). In the Manchester community, the majority seem to improve with time (Macfarlane et al. 1996). About a third don't improve in spite of whatever benefit they derive from their propensity to seek medical care, a propensity driven by psychosocial variables as much as the physical perception of pain (Kersh et al. 2001). They are the population that the World Health Organization took note of. A quarter of these people manifest serious anxiety or mood disorder prior to consultation (Macfarlane et al. 1999), which qualifies for a primary psychiatric disease label in nearly 17 percent of those who seek care (Benjamin et al. 2000).

What is their diagnosis? There is clearly a relationship between medically unexplained somatic symptoms and affective disorders; however, the labeling is extremely variable depending on characteristics of physicians, health-care systems, and cultures (Simon et al. 1999). The labeling is also rife with controversy (Sharpe 2002). I am comfortable with "an overwhelming loss of the sense of well-being," of which I think the pain is but one manifestation. I am furthermore comfortable asserting that this state of mind is on the tail end of the spectrum of normal (Wolfe and Rasker 2006) and not an abnormal state of mind. The psychiatric literature struggles with this large group of patients because most have no overt thought disorder (McWhinnet et al. 1997). "Functional somatic syndromes" is the appellation of leading psychiatrists in the United States in this field (Barsky and Borus 1999), which is meant to capture the heightened awareness and amplification of physical symptoms. "Hypochondriasis" is set off as a refractory subset with an unshakable conviction that they harbor a serious disease (Barsky 2001). There are rheumatologists who insist that the widespread pain is not so widespread but relates to tender points, and they apply the fibromyalgia label. However, tender points require the finger of faith (Croft 2000). They are often present in women who do not suffer and are not likely to develop persistent widespread pain (Forseth et al. 1999). In the setting of persistent widespread pain, tender points are related to generalized pain and pain behavior when studied carefully (Nicassio et al. 2000); they are nothing more than a measure of distress. The label applied to these patients reflects the "chief complaint" that is offered, elicited, or heard and not a valid categorization (Hadler 1999; Sullivan et al. 2002). FM, CFS, IBS, TMJ, and other acronyms denote this single spectrum of functional somatic syndromes.

There is much information about the plight and fate of these people. But no reliable hint, let alone common thread, is emerging as to a biological cause. Genetic influences can be discerned in analyses of twins, but they are slight. Nearly 10 percent of eleven-year-old Finnish twins had persistent widespread pain, but minimal genetic influence was discerned (Mikkelsson et al. 2001). The result was similar when Swedish twins were surveyed for chronic widespread pain (Kato et al. 2006) or chronic fatigue (Sullivan et al. 2005). Other investigators have sought associations with unusual psychological or physical traumatic events, but the results are inconsistent at best. The best of these studies come up with somewhat conflicting results. Viner and Hotopf (2004) could identify no association between psychological stress in childhood or maternal psychopathology and the likelihood of developing a functional somatic syndrome as an adult. However, Mallen et al. (2006) found that young adults with chronic persistent pain were more likely to recall from childhood having two or more relatives who suffered chronic pain or having suffered such themselves.

Most patients with these labels attribute the onset of their illness to something. In one tertiary-care setting (Neerinckx et al. 2000), the attributions heard most frequently were "chemical imbalance," "virus," "stress," and "emotional confusion." In Canada, most physiatrists, orthopedists, and general practitioners are not convinced that FM can be a consequence of or "reactive" to discrete events, including discrete traumatic events. Only some Canadian rheumatologists are comfortable with that hypothesis (White et al. 2000) despite British data that there is no important increment in the incidence of persistent widespread pain in the six months after a motor vehicle accident (Wynne-Jones et al. 2005). We do know that patients with this spectrum of illness in tertiary settings who manifest an attributional style have the worse prognosis (Vercoulen et al. 1996; Wilson et al. 1994). But then again, the prognosis is dismal even for the others, in that relatively few return to a sense of well-being. Pharmaceutical agents and most rehabilitative schemes are minimally effective, if at all. Given the tendency of these patients to "catastrophize" (Hassett et al. 2000), psychotherapy aimed at improving coping skills has been advocated. There is a suggestion that cognitive behavior therapy might help (Allen et al. 2006), particularly when fatigue is the dominant symptom (Price and Crouper 1998; Whiting et al. 2001). The data are not that impressive, which may not bode well for effectiveness outside the research-study setting, or when persistent widespread pain dominates the illness (Williams et al. 2001). Patients with functional somatic disorders generally find support groups helpful, though the price of this support is an escalation in symptom severity; they would have done better to stay away (Friedberg et al. 2005).

Patients labeled with the functional somatic disorders, particularly those who perceive themselves incapable of working, are characterized by the intensity of their idioms of distress and the dispassionate fashion in which they communicate their narrative of illness (Garro 1992). They are the most ill people ever described who are spared any end-organ damage, demonstrable organ dysfunction, or specific biochemical abnormality (Showalter 1996). In that regard they are fortunate. But that is not to belittle the pall under which they subsist (Greenhalgh 2001; Barker 2005). Nor is it to deny the Kafkaesque nature of a disability-determination process that must question the veracity of their perception of illness (Hadler 1999). Fibromyalgia is a social construction. It is the fashion in which our society has come to medicalize woefulness (Hadler and Greenhalgh 2005).

The classic treatise on suffering is by Eric Cassell (2004). Why do these patients suffer so? Pain can be unspeakable (Scarry 1985). However, those who are burdened with persistent widespread pain feel the need to defend the veracity of their experience (Hadler 1996). For a comprehensive treatment of the "mind-body" split, I suggest the monograph by Rey (1995) and the volume edited by Wright and Potter (2000). I am not alone in calling for a revision and modernization of this social construction (Bracken and Thomas 2002). However, my revision would countenance more than the fact that mind, suffering, and illness are socially constructed; it would emphasize the degree to which pain, body, and disease are also socially constructed. As it stands, the medical management of these patients with inexplicable health problems is difficult (Fischoff and Wessely 2003), often impossible, and rife with the potential for iatrogenesis.

Chapter 11

For a discussion of geriatric back disease, I'm partial to my chapter in the *Oxford Textbook of Geriatric Medicine* (Hadler 2000). For a discussion of the course and management of the acute compression-fracture syndrome, I'd suggest Joines and Hadler (2005), and for the prevalence of back symptoms in elders, see Edmond and Felson (2000) and Bressler et al. (1999). Because of all the randomized controlled trials, there is an extensive literature exploring the incidence and prevalence of compression fractures. The figures I am using are representative (Nevitt et al. 1998; Lindsay et al. 2001). About 20 percent of women over age fifty have at least one subtle compression fracture (Jackson et al. 2000). There is a suggestion that disc-space narrowing but not osteophytosis predisposes to adjacent thoracic fragility fractures independent of BMD (Sornay-Rendu et al. 2006), suggesting that the biomechanics of the spine rather than external forces alone may be at play.

Individuals who suffer an osteoporotic hip fracture face higher in-hospital mortality (Goldacre et al. 2002) and leave the hospital to face a high likelihood of compromised longevity and functionality (Hannan et al. 2001; Cree et al. 2000; March et al. 2000). This is particularly true of women suffering from co-morbidities and postoperative complications (Roche et al. 2005). Elderly women are aware of this and feel profoundly threatened by falls and the likelihood that a hip fracture will signal the end of their independence (Salkeld et al. 2000). In terms of the likelihood of suffering an osteoporotic hip fracture from a fall, both the degree of osteopenia (de Laet et al. 1998) and the severity of the fall (Greenspan et al. 1994) are well-documented determinants. The most produc-tive approach to decreasing the likelihood of osteoporotic hip fractures takes advantage of the latter observation. Fall-induced injuries are increasing in older adults at a rate that cannot be explained by demographic changes (Kannus et al. 1999). This may reflect the frailty of the elderly, including compromised vision (Pedula et al. 2006), which predicts hip fracture as well as hospitalization and death (Woods et al. 2005). Many consume pharmaceuticals with side effects that can compromise mobility, stability, and alertness (Leipzig et al. 1999). Much effort is being expended to decrease the likelihood of falls. Exercise (Feskanich et al. 2002) and exercise programs (Rubenstein et al. 2000) are beneficial. Hip protectors proved very effective in some studies (Rubenstein 2000; Parker et al. 1999), even cost-effective in nursing-home residents (Singh et al. 2004), but the results have not been consistent (Parker et al. 2006). Hip protectors may be at odds with the vanity of many an elderly woman (Kannus et al. 2000), but they are preferred over bisphosphonates nonetheless (Fraenkel et al. 2006). Families and managers of residential facilities for the elderly need to be aware that com-plex interventions that are based on individual health assessments can reduce falls. These should include behavioral interventions and modifications of envi-ronmental hazards (Gillespie et al. 1998).

The controversy about recommending dairy foods for bone health is nicely reviewed by Weinsier and Krumdieck (2000). There is evidence that the frail individuals most likely to suffer osteoporotic hip fractures are likely to be mal-nourished generally (Hanger et al. 1999), including calcium (Ensrud et al. 2000) and vitamin D (LeBoff et al. 1999) deficient, but these tend to be debilitated, in-stitutionalized elderly. There are randomized controlled trials, over a decade old now, suggesting that supplementation with vitamin D and calcium has demon-strable benefit in terms of hip fracture risk (M. C. Chapuy et al. 1992), not just improving osteopenia. However, this benefit was small and has proved difficult to reproduce. Several large randomized-controlled trials can discern no benefit in terms of fragility fractures from calcium and vitamin D supplementation in elderly women (Porthouse et al. 2005; Jackson et al. 2006; Prince et al. 2006), even elderly women who had already suffered a fragility fracture (RECORD Trial Group 2005). Perhaps, if higher doses of vitamin D are consumed — 800 IU per day rather than the customary 400 IU per day — there would be an effect on the incidence of fragility fractures (Bischoff-Ferrari et al. 2005), but not much of an effect. One can demonstrate an increase in BMD, even in healthy children (Winzenbert et al. 2006). Clearly, nutrition in general and adequacy of dietary calcium and vitamin D deserve attention, but they pale next to the environmental modifications and behavioral interventions discussed above in designing a milieu that promotes bone health in the elderly (Wallace 2000) and thereby facilitates the enjoyment of a ripe old age. For upper limb fractures, Colles fractures in particular, that assertion is irrefutable. The European Prospective Osteoporosis Study (Kaptoge et al. 2005) can barely detect a relationship between BMD and the incidence of fragility fractures when the history of frequent falls is taken into account.

Fuller Albright first recognized the association of menopause and osteoporosis and first recommended estrogen therapy for women with pathologic fractures (Albright et al. 1941). The observation that HRT had little effect on quality of life, aside from perimenopausal symptoms, was an offshoot of the "HERS" study, a study assessing the effect of HRT on heart disease (Hlatky et al. 2002). The study came up with the surprising result that women on HRT have more back pain (Musgrave et al. 2001). The two recent meta-analyses of the health outcomes consequent to HRT were by Nelson et al. (2002) and Humphrey et al. (2002). The Writing Group for the Women's Health Initiative published their results shortly thereafter (2002). The discussion by Fletcher and Colditz (2002) followed, from which I garnered the data in the table. The U.S. Preventive Services Task Force issued their cautionary recommendations in 2002 and reiterated it in 2005. Recent editorializing calls for caution in the use of HRT because the potential harm outweighs the potential benefit, even though neither harm nor benefit is impressive in magnitude (Solomon and Dluhy 2003). Torturing the data from the Women's Health Initiative has produced suggestions that HRT is responsible for a slight increase in the likelihood of gallbladder disease (Cirillo et al. 2005) as well as venous thrombosis (Cushman et al. 2004).

Some are belaboring the inconsistencies between trials and observational cohort studies as to the cardiovascular risks of exposure to HRT. These differences might be ascribed to limitations in the study methodologies, as well as to differences in the pharmacological preparations for HRT. The consensus seems to be that there must be a better way than traditional HRT (Grodstein et al. 2003).

That consensus has gained adherents, with the further analysis of the data from the Women's Health Initiative reiterating the stroke risk (Wasertheil-Smoller et al. 2003; Anderson et al. 2004) and suggesting some hazard in terms of cognitive impairment (Rapp et al. 2003; Shumaker et al. 2003 and 2004; Schneider 2004). Perhaps the death knell for treating postmenopausal women with HRT will come less from the litany of tiny hazards than from the analysis of the quality of life of the women who participated in the Women's Health Initiative. Remember that this was a placebo-controlled randomized trial. It turned out that the women on HRT and the women on placebo were indistinguishable in terms of general health, vitality, mental health, depressive symptoms, or sexual satisfaction (Hays et al. 2003). That was true if they were prescribed estrogens without progestin replacement (Brunner et al. 2005). Even more fascinating is the experience of these women when treatment was discontinued after the putative hazard was uncovered. About 63 percent of women who had been on HRT reported moderate or severe symptoms, such as hot flashes, night sweats, or pain and stiffness. But 41 percent of the women on placebo also experienced these symptoms to the same degree (Petitti 2005). The symptomatic benefit of placebo and the "placebo withdrawal effect" should inform us as to another social construction, which is that menopause is an "illness." An NIH State-of-the-Science Panel (2005) concluded that low-dose estrogen should be reserved for perimenopausal symptoms, but HRT has a tenuous role if any in the management of any symptoms that occur during menopause. Sic transit the HRT social construction.

The raloxifene trial proudly wears its acronym, not to be outdone by all the acronyms in the cardiovascular literature. It was the MORE trial, for "Multiple Outcomes of Raloxifene Evaluation" (Ettinger et al. 1999; Barrett-Connor et al. 2002). Interestingly, it was noted that women with low BMD and/or compression fractures were more likely to be depressed (Silverman et al. 2007). This need not be cause and effect, nor could such be tested given the design of MORE. However, I suspect that "depression" is a manifestation of frailty. In another raloxifene trial, no risk for primary coronary events could be discerned (Barrett-Connor et al. 2006). The upshot is that the tiny benefit in terms of fragility fractures must be weighed only against the increased risks of venous thromboembolism and stroke. Riggs and Hartmann (2003) have reviewed the biology and pharmacology of the SERMs.

There is a Cochrane Collaboration systematic review of the effectiveness of etidronate in thwarting osteoporotic vertebral fractures (Cranney et al. 2001). The pivotal risedronate trial was by Harris et al. (1999). In a follow-up, industry-supported three-year trial (McClung et al. 2001), the incidence of hip fracture in women who were seventy to seventy-nine years old and chosen because they were at high risk for osteoporotic fractures (exceedingly low BMD, often with disordered gait), was reduced from 3.2 percent to 1.9 percent by daily dosing with risedronate. In eighty-year-old women, also at high risk, the reduction was from 5.1 to 4.2 percent. This reduction is neither statistically or clinically significant. The authors and the pharmaceutical firm want us to consider the reduction from 3.2 to 1.9 percent in high-risk women age seventy to seventy-nine as clinically significant. Really? All these women are to be treated to effect an absolute reduction in radiographic compression of a vertebral body of 1.3 percent? I don't believe such a small health effect can be reliably measured. Even if it can, realize that only those exceedingly rare individuals who suffer dramatic fractures, so-called Grade 3, have a measurable decrease in their quality of life (Crans et al. 2004). For the vast majority of elderly women, the radiographic vertebral compression fractures are irrelevant.

The alendronate data is pretty much the same. The pivotal trial bore the acronym "FIT" for "Fracture Intervention Trial," published by Black et al. (1999) after three years of follow-up and by Cummings et al. (1998) after four. Merck has even underwritten trials in men with low BMD (Orwoll et al. 2000), and, lo and behold, alendronate thwarts osteopenia and may even thwart spinal compression fractures. Another Merck-sponsored trial must have warmed the hearts of their marketing division. If you stop alendronate, as opposed to stopping HRT, the rate of bone loss does not accelerate (Greenspan et al. 2002). I am troubled that none of this makes an important difference for well people or patients with primary osteopenia, even primary osteoporosis. Even a cost-effectiveness analysis of the FIT trial failed to justify alendronate for osteopenia (Schousboe et al. 2005). Investigators who performed that analysis declared potential conflicts of interest in that grants were received from pharmaceutical firms in competition with Merck but not from Merck, the manufacturer of alendronate. In an accompanying editorial, McClung (2005) argued that osteopenia should be sought in women who are more likely to suffer a fragility fracture — older women, women who have discontinued HRT, women with earlier menopause, and the like. Furthermore, he argued, the issue is not one of alternative treatments, since "no other antiresorptive drug is more effective than alendronate in reducing fracture risk." Dr. McClung is among several consultants for Merck and has received a number of "grants" from the firm. McClung is in good company — or at least he has prominent fellow travelers publishing similar conclusions in invited commentaries in similarly prominent journals (Rosen 2005; Raisz

TABLE 12. Incidence of Vertebral Fractures (VF) over Four Years of Treatment with Alendronate versus Placebo

Outcomes	Percentage of Incidence with Alendronate	Percentage of Incidence with Placebo	Number Needed to Treat
Clinical VF with baseline VF	0.3	0.9	185
Clinical VF without baseline VF	0.3	0.7	Not significant
Radiographic VF with baseline VF	1.5	2.7	83
Radiographic VF without baseline VF	1.2	1.9	Not significant

Source: Adapted from Quandt et al. (2005).

2005). There is another trial testing whether alendronate can reduce the incidence of vertebral fractures (VF) over the course of nearly four years. Postmenopausal women with osteopenia, defined as mildly reduced BMD, were recruited (Quandt et al. 2005). The principal findings are presented in Table 12.

Is any reader of *Worried Sick* prepared to argue that treatment really matters? Even for the higher risk elderly women, women who already had a vertebral fracture, do you think swallowing this pill for four years mattered? It reduced the absolute incidence of a new VF by a fraction of a percent. Is that even measurable? So what if alendronate can increase BMD? So what if it is relatively safe to take it for many years? There is nothing to be gained from taking it for more than a few years (Black et al. 2006), and I'd argue there's nothing to be gained of substance from taking it at all.

The notion that the bisphosphonates are safe has had something of a comeuppance. A rare but devastating side effect has been described: osteonecrosis of the jaw (Woo et al. 2006). True, most of the cases occurred with the longer-acting agents that have been used as chemotherapy for neoplasia — myeloma, for example. This tragic complication casts a pall on the remarkable biochemical achievements that produced a bisphosphonate to be administered annually (Reid et al. 2002; Black et al. 2007). However, it is also described with the agents I've just discussed that are used to treat osteoporosis. It's not an issue for me; I find the benefit so ephemeral that I'd tolerate no toxicity.

Furthermore, since I'm not going to treat, screening is unnecessary. For a discussion of the technical shortcomings of DEXA scanning, I'd suggest the paper by Nielsen et al. (1998). For a discussion of the discordance between the hip and spine DEXA measurements, I suggest Woodson (2000). For a discussion of the push toward densitometry and its shortcomings, I suggest Masud and Francis (2000). The U.S. Preventive Services Task Force came out with recommendations for screening for osteoporosis in 2002. The recommendations were accompanied by an extensive discussion of the literature upon which they are based (Nelson et al. 2002). Another literature review (Cummings et al. 2002) with complementary recommendations (Bates et al. 2002) was published in *JAMA* by investigators who had major roles in the alendronate trials. The NIH Consensus Statement (2000) did not advocate universal screening even after age sixty-five and stood by that conclusion in a paper published a year later (National Institutes of Health Consensus Development Panel on Osteoporosis 2001). The U.S. Agency for Healthcare Research and Quality (2001) shares my perspective on these data. The precursor to that agency ran into the fatal, behind-the-scenes sword of "criticism" I discussed previously (chapter 9) and was eliminated. So far, I'm able to parry that sword. If any reader is laboring under the premise that science, clinical research, clinical trials, and data interpretation are not subject to the vicissitudes of realpolitik, let me disabuse you, hopefully for now and forever.

The "market" for osteoporosis prevention is a promised land for Big Pharma and the equities markets. Without even a hesitation, the medical literature is rationalizing screening white and Asian women who are aging, particularly if they are thin. There is an argument that since black women have a lower fracture risk than white women at every level of BMD (Cauley et al. 2005), race-specific normative data must be established so that screening can be race specific (Acheson 2005). There are similar arguments afoot for screening men. New and "better" drugs are trickling into this market, in particular biologic agents that are impressively priced. Teriparatide is a fragment of human parathyroid hormone that was licensed by the FDA. It is touted because it causes bone accretion, as opposed to bisphosphonates, which slow resorption. It works about as well, or as poorly, as the bisphosphonates (Neer et al. 2001; Cranney et al. 2006). Enamored with the molecular biology, a trial was undertaken of serial use demonstrating that the gains of a year of teriparatide can be maintained by two subsequent years of alendronate (Black et al. 2005). That's good news for the BMD, but does it matter to the patient? Certainly it will not advantage those with asymptomatic osteopenia in any meaningful way. Perhaps combination or serial therapy (Heaney and Recker 2005) will prove useful for those rare younger individuals who have catastrophic osteoporosis. If only the marketing world understood that.

Teriparatide is not the only inventiveness driven by the potential of an aging spine as a market. There is a human monoclonal antibody, denosumab, that rattles osteoclast function by a mechanism entirely different from the bisphosphonates and results in increased BMD (McClung et al. 2006). Denosumab binds RANKL, the receptor that activates a molecule that in turn activates critical genes. But it'll have to do a lot more for my patient before I'm willing to prescribe it.

It should come as no surprise, after chapters 2, 6, and 7, that the surgical community would feel left out of the race to medicalize the aging spine. Spine surgeons and invasive radiologists have come up with procedures for compression fractures that are deemed symptomatic and unremitting. There are attempts to "stabilize" this fracture by injecting the same cements used for joint replacements into the collapsed vertebral body. That's not all. Vertebral compression fracture causes a wedge-like deformity of the vertebral body that tends to bend the spine forward, a deformity termed "kyphosis." So, "kyphoplasty" has been invented. A balloon is inserted into the collapsed vertebral body, inflated to reduce the wedge, and stabilized with cement. There is no science supporting the effectiveness of either procedure. There are anecdotes. Furthermore, since the FDA has a different test for devices than for pharmaceuticals, kyphoplasty balloons are sold and the cements used "off label." Others are highly skeptical (Jarvik et al. 2006); I'm outraged.

The most entertaining discussion of social constructions I have come across is the monograph by Hocking (2000). Likewise, I recommend the monograph by Blackmore (1999) for a discussion of the meme. These treatises will enable any perplexed reader to productively revisit this and the previous chapter.

Chapter 12

I cited some of the literature on SES and health in countries that are not resource constrained in the supplementary reading for chapter 1. In addition, I'd suggest Kawachi et al. (1999), Marmot and Wilkinson (1999), Kawachi and Berkman (2003), and Marmot (2004). Several years ago, the U.S. National Center for Health Statistics produced a compendium of health data that considered the influence of SES (Pamuk et al. 1998) that remains an important resource. The realization continues to grow that the relationship between SRH and mortality has less to do with "health needs" than with employment (O'Reilly et al. 2005).

For a discussion of the health consequences of destitution in countries that are resource constrained, see the classic theoretical treatise by Dasgupta (1993). But if you want a sense what life is like on the cusp of poverty in the urban United States, I'd suggest the monograph by the anthropologist K. Newman (1999). The volume of *People of the Abyss* I read was a "rare book" (London 1903), but there are more recent publications. The essay by McCally et al. (1998) tackles the issue of the influence of SES on health outcomes from a medical perspective, concluding that there may be a medical solution in increased access. That is not the conclusion of most of the authors I am citing; neither is it mine (Hadler 1999b).

The thrust of this chapter is an understanding of the critical influence of an adverse psychosocial context at work on health and longevity, and the fashion in which disabling regional musculoskeletal disorders serve as a surrogate indicator of this adversity. The thrust of this chapter is also the thrust of my career as a clinical investigator for nearly thirty years. The topic is the centerpiece of many of my earlier books, most recently the third edition of *Occupational Musculoskeletal Disorders* (Hadler 2005). Much progress has been made since I started my quest for understanding and coined the term "Industrial Rheumatology" in the mid-1970s. Of course, the state of the science then was primitive. There was no way but up. The first edition of *Occupational Musculoskeletal Disorders*, published in 1994, was a state-of-the-art exercise, relying on inferential reasoning and a scant science to provide an approach to the complex issues that had evolved to engulf the worker disabled with a regional musculoskeletal disorder. The second edition was an exercise in picking through a literature that was rapidly evolving from the anecdotal to the systematic. The third edition offers much more than a window on the revolution in life-course science. The study of occupational musculoskeletal disorders is the cutting edge of the revolution. I have tried to capture some of this excitement in chapter 9. It required constraint not to have this topic commandeer the book. If that happened, I would be doing a disservice to the thesis of *Worried Sick*, which is to provide the reader with the information and mind-set necessary to confront medicalization in contemporary society. Chapter 9 is meant to perform that service for the reader whenever she or he is performing in the role of employee.

A work setting that feels "bad" renders all of us more vulnerable, less secure, and less self-assured. In such a state, our next morbidity can feel like the last straw. Cultural constraints and the realities of workers' compensation indemnity schemes make it more likely that our next regional musculoskeletal disorder will feel dreadfully dire. The consequences of pursuing recourse in workers' compensation for regional musculoskeletal disorders are Kafkaesque, iatrogenic, and replete with false promise. I suggest the third edition of *Occupational Musculoskeletal Disorders* for a discussion and defense of that purple assertion. I am not alone in recognizing the iatrogenicity inherent in the workers' compensation algorithm for back injury (Hadler 2001; Johnston et al. 2003). Furthermore, we have been able to do more than recognize the iatrogenicity: we have managed to document it (Tait et al. 2004, 2006; Chibnall et al. 2005, 2006a, 2006b). And we have published a commentary on the "injury" construction in *JAMA* (Hadler et al. 2007). A review from the Cochrane Collaboration (Martimo et al. 2007) is complementary. The "injury" construct is untenable and, I hope, history.

The literature that implicates the psychosocial context of work as the prime mover in this dialectic has matured apace since I wrote the third edition of *Occupational Musculoskeletal Disorders*. Papers by Jarvik et al. (2005) and IJzelenberg and Burdorf (2005) are two of many examples. Kaila-Kangas et al. (2006), studying the Finnish workforce, noted that the effect of an adverse psychosocial context on the incidence of disabling back pain does not distinguish socioeconomic differences. Absenteeism for regional musculoskeletal disorders is not the only consequence of an adverse psychosocial work context (Cheng et al. 2000). It may be the prodrome, or the canary in the mineshaft. The latest insight, derived from the Whitehall study, relates to the increased incidence of cardiac disease when workers consider the work context unjust (Kivimäki et al. 2005); in the short term, an unjust work context can drive you "nuts" (Ferrie et al. 2006). The concept of "justice at work" is a component of what I term the psychosocial context. It relates to whether you feel your supervisor values you and your opinions, treats you fairly, and is trustworthy. This is but one of myriad factors that can contribute to the adverse nature of the context of work. There are elements of work architecture such as breaks, work latitude, work autonomy, effort-reward imbalance, task alteration, job security, and the like that can take a toll. There are interpersonal challenges such as supervisor support and coworker interactions. There are personal factors such as affective disorders also at play. All of this complexity influences the likelihood of short- and long-term sickness absences from all causes, but notably from disabling regional musculoskeletal disorders. Since feeling valued is a common denominator, it is no surprise that blue-collar (manual) workers are more likely to find their backache disabling (Kaila-Kangas et al. 2006).

The historiography that I offered can be pursued in Hadler 1978, 1998, 2005; and Denbe 1996. Erichsen was surgeon to Queen Victoria and published a collection of essays titled *Railway and Other Injuries of the Nervous System* (1866), which I am fortunate to own. Keller and Chappel (1996) offer a more readily available discussion of "Erichsen's disease." Mixter and Barr invented the semiotic "ruptured disc" in a paper in 1934. The Johnstone quote is on page 381 of his textbook (1941).

Industrial psychology is making inroads into defining the elements of an adverse psychosocial context of working. The pioneering work on job stress and strain is by Karasek and Theorell (1990). "Allostatic load" (Kubzhansky et al. 1999) and motivational "flow" (Guastello et al. 1999) seem to be attempting to measure the state of feeling comfortable in one's skin. Monotony and isolation seem to be less adverse circumstances at work than disapproval or lack of a feeling of control. The latter are harder to live with day after day.

The epidemiological evidence supporting my contention that an adverse psychosocial work context is bad for your health is considerable. It is even possible to demonstrate that workers experiencing job insecurity are more likely to recall and record all manner of health complaints (Mohren et al. 2003). The frequency of short- and long-term absences regardless of the reason is associated with the adverse nature of the psychosocial context of work. The literature grows apace: Bültmann et al. (2005), Hanebuth et al. (2006), Head et al. (2006), Li et al. (2006), Lund et al. (2005), and Nielsen et al. (2006). The adverse psychosocial context of work is even the secret to "burnout" (Borritz et al. 2005). However, I am emphasizing the studies that demonstrate the high likelihood of finding regional musculoskeletal disorders disabling when faced with an adverse psychosocial context of work. The Finnish experience a decade ago is telling (Vahtera et al. 1997). The Whitehall studies document the influence of an adverse psychosocial work environment on mortality (Bosma et al. 1998), as well as disabling backache (Hemingway et al. 1997) and the malignant influence of downsizing (Ferrie et al. 1998). Downsizing has a powerful negative effect on self-reported health status (Reissman et al. 1999; Borg et al. 2000), a measure that rivals SES as a predictor of all-cause mortality.

The analysis of regional variations in Medicare spending, health outcomes, and patient satisfaction is by Fisher et al. (2003a, 2003b). As for iatrogenicity in octogenarians, the Swiss TIME Trial of medical versus surgical interventions should quash the zeal for invasive strategies (Pfisterer et al. 2003). There was no difference in survival at one year or quality of life at one year. There were some improvements in quality of life early on in the year for the survivors of CABGs, but that's a high price to pay (figuratively, let alone literally). I wonder how many octogenarians would pay that price without substantive gain at a year?

The literature on polypharmacy in octogenarians is rich. It is complemented by an analysis documenting the toxicities of this practice (Gurwitz et al. 2003). There is some evidence that participation in physically and mentally challenging leisure activities will advantage the elderly both in terms of cognitive status (Verghese et al. 2003) and longevity (Gregg et al. 2003a). Of course these inferences derive from observational cohort studies and are based on very weak associations that are likely to be confounded by unmeasured variables (SES is ignored, yet again, for example). However, the message to participate has such face value as to be worthy of trumpeting. If nothing else, such participation can enrich your life until it is your time (Hadler 2003b).

Chapter 13

The trial designed to compare a placebo pill with sham acupuncture was conducted by Kaptchuk et al. (2006). The subjects had regional arm pain, which was ascribed to repetitive usage. This is a very special circumstance, sharing many of the features of the regional back "injury" I detailed in chapter 12 and discussed at great length in the most recent edition of *Occupational Musculoskeletal Disorders* (Hadler 2005). It is also discussed by Lucire in her brilliant monograph *Constructing RSI: Belief and Desire* (2003).

For an engaging romp through the false starts of the Western medical tradition since Hippocrates, read Wootton (2006). Sectarian medicine (Gevitz 1987) is now called "complementary and alternative" to avoid any hint of chauvinism. For a discussion of the history of homeopathy, I'd suggest Kaufman (1988), Jonas et al. (2003), or Dooley (2002). Wardwell (1988) discussed the early history of the chiropractic; Meeker and Haldeman (2002) discuss its current status, which they argue is at the crossroads of mainstream and alternative medicine. I am less charitable in my assessment (Hadler 2000). Starr (1982) describes the politics that led to the absorption of homeopathy into mainstream medicine. The quote from Oliver Wendell Holmes can be found in his collected essays (1899). One form of New Age magnet therapy, bipolar permanent magnets, was tested for chronic low back pain (Collacott et al. 2000) without discernible effect. I find the fact that the trial was undertaken and published in *JAMA* more illuminating than the actual science. There is absolutely no physical basis that allows one to even imagine a biological effect. It is as ludicrous as suggesting that using cell phones causes brain cancer or living near power lines causes leukemia. Social constructions pop up like weeds; ignore them and they seldom go away.

Carey et al. (1995) and my other colleagues at UNC published a study comparing costs of treating backache between chiropractors, primary-care physicians, and orthopedists. That study suggested that patients with regional back pain who were attended by chiropractors were more satisfied with their care, even though there was no differential in benefit. The fact that patients with back pain attended by chiropractors are more pleased with the service than patients of other providers has been demonstrated in many other studies, including randomized trials from UCLA (Hertzman-Miller et al. 2002; Hurwitz et al. 2006). This differential is generally ascribed to the proclivity of chiropractors to speak with their patients and explain their therapeutic premises empathetically and definitively. They are expounding on a belief system as to the cause and cure of back pain that is unproved and not readily amenable to testing. For their patients to be satisfied, these explanations must seem sufficient and not beyond reason. For me, since they ignore the psychosocial confounders and focus on sophistical anatomical considerations, these empathetic explanations are unconscionable. Yet, the patients are "satisfied" and remain "satisfied" while contending with relentless symptomatology. Some call this the placebo effect and defend it as such (Kaptchuk 2002). I am unwilling to condone — perhaps incapable of condoning on philosophical grounds — such a defense.

Coulehan (1991) discusses the chiropractic treatment act. Several authors speak to therapeutic envelopes, usually under a different rubric, such as "matrix" (Hacking 2000) or "domain" (Hazemeijer and Rasker 2003).

Discussions of the pharmacology of herbal remedies are now commonplace in the mainstream medical literature (de Smet 2002). So too are discussions of the consequences of an absence of standards for purity (Straus 2002; Fontanarosa et al. 2003) and of the decision by Congress to consider these agents foodstuff and forego regulations as to their safety and effectiveness (Marcus and Grollman 2002). There are those who argue that considering these supplements to be "food" and not nutrients serves the public health (Lichtenstein and Russell 2005). Believers in and purveyors of herbal preparations take refuge from critics (such as me) in the tremendous variability in the constituents of the various manufactured preparations, let alone all the patent preparations sold by venders of many an ilk. Even a review from the Cochrane Collaboration (Gagnier et al. 2007) could not dismiss all herbal remedies for low back pain. Willow bark, devil's claw, and cayenne may offer short-term benefits. However, there is no need to bother with willow bark; the active ingredient was isolated a century ago and modified as aspirin (chapter 9). Cayenne is a pepper preparation that is a counterirritant if you prefer a burning sensation in your skin to backache. But these few preparations that may be rational are exceptional. Most herbs have naught but conviction to recommend them based on trials.

Believers and purveyors claim their preparation is different from and better than the preparation that fared so poorly in the latest randomized controlled trial. There is no rational counterargument, nor is there a feasible way to formally study everyone's pet remedy. The same argument pertains in defense of all the variations in manual medicine (see below). For that matter, it pertains to all the variations in the violence we do to coronary arteries discussed in chapter 2. Some rely on systematic reviews and meta-analyses of similar trials, usually similar trials with varying but marginal outcomes, to test assertions of effectiveness. It is assumed some greater truth will emerge. Even with such an exercise, a claim of "no effect" should be read as a claim of no discernible effect (Alderson and Chalmers 2003). No one can prove a negative; benefit could well be missed. Some will argue "Why not?" and call for more studies, as Turner (2002) does for echinacea and the common cold. My response is that we're not likely to be missing much benefit and as likely to be missing some toxicity. I'll pass. Turner et al. learned that for echinacea in his much more comprehensive RCT (2005).

The FDA's list of toxicities from dietary supplements can be accessed online at ‹http://www.cfsan.fda.gov/~dms/ds-ill.html›. Haller and Benowitz (2000) discuss ephedra alkaloids and their toxicities. Ang-Lee et al. (2001) discuss the need for concern about herbal medicines in the surgical arena. As for the benefit/risk ratio of dietary supplements, Ernst (2002) does it justice. Examples of the science include the papers published by Barrett et al. (2002) and Turner et al. (2005) on echinacea, Wilt et al. (1998) and Bent et al. (2006) on saw palmetto, and Linde and Mulrow on St. John's wort (1998).

Drazen's lament about egregious advertising practices for dietary supplements was published in 2003 in the *New England Journal of Medicine*. I would recommend ‹http://www.citizen.org/hrg› for well-referenced discussions of the toxicity of ephedra, and much more that speaks to the excesses of the pharmaceutical industry and the dietary supplement injury. This is the website for Sidney Wolfe's Health Research Group in Public Citizen. This is a public advocacy group, and in keeping with that credential it is predisposed to aggressive language, if not tactics. But they do their homework and are a worthy source of information.

Fairfield and Fletcher (2002) reviewed the scientific literature exploring the effects of vitamin supplementation on chronic disease prevention in adults. The review is outstanding and both reiterated and updated in an NIH "State-of-the-Science" conference (Huang et al. 2006). It is very difficult to convince oneself that the science supports any contention that vitamin supplementation prevents common chronic disease. There is little suggestion that antioxidants offer any protection against stroke (Ascherio et al. 1999), respiratory tract infections (Graat et al. 2002), or cardiovascular events (Heart Outcomes Prevention Evaluation Study Investigators [HOPE] 2000; Lee et al. 2005). There are suggestions from cohort studies that vitamin E may have a discernible effect on the likelihood of dementia, but they are barely suggestions (Engelhart et al. 2002; Morris et al. 2002; Foley and White 2002) and difficult to reproduce (McMahon et al. 2006). Antioxidants may decrease the risk of macular degeneration in the elderly (van Leeuwen et al. 2005). But they offer nothing for mortality (Bjelakovic et al. 2007). There is a suggestion that patients with type 2 diabetes will have fewer upper respiratory infections if they consume a daily multivitamin (Baringer et al. 2003; Fawzi and Stampfer 2003). This study recruited patients from two urban clinics in North Carolina, a state with a well-documented, impressive income gap. Perhaps this population suffers from micronutrient deficiency in addition to social deprivation and its handmaiden, the Metabolic Syndrome. However, all of these suggestions of benefit must be weighed against the more consistent data that antioxidant supplementation can be harmful. The argument that high-dose vitamin E supplementation is associated with increased all-cause mortality is tenable (Miller et al. 2005; Hanley and Miller 2005; Bjelakovic et al. 2007). And subtle hypervitaminosis A increases fracture risk (Michaëlsson et al. 2003; Lips 2003). As for lowering homocysteine with folic acid, it's no longer a good idea since it doesn't prevent vascular disease (Lonn et al. 2006). That being the case, why bother measuring homocysteine (Rosenberg and Mulrow 2006)? A recent British trial suggests that intermittent vitamin D dosing is as effective as any pharmaceutical in preventing vertebral fractures (Trivedi et al. 2003). However, that is much ado about the miniscule (chapter 11).

Wolsko et al. (2003) performed the national telephone survey probing the recourse taken by Americans who recalled back or neck pain in the past year. The table of the frequency of use is taken from this reference. The results of the National Health Interview Survey were published by Quandt et al. (2005b). In Washington State, about 40 percent of patients with back pain saw a non-physician exclusively, while another 40 percent saw a physician exclusively in 2002 (Lind et al. 2005). Such discrimination is not the rule. Druss et al. (2003) discusses the implications for patient care of the growing trend to seek care from both physician and nonphysician providers simultaneously. Astin (1998) published the complementary national survey suggesting that the effectiveness relates to the "therapeutic envelope" — the beliefs shared by the purveyor of the treatment act and the recipient. That pertains to the patients of the chiropractic, although surveys suggest that this patient population burdens more than impaired self-reported health status; they burden impaired "mental health" (Coulter et al. 2002), an observation that harkens to my discussion in chapters 9 and 12 of factors that impair one's effectiveness in coping with back pain, which I reiterated in my commentary (Hadler 2002) published with the paper by Coulter et al. A study by Eisenberg et al. (2007) speaks to the complexity of the notion of a therapeutic envelope. The study population was comprised of adults who sought care for low back pain at the Harvard Vanguard multispecialty clinic. By definition, they sought care from physicians. They were randomized to whatever that care entailed or the ability to choose from a menu of CAM. After five weeks, those who added some form of CAM to their medical therapy were no better off for the choosing in terms of symptoms or function. They were more "satisfied" with their choice, but that came at considerable additional expense. This must speak to preconceived notions, to beliefs. The power of belief on illness, disability, and medicine is one of the major themes of this volume. It is also the topic of a fascinating collection of essays (Halligan and Aylward 2006).

The science that has tested the benefits of complementary and alternative modalities is extensive. So much effort has been expended on physical modalities that multiple systematic reviews and meta-analyses are available for backache: acupuncture (van Tulder et al. 1999), "distant healing" (Astin et al. 2000), and spinal manipulation (Bronfort 1999; Koes et al. 1996). Several individual trials are worth reading. Our trial of spinal manipulation for low back pain (Hadler 1987) has been reproduced several times, including by Andersson et al. (1999). However, manipulation offers nothing when compared to mobilization for neck pain (Gross et al. 2004). Homeopathy proved no match for sore muscles (Vickers et al. 1997).

Acupuncture seems to be the modality du jour. The sham acupuncture versus placebo pill study that introduced this chapter helps us come to grips with this literature, which seems to be exhibiting unbridled growth. There are numerous randomized controlled trials. For persistent low back pain, the benefit is minimal if it is real (Ratcliffe et al. 2006; Thomas et al. 2006). Acupuncture proved no match for neck pain in two reasonably designed studies (Irnich et al. 2001; White et al. 2004), although, of course, it is not a sham (Trinh et al. 2007).

Acupuncture is no match for migraine (Linde et al. 2005), but the acupuncturists can take solace in the systematic review that failed to find an advantage for any manual therapy for tension-type headaches (Fernández-de-las-Peñas et al. 2006). Acupuncture seemed to offer a tiny advantage as adjunctive therapy in trials of knee pain (Berman et al. 2004; Foster et al. 2007), but I'm not that gullible (Zochling et al. 2003; Manheimer et al. 2007); sham acupuncture works as well (Scharf et al. 2006). Maybe the answer is to do away with the needle and just press on the spots that one believes to be important. Acupuncture may give way to acupressure. It worked well enough in Taiwan (Li-Chen et al. 2006) to tantalize some in Britain (Frost and Stewart-Brown 2006). I am bemused. Pressing on the tender spots of patients with back pain was considered diagnostic of disease by Osler and by many who welcome "fibromyalgia" into their belief systems and therapeutic envelopes (chapter 10). But then again, there are those who think that small and inconsistent effects in multiple randomized trials justify the use of some herbs to treat low back pain (Gagnier et al. 2007).

Many of the techniques involved in these CAM modalities are based on physical findings that require some finger of faith on the part of the therapist; interobserver variability is enormous. That pertains to the "energy field" in therapeutic touch (Rosa et al. 1998) and needle placement in acupuncture (Kalauokalani et al. 2001), as well as many of the signs relied upon by chiropractors.

There are those that argue that alternative medicine is scientifically grounded, given that no refutation can be incontrovertible and all refutations have a subjective element (Vandenbroucke and de Craen 2001). There are those who argue that a healing ritual can have clinical significance to the extent it magnifies the placebo effect (Kaptchuk 2002). The argument is carried further in that the themes of vitalism and spirituality can be empowering and authenticating (Kaptchuk and Eisenberg 1998). This line of argument, it seems to me, pales if empowerment and authentication require living in a contrived therapeutic envelope. That's a sad fate.

To be effective, any treatment act must consider the preconceived notions the patient/client carries to the encounter. These belief systems are part of the persona of the patient and influence participation in the treatment act and its outcome. Value judgments have little place in this consideration. However, to turn belief systems into therapeutic tools is to walk a fine line between the ranks of the clerics and the ranks of the charlatans. Understanding the fashion in which the patient-client's religious and spiritual beliefs influence the illness narrative and the treatment act is the art of medicine. Prescribing spirituality or religion as part of the treatment act may be comforting, palliative if you will, but it is not the act of a physician — it is the act of a priest. The former is the art of healing; the latter is not (Sloan et al. 2000).

Chapter 14

Baker's (1996) treatise on the genealogy of "moral hazard" was published in the *Texas Law Review*. My discussions are complementary (Hadler 1999a).

This "Health Assurance, Disease Insurance Plan" has been presented to many professional groups. A version was published (Hadler 2005).

Bodenheimer (2005) offers a nice summary of the high and rising costs of "health care" in the United States, illustrating how these costs outstrip all other countries in magnitude and lag behind all others in cost-effectiveness. The health-policy world, of which RAND Corporation is a leader (McGlynn et al. 2003), is wedded to the notion that much of the ineffectiveness and therefore waste can be ascribed to the impressive variability in the quality of the care delivered across the country. The usual measures of "quality" relate to adherence to guidelines for appropriate care (Romano 2005). This belief persists despite the fact that it is as difficult to enforce adherence to such guidelines (Snyder and Anderson 2005) as it is to show that adherence really matters in terms of in-patient mortality and the like (Williams et al. 2005). There is a very extensive "quality literature" and much advocacy, including in the current political debate. All of this should be brought up short by the results of the pay-for-performance project launched by the Centers for Medicare and Medicaid Services in 2003. The project targeted the treatment of over 100,000 patients treated for acute myocardial infarctions in fifty-four hospitals, which were offered financial incentives to adhere to the treatment guidelines promulgated by the American College of Cardiology and American Heart Association. The clinical outcomes in these pay-for-performance hospitals were compared with the outcomes in 446 control hospitals. The pay-for-performance program led to slight but measurable change in performance but to no significant incremental improvement in outcomes (Glickman et al. 2007).

Of course, the reader of *Worried Sick* is not surprised by any of this.

bibliography

Abbreviations

Am J Med	*American Journal of Medicine*
Am J Public Health	*American Journal of Public Health*
Ann Intern Med	*Annals of Internal Medicine*
Ann Rheum Dis	*Annals of Rheumatic Diseases*
Arch Intern Med	*Archives of Internal Medicine*
Arthritis Care Res	*Arthritis Care and Research*
Arthritis Rheum	*Arthritis and Rheumatism*
BMJ	*British Medical Journal*
Can Med Assoc J	*Canadian Medical Association Journal*
Clin J Pain	*Clinical Journal of Pain*
Clin Med JRCPL	*Clinical Medicine, the Journal of the Royal College of Physicians (London)*
JAMA	*Journal of the American Medical Association*
J Am Coll Cardiol	*Journal of the American College of Cardiology*
J Am Geriatr Soc	*Journal of the American Geriatrics Society*
J Gen Intern Med	*Journal of General Internal Medicine*
J Natl Cancer Inst	*Journal of the National Cancer Institute*
J Occup Environ Med	*Journal of Occupational and Environmental Medicine*
J Rheumatol	*Journal of Rheumatology*
N Engl J Med	*New England Journal of Medicine*
Psychol Med	*Psychological Medicine*

Abrahamson, M. J. Clinical Crossroads: A 74-year-old woman with diabetes. *JAMA* 297 (2007): 196–202.

Abramson, J., and J. M. Wright. Are lipid-lowering guidelines evidence-based? *Lancet* 369 (2007): 168–69.

Acheson, L. S. Bone density and the risk of fractures: Should treatment thresholds vary by race? *JAMA* 293 (2005): 2151–54.

Ackerknecht, E. H. *Rudolf Virchow: Doctor, Statesman, Anthropologist.* Madison: University of Wisconsin Press, 1953.

Adams, K. F., A. Schatzkin, T. B. Harris et al. Overweight, obesity, and mortality in a large prospective cohort of persons 50 to 71 years old. *N Engl J Med* 355 (2006): 763–78.

Adler, A. I., I. M. Stratton, H. Andrew et al. Association of systolic blood pressure with macrovascular and microvascular complications of type 2 diabetes (UKPDS 36): Prospective observational study. *BMJ* 321 (2000): 412–19.

Agency for Healthcare Research and Quality (AHRQ). Osteoporosis in postmenopausal women: Diagnosis and monitoring: Summary. Evidence Report/Technology Assessment Number 28. AHRQ Publication 01-E031. Rockville, Md.: Agency for Healthcare Research and Quality, February 2001. ‹http://ahrq.gov//clinic/osteosum.htm›.

Albertsen, P. C. PSA testing: public policy or private penchant? *JAMA* 296 (2006): 2371–73.

Albertsen, P. C., J. A. Hanley, and J. Fine. 20-year outcomes following conservative management of clinically localized prostate cancer. *JAMA* 293 (2005): 2095–101.

Albright, F., P. H. Smith, and A. M. Richardson. Menopausal osteoporosis. *JAMA* 22 (1941): 2465–74.

Alderson, P., and I. Chalmers. Survey of claims of no effect in abstracts of Cochrane reviews. *BMJ* 326 (2003): 475.

Allen, L. A., F. L. Woolfolk, J. I. Escobar et al. Cognitive-behavioral therapy for somatization disorder: A randomized controlled trial. *Arch Intern Med* 166 (2006): 1512–18.

Alsheikh-Ali, A. A., M. S. Ambrose, J. T. Kuvin, and R. H. Karas. The safety of resuvastatin as used in common clinical practice: A postmarketing analysis. *Circulation* 111 (2005): 3051–57.

Alter, D. A., A. Chong, P. C. Austin et al. Socioeconomic status and mortality after acute myocardial infarction. *Ann Intern Med* 144 (2006): 82–93.

American College of Rheumatology Subcommittee on Osteoarthritis Guidelines. Recommendations for the medical management of osteoarthritis of the hip and knee: 2000 update. *Arthritis Rheum* 45 (2000): 1905–15.

American Diabetes Association. Standards of medical care in diabetes — 2006. *Diabetes Care* 29, supp. 1 (2006): 24–42.

Andersen, L. B., P. Schnohr, M. Schroll, and H. O. Hein. All-cause mortality associated with physical activity during leisure time, work, sports, and cycling to work. *Arch Intern Med* 160 (2000): 1621–28.

Andersen, M., J. Kragstrup, and J. Søndergaard. How conducting a clinical trial affects physicians' guideline adherence and drug preferences. *JAMA* 295 (2006): 2759–64.

Anderson, C. A. M., and L. J. Appel. Dietary modification and CVD prevention: A matter of fat. *JAMA* 295 (2006): 693–96.

Anderson, G. L., M. Limacher, A. R. Asaf et al. Effects of conjugated equine estrogen in postmenopausal women with hysterectomy: The Women's Health Initiative randomized controlled trial. *JAMA* 291 (2004): 1701–12.

Andersson, G. B. J., T. Lucente, A. M. Davis et al. A comparison of osteopathic spinal manipulation with standard care for patients with low back pain. *N Engl J Med* 341 (1999): 1426–31.

Angell, M. Is academic medicine for sale? *N Engl J Med* 342 (2000): 1516–18.

———. The pharmaceutical industry — to whom is it accountable? *N Engl J Med* 342 (2000): 1902–4.

Ang-Lee, M. K., J. Moss, and C. S. Yuan. Herbal medicines and perioperative care. *JAMA* 286 (2001): 208–16.

Antihypertensive and Lipid-Lowering Treatment to Prevent Heart Attack Trial (ALLHAT). Major outcomes in high-risk hypertensive patients randomized to angiotensin-converting enzyme inhibitor or calcium channel blocker vs. diuretic. *JAMA* 288 (2002): 2981–97.

Antihypertensive and Lipid-Lowering Treatment to Prevent Heart Attack Trial — Lipid-Lowering Treatment (ALLHAT-LLT). Major outcomes in moderately hypercholesterolemic, hypertensive patients randomized to pravastatin vs. usual care. *JAMA* 288 (2002): 2998 – 3007.

Appel, L. J., T. J. Moore, E. Obarzanek et al. A clinical trial of the effects of dietary patterns on blood pressure. *N Engl J Med* 336 (1997): 1117 – 24.

Appel, L. J., F. M. Sacks, V. J. Care et al. Effects of protein, monounsaturated fat, and carbohydrate intake on blood pressure and serum lipids. *JAMA* 294 (2006): 2455 – 64.

Applegate, W. B., S. Pressel, J. Wittes et al. Impact of the treatment of isolated systolic hypertension on behavioral variables: Results from the Systolic Hypertension in the Elderly Program. *Arch Intern Med* 154 (1994): 2154 – 60.

Arky, R. A. "Doctor, is my sugar normal?" *N Engl J Med* 353 (2005): 1511 – 12.

Armstrong, K., E. Moye, S. Williams et al. Screening mammography in women 40 to 49 years of age: A systematic review for the American College of Physicians. *Ann Intern Med* 146 (2007): 516 – 26.

Arpino, G., R. Laucirica, and R. M. Elledge. Pre-malignant and in situ breast disease: Biology and implications. *Ann Intern Med* 143 (2005): 446 – 57.

Ascherio, A., E. B. Rimm, M. A. Hernán et al. Relation of consumption of vitamin E, vitamin C, and carotenoids to risk for stroke among men in the United States. *Ann Intern Med* 130 (1999): 963 – 70.

Ascherio, A., E. B. Rimm, M. J. Stampfer et al. Dietary intake of marine n-3 fatty acids, fish intake and the risk of coronary artery disease among men. *N Engl J Med* 332 (1995): 977 – 82.

Assenfeldt, W. J. J., S. C. Morton, E. I. Yu, M. J. Suttorp, and P. G. Shekelle. Spinal manipulative therapy for low back pain. *Ann Intern Med* 138 (2003): 871 – 81.

Astin, J. A. Why patients use alternative medicine. *JAMA* 279 (1998): 1548 – 53.

Astin, J. A., E. Harkness, and E. Ernst. The efficacy of "distant healing": A systematic review of randomized trials. *Ann Intern Med* 132 (2000): 903 – 10.

Atkin, P. A. A paradigm shift in the medical literature. *BMJ* 325 (2002): 1450 – 51.

Avorn, J. Torcetrapib and atorvastatin — should marketing drive the research agenda? *N Engl J Med* 352 (2005): 2573 – 76.

Babcock, L. J., M. Lewis, E. M. Hay et al. Chronic shoulder pain in the community: A syndrome of disability or distress? *Ann Rheum Dis* 61 (2002): 128 – 31.

Baigent, C., and C. Patrono. Selective cyclooxygenase 2 inhibitors, aspirin, and cardiovascular disease. *Arthritis Rheum* 48 (2003): 12 – 20.

Baines, C. J. The Canadian National Breast Screening Study: A perspective on criticisms. *Ann Intern Med* 120 (1994): 326 – 34.

Baker, K. R., M. E. Nelson, D. T. Felson et al. The efficacy of home-based progressive strength training in older adults with knee osteoarthritis: A randomized controlled trial. *J Rheumatol* 28 (2001): 1655 – 65.

Baker, T. On the genealogy of moral hazard. *Texas Law Review* 75 (1996): 237 – 92.

Bamshad, M. Genetic influences on health: Does race matter? *JAMA* 294 (2005): 937 – 46.

Banks, E., G. Reeves, V. Beral et al. Influence of personal characteristics of individual women on sensitivity and specificity of mammography in the Million Women Study: Cohort study. *BMJ* 329 (2004): 477 – 82.

Banks, J., M. Marmot, Z. Oldfield, and J. P. Smith. Disease and disadvantage in the United States and in England. *JAMA* 295 (2006): 2037–45.

Barclay, R. L., J. J. Vicari, A. S. Doughty et al. Colonoscopic withdrawal times and adenoma detection during screening colonoscopy. *N Engl J Med* 355 (2006): 2533–41.

Barker, K. K. *The Fibromyalgia Story: Medical Authority and Women's Worlds of Pain.* Philadelphia: Temple University Press, 2005.

Baron, J. A., B. F. Cole, R. S. Sandler et al. A randomized trial of aspirin to prevent colorectal adenomas. *N Engl J Med* 348 (2003): 891–99.

Barr, R. G., D. M. Nathan, J. B. Meigs, D. E. Singer. Tests of glycemia for the diagnosis of type 2 diabetes mellitus. *Ann Intern Med* 137 (2002): 263–72.

Barratt, A., K. Howard, L. Irwig et al. Model of outcomes of screening mammography: Information to support informed choices. *BMJ* 330 (2005): 936–38.

Barrett, B. P., R. L. Brown, K. Locken et al. Treatment of the common cold with unrefined Echinacea. *Ann Intern Med* 137 (2002): 939–46.

Barrett-Connor, E., D. Grady, A. Sashegyi et al. Raloxifene and cardiovascular events in osteoporotic postmenopausal women. *JAMA* 287 (2002): 847–57.

Barrett-Connor, E., L. Mosca, P. Collins et al. Effects of raloxifene on cardiovascular events and breast cancer in postmenopausal women. *N Engl J Med* 355 (2006): 125–37.

Barringer, T. A., J. K. Kirk, A. C. Santaniello, K. L. Foley, and R. Michielutte. Effect of a multivitamin and mineral supplement on infection and quality of life. *Ann Intern Med* 138 (2003): 365–71.

Barsky, A. J. The patient with hypochondriasis. *N Engl J Med* 345 (2001): 1395–99.

Barsky, A. J., and J. F. Borus. Functional somatic syndromes. *Ann Intern Med* 130 (1999): 910–21.

Barsky, A. J., J. Orav, and D. W. Bates. Somatization increases medical utilization and costs independent of psychiatric and medical comorbidity. *Archives of General Psychiatry* 62 (2005): 903–10.

Bates, D. W., D. M. Black, and S. R. Cummings. Clinical use of bone densitometry: Clinical applications. *JAMA* 288 (2002): 1898–900.

Batty, G. D., G. Der, S. MacIntyre, and I. J. Deary. Does IQ explain socioeconomic inequalities in health? Evidence from a population-based cohort study in the west of Scotland. *BMJ* 332 (2006): 580–84.

Bavry, A. A., D. J. Kumbhani, T. J. Helton et al. Late thrombosis of drug-eluting stents: A meta-analysis of randomized clinical trials. *Am J Med* 119 (2006): 1056–61.

Beattie, M. S., N. E. Lane, Y. Y. Hung, and M. C. Nevitt. Association of statin use and development and progression of hip osteoarthritis in elderly women. *J Rheumatol* 32 (2005): 106–10.

Beckles, G. L. A., and P. E. Thompson-Reid. Socioeconomic status of women with diabetes — United States, 2000. *Morbidity and Mortality Weekly Report* 51 (2002): 147–59.

Bekelman, J. E., Y. Li, and C. P. Gross. Scope and impact of financial conflicts of interest in biomedical research: A systematic review. *JAMA* 289 (2003): 454–65.

Benjamin, S., S. Morris, J. McBeth et al. The association between chronic widespread pain and mental disorder. *Arthritis Rheum* 43 (2000): 561–67.

Benson, K., and A. J. Hartz. A comparison of observational studies and randomized controlled trials. *N Engl J Med* 342 (2000): 1878–86.

Bent, S., C. Kane, K. Shinohara et al. Saw palmetto for benign prostatic hyperplasia. *N Engl J Med* 354 (2006): 557–66.

Beresford, S. A. A., K. C. Johnson, C. Ritenbaugh et al. Low-fat dietary pattern and risk of colorectal cancer. *JAMA* 295 (2006): 643–54.

Bergman, S., P. Herrström, L. T. H. Jacobsson, and I. F. Petersson. Chronic widespread pain: A three-year follow-up of pain distribution and risk factors. *J Rheumatol* 29 (2002): 818–25.

Berkman, L., and I. Kawachi, eds. *Social Epidemiology*. Oxford: Oxford University Press, 2000.

Berlin, J. A., and D. Rennie. Measuring the quality of trials. *JAMA* 282 (1999): 1083–85.

Berman, B. M., L. Lao, P. Langenberg et al. Effectiveness of acupuncture as adjunctive therapy in osteoarthritis of the knee. *Ann Intern Med* 141 (2004): 901–10.

Bhatt, D. L. To cath or not to cath: That is no longer the question. *JAMA* 293 (2005): 2935–37.

Bialar, J. C., and H. L. Gornik. Cancer undefeated. *N Engl J Med* 336 (1997): 1569–74.

Bigger, J. T. Diuretic therapy, hypertension, and cardiac arrest. *N Engl J Med* 330 (1994): 1899–1900.

Bigos, S. J., O. R. Bowyer, G. R. Braen et al. Acute low back problems in adults. U.S. Department of Health and Human Services, AHCPR publication no. 95-0642, 1994.

Bill-Axelson, A., L. Holmberg, M. Ruutu et al. Radical prostatectomy versus watchful waiting in early prostate cancer. *N Engl J Med* 352 (2005): 1977–84.

Billroth, T. *The Medical Sciences in the German Universities: A Study in the History of Civilization*. New York: Macmillan, 1924.

Bischoff-Ferrari, H. A., W. C. Willett, J. B. Wong, et al. Fracture prevention with vitamin D supplementation: A meta-analysis of randomized controlled trials. *JAMA* 293 (2005): 2257–64.

Bjelakovic, G., D. Nikolova, L. L. Gluud et al. Mortality in randomized trials of antioxidant supplements for primary and secondary prevention. *JAMA* 297 (2007): 842–57.

Black, D. M., A. V. Schwartz, K. E. Ensrud et al. Effects of continuing or stopping alendronate after 5 years of treatment: The fracture intervention trial long-term extension (FLEX)—a randomized trial. *JAMA* 296 (2006): 2927–38.

Black, D. M., J. P. Bilezikian, K. E. Ensrud et al. One year of alendronate after one year of parathyroid hormone (1-84) for osteoporosis. *N Engl J Med* 353 (2005): 555–65.

Black, D. M., P. D. Delmas, R. Eastell et al. Once-yearly zoledronic acid for treatment of postmenopausal osteoporosis. *N Engl J Med* 356 (2007): 1809–22.

Black, D. M., S. R. Cummings, D. B. Karpf et al. Randomized trial of effect of alendronate on risk of fracture in women with existing vertebral fractures. *Lancet* 348 (1996): 1535–41.

Blackmore, S. *The Meme Machine*. Oxford: Oxford University Press, 1999.

Boden, W. E., R. A. O'Rourke, K. K. Teo et al. Optimal medical therapy with or without PCI for stable coronary disease. *N Engl J Med* 356 (2007): 1503–16.

Bodenheimer, T. High and rising health care costs, part 1: Seeking an explanation. *Ann Intern Med* 142 (2005): 847–54.

———. Uneasy alliance: Clinical investigators and the pharmaceutical industry. *N Engl J Med* 342 (2000): 1539–43.

Bombardier, C., L. Laine, A. Reicin et al. Comparison of upper gastrointestinal toxicity of refecoxib and naproxen in patients with rheumatoid arthritis. *N Engl J Med* 343 (2000): 1520 – 28.

Bonadonna, G., A. Moliterni, M. Zambetti et al. Thirty years' follow-up of randomized studies of adjuvant CMF in operable breast cancer: Cohort study. *BMJ* 330 (2005): 217 – 20.

Bonadonna, G., P. Valagussa, A. Moliterni et al. Adjuvant cyclophosphamide, methotrexate and fluorouracil in node-positive breast cancer. *N Engl J Med* 332 (1995): 901 – 6.

Borg, V., T. S. Kristensen, H. Burr. Work environment and changes in self-rated health: A five year follow-up study. *Stress Medicine* 16 (2000): 37 – 47.

Borritz, M., U. Bültmann, R. Rugulies et al. Psychosocial work characteristics as predictors for burnout: Findings from 3-year follow up of the PUMA study. *J Occup Environ Med* 47 (2005): 1015 – 25.

Bosma, H., R. Peter, J. Siegrist, and M. Marmot. Two alternative job stress models and risk of coronary heart disease. *Am J Public Health* 88 (1998): 68 – 74.

Bot, S. D. M., J. M. Van der Waal, C. B. Terwee et al. Predictors of outcome in neck and shoulder symptoms. *Spine* 30 (2005): E459 – 70.

Boutitie, F., F. Gueyffier, S. Pocock et al. J-shaped relationship between blood pressure and mortality in hypertensive patients: New insights from a meta-analysis of individual-patient data. *Ann Intern Med* 136 (2002): 438 – 48.

Boyd, N. F., G. S. Dite, J. Stone et al. Heritability of mammographic density, a risk factor for breast cancer. *N Engl J Med* 347 (2002): 886 – 94.

Bracken, P., and P. Thomas. Time to move beyond the mind-body split. *BMJ* 325 (2002): 1433 – 34.

Brancati, F. L., W. H. L. Kao, A. R. Folsom et al. Incident type 1 diabetes mellitus in African American and white adults. *JAMA* 283 (2000): 2253 – 59.

Brandt, K. D., and J. D. Bradley. Should the initial drug used to treat osteoarthritis pain be a nonsteroidal anti-inflammatory drug? *J Rheumatol* 28 (2001): 467 – 73.

Brandt, K. D., D. K. Heilman, C. Slemenda et al. A comparison of lower extremity muscle strength, obesity, and depression scores in elderly subjects with knee pain with and without radiographic evidence of knee osteoarthritis. *J Rheumatol* 27 (2000): 1937 – 46.

Braunwald, E. Effects of coronary-artery bypass grafting on survival: Implications of the randomized coronary-artery surgery study. *N Engl J Med* 309 (1983): 1181 – 84.

Braveman, P. A., C. Cubbin, S. Egerter et al. Socioeconomic status in health research: One size does not fit all. *JAMA* 294 (2005): 2879 – 88.

Brennan, T. A., D. J. Rothman, L. Blank et al. Health industry practices that create conflicts of interest. *JAMA* 295 (2006): 429 – 33.

Bressler, H. B., W. J. Keyes, P. A. Rochon, and E. Badley. The prevalence of low back pain in the elderly. *Spine* 24 (1999): 1813 – 19.

Brett, A. S. Psychologic effects of the diagnosis and treatment of hypercholesterolemia: Lessons from case studies. *Am J Med* 91 (1991): 642 – 47.

Brewer, N. T., T. Salz, and S. E. Little. Systematic review: The long-term effects of false-positive mammograms. *Ann Intern Med* 146 (2007): 502 – 10.

Bronfort, G. Spinal manipulation: Current state of research and its indications. *Neurologic Clinics* 17 (1999): 91 – 111.

Brosseau, L., S. Milne, V. Robinson et al. Efficacy of the transcutaneous electrical nerve stimulation for the treatment of chronic low back pain. *Spine* 27 (2002): 596 – 603.

Brouwer, I. A., P. L. Zock, A. J. Camm et al. Effect of fish oil on ventricular tachyar-rhythmia and death in patients with implantable cardioverter defibrillators. *JAMA* 295 (2006): 2613–19.

Brownlee, S. *Overtreated: Why Too Much Medicine Is Making Us Sicker and Poorer.* New York: Bloomsbury, 2007.

Brunner, R. L., M. Gass, A. Aragaki et al. Effects of conjugated equine estrogen on health-related quality of life in postmenopausal women with hysterectomy. *Arch Intern Med* 165 (2005): 1976–86.

Bruyere, O., A. Honore, L. C. Rovati et al. Radiologic features poorly predict clinical out-comes in knee osteoarthritis. *Scandinavian Journal of Rheumatology* 31 (2002): 13–16.

Buchbinder, R., and D. Jolley. Effects of a media campaign on back beliefs is sustained 3 years after its cessation. *Spine* 30 (2005): 1324–30.

Bültmann, U., M. J. H. Huibers, L. P. G. M. Van Amelsvoort et al. Psychological distress, fatigue and long-term sickness absence: Prospective results from the Maastricht cohort study. *J Occup Environ Med* 47 (2005): 941–47.

Burgess, C., V. Cornelius, S. Love et al. Depression and anxiety in women with early breast cancer: Five-year observational cohort study. *BMJ* 330 (2005): 702–5.

Burstein, H. J., K. Polyak, J. S. Wong et al. Ductal carcinoma in situ of the breast. *N Engl J Med* 350 (2004): 1430–41.

Campbell, E. G., J. S. Weissman, C. Vogeli et al. Financial relationships between institu-tional review board members and industry. *N Engl J Med* 355 (2006): 2321–29.

Cannon, W. B. *The Wisdom of the Body.* New York: W. W. Norton, 1932.

Carandang, R., S. Seshadri, A. Beiser et al. Trends in incidence, lifetime risk, severity and 30-day mortality of stroke over the past 50 years. *JAMA* 296 (2006): 2939–46.

Carey, T. S., J. Garrett, A. Jackman et al. The outcomes and costs of care for acute low back pain among patients seen by primary care practitioners, chiropractors and orthopedic surgeons. *N Engl J Med* 333 (1995): 913–17.

Caro, J., W. Klittich, A. McGuire et al. The West of Scotland coronary prevention study: Economic benefit analysis of primary prevention with pravastatin. *BMJ* 315 (1997): 1577–82.

Carter, H. B. Prostate cancers in men with low PSA levels — Must we find them? *N Engl J Med* 350 (2004): 2292–94.

CASS Principal Investigators. Myocardial infarction and mortality in the coronary artery surgery study (CASS) randomized trial. *N Engl J Med* 310 (1984): 750–58.

Cassel, E. J. *The Nature of Suffering and the Goals of Medicine.* 2nd ed. Oxford: Oxford University Press, 2004.

Catalona, W. J., S. Loeb, and M. Han. Viewpoint: Expanding prostate cancer screening. *Ann Intern Med* 144 (2006): 441–43.

Cauley, J. A., L. Y. Lui, K. E. Ensrud et al. Bone mineral density and the risk of incident nonspinal fractures in black and white women. *JAMA* 293 (2005): 2102–8.

Cayley, D. *Ivan Illich: In Conversation.* Concord, Ontario: Anansi Press, 1992.

Chan, A. W., A. Hróbjartsson, M. T. Haahr et al. Empirical evidence for selective report-ing of outcomes in randomized trials. *JAMA* 291 (2004): 2457–65.

Chan, E. C. Y., M. J. Barry, S. W. Vernon, and C. Ahn. Physicians and their personal prostate cancer-screening practices with prostate-specific antigen. *J Gen Intern Med* 21 (2006): 257–59.

Chandola, T., E. Brunner, and M. Marmot. Chronic stress at work and the metabolic syndrome: Prospective study. *BMJ* 332 (2006): 521–25.

Chapple, A., S. Ziebland, S. Shepperd et al. Why men with prostate cancer want wider access to prostate specific antigen testing: Qualitative study. *BMJ* 325 (2002): 737–39.

Chapuy, M. C., M. E. Arlot, F. Duboeuf et al. Vitamin D3 and calcium to prevent hip fractures in elderly women. *N Engl J Med* 327 (1992): 1637–42.

Cheng, Y., I. Kawachi, E. H. Coakley et al. Association between psychosocial work characteristics and health functioning in American women: Prospective study. *BMJ* 320 (2000): 1432–36.

Cherkin, D. C., K. J. Sherman, R. A. Deyo, and P. G. Shekelle. A review of the evidence for the effectiveness, safety, and cost of acupuncture, massage therapy, and spinal manipulation for back pain. *Ann Intern Med* 138 (2003): 898–906.

Chibnall, J. T., R. C. Tait, E. M. Andresen, and N. M. Hadler. Clinical and social predictors of application for Social Security Disability Insurance by Workers' Compensation claimants with low back pain. *J Occup Environ Med* 48 (2006b): 733–40.

———. Race and socioeconomic differences in post-settlement outcomes for African American and Caucasian Workers' Compensation claimants with low back injuries. *Pain* 114 (2005): 462–72.

———. Race differences in diagnosis and surgery for occupational low back injuries. *Spine* 31 (2006a): 1272–75.

Chobanian, A. V., G. L. Bakris, H. R. Black et al. The seventh report of the Joint National Committee on Prevention, Detection, Evaluation, and Treatment of high blood pressure: The JNC 7 report. *JAMA* 289 (2003): 2560–72.

Cholesterol Treatment Trialists' (CCT) Collaborators. Efficacy and safety of cholesterol-lowering treatment: Prospective meta-analysis of data from 90,056 participants in 14 randomized trials of statins. *Lancet* 366 (2005): 1267–78.

Chren, M. M., and S. Landefeld. Physicians' behavior and their interactions with drug companies. *JAMA* 271 (1994): 684–89.

Cirillo, D. J., R. B. Wallace, R. J. Rodabough et al. Effects of estrogen therapy on gallbladder disease. *JAMA* 293 (2005): 330–39.

Clegg, D. O., D. J. Reda, C. L. Harris et al. Glucosamine, chondroitin sulfate, and the two in combination for painful knee osteoarthritis. *N Engl J Med* 354 (2006): 795–808.

Collacott, E. A., J. T. Zimmerman, D. W. White, and J. P. Rindone. Bipolar permanent magnets for the treatment of chronic low back pain. *JAMA* 283 (2000): 1322–25.

Collins, J. F., D. A. Lieberman, T. E. Durbin et al. Accuracy of screening for fecal occult blood on a single stool sample obtained by digital rectal examination: A comparison with recommended sampling practice. *Ann Intern Med* 142 (2005): 81–85.

Concato, J., C. K. Wells, R. I. Horwitz et al. The effectiveness of screening for prostate cancer. *Arch Intern Med* 166 (2006): 38–43.

Cooper, R. S., J. S. Kaufman, and R. Ward. Race and genomics. *N Engl J Med* 348 (2003): 1166–70.

Cope, O. *Man, Mind & Medicine.* Philadelphia: Lippincott, 1968.

Coulehan, J. L. The treatment act: An analysis of the clinical art in chiropractic. *Journal of Manipulative and Physiological Therapeutics* 14 (1991): 5–13.

Coulter, I. D., E. L. Hurwitz, A. H. Adams et al. Patients using chiropractors in North America. *Spine* 27 (2002): 291–98.

Cranney, A., V. Welch, J. D. Adachi et al. Etidronate for treating and preventing post-menopausal osteoporosis. Cochrane Database of Systematic Reviews 4 (CD003376), 25 March 2001.

Cranney, A., Z. Papaioannou, N. Zytaruk et al. Parathyroid hormone for the treatment of osteoporosis: A systematic review. Can Med Assoc J 175 (2006): 52–59.

Crans, G. G., S. L. Silverman, H. K. Genant et al. Association of severe vertebral fractures with reduced quality of life. Arthritis Rheum 50 (2004): 4028–34.

Cree, M., C. L. Solkolne, E. Belseck et al. Mortality and institutionalization following hip fracture. J Am Geriatr Soc 48 (2000): 283–88.

Croft, P. Testing for tenderness: What's the point? J Rheumatol 27 (2000): 2531–33.

Cummings, S. R., D. B. Bates, and D. M. Black. Clinical use of bone densitometry: Scientific review. JAMA 288 (2002): 1889–97.

Cummings, S. R., D. M. Black, D. E. Thompson et al. Effect of alendronate on risk of fracture in women with low bone density but without vertebral fractures. JAMA 280 (1998): 2077–82.

Curb, J. D., S. L. Pressel, J. A. Cutler et al. Effect of diuretic-based antihypertensive treatment on cardiovascular disease risk in older diabetic patients with isolated systolic hypertension. JAMA 276 (1996): 1886–92.

Curfman, G. D., S. Morrissey, and J. M. Drazen. Expression of concern: Bombardier et al., "Comparison of upper gastrointestinal toxicity of rofecoxib and naproxen in patients with rheumatoid arthritis." N Engl J Med 343 (2000): 1520–28; N Engl J Med 353 (2005): 2813–14.

———. Expression of concern reaffirmed. N Engl J Med 354 (2006): 1193.

Cushman, M., L. H. Kuller, R. Prentice et al. Estrogen plus progestin and risk of venous thrombosis. JAMA 292 (2004): 1573–80.

D'Amico, A. V., M. H. Chen, K. A. Roehl et al. Preoperative PSA velocity and the risk of death from prostate cancer after radical prostatectomy. N Engl J Med 351 (2004): 125–35.

Dasgupta, P. An Inquiry into Well-being and Destitution. Oxford: Clarendon Press, 1993.

Davey Smith, G., and S. Ebrahim. Data dredging, bias, or confounding. BMJ 325 (2002): 1437–38.

Davey Smith, G., J. D. Neaton, D. Wentworth et al. Mortality differences between black and white men in the USA: Contribution of income and other risk factors among men screened for the MR FIT. Lancet 351 (1998): 934–39.

Davey Smith, G., Y. Bracha, K. H. Svendsen et al. Incidence of type 2 diabetes in the randomized multiple risk factor intervention trial. Ann Intern Med 142 (2005): 313–22.

De Laet, C. E. D. H., B. A. Van Hout, H. Burger et al. Hip fracture prediction in elderly men and women: Validation in the Rotterdam Study. Journal of Bone and Mineral Research 13 (1998): 1587–93.

Dembe, A. E. Occupation and Disease: How Social Factors Affect the Conception of Work-Related Disorders. New Haven: Yale University Press, 1996.

De Smet, P. A. G. M. Herbal remedies. N Engl J Med 374 (2002): 2046–56.

De Winter, R. J., F. Windhausen, J. H. Cornel et al. Early invasive versus selectively invasive management for acute coronary syndrome. N Engl J Med 353 (2005): 1095–104.

Deyo, R. A., D. T. Gray, W. Kreuter et al. United States trends in lumbar fusion surgery for degenerative conditions. Spine 30 (2005): 1441–45.

Diabetes Control and Complications Trial (DCCT) Research Group. The effect of intensive treatment of diabetes on the development and progression of long-term complications of insulin-dependent diabetes mellitus. *N Engl J Med* 329 (1993): 977–86.

Diabetes Control and Complications Trial/Epidemiology of Diabetes Interventions and Complications (DCCT/EDIC) Study Research Group. Intensive diabetes treatment and cardiovascular disease in patients with type 1 diabetes. *N Engl J Med* 353 (2005): 2643–53.

Diabetes Prevention Program Research Group. Reduction in the incidence of type 2 diabetes with lifestyle intervention or metformin. *N Engl J Med* 346 (2002): 393–403.

Diamond, B. Money matters roil Cleveland Clinic's reputation. *Nature Medicine* 12 (2006): 257.

Diepenmaat, A. C. M., M. F. van der Wal, H. C. W. de Vet et al. Neck/shoulder, low back and arm pain in relation to computer use, physical activity, stress and depression among Dutch adolescents. *Pediatrics* 117 (2006): 412–16.

Diez Roux, A. V., S. S. Merkin, D. Arnett et al. Neighborhood of residence and incidence of coronary heart disease. *N Engl J Med* 345 (2001): 99–106.

Dixon, J. M. Screening for breast cancer. *BMJ* 332 (2006): 499–500.

Djulbegovic, B., M. Lacevic, A. Cantor et al. The uncertainty principle and industry-sponsored research. *Lancet* 356 (2000): 635–38.

Domanski, M. J. Primary prevention of coronary artery disease. *N Engl J Med* 357 (2007): 1543–45.

Donohue, J. M., M. Cevasco, and M. B. Rosenthal. A decade of direct-to-consumer advertising of prescription drugs. *N Engl J Med* 357 (2007): 673–81.

Dooley, T. R. *Homeopathy: Beyond Flat Earth Medicine*. San Diego: Timing Publication, 2002.

Downs, J. R., M. Clearfield, S. Weis et al. Primary prevention of acute coronary events with lovastatin in men and women with average cholesterol levels: Results of AFCAPS/ TexCAPS: Air Force/Texas Coronary Atherosclerosis Prevention Study. *JAMA* 279 (1998): 1615–22.

Drazen, J. M. Inappropriate advertising of dietary supplements. *N Engl J Med* 348 (2003): 777–78.

Drazen, J. M., and G. D. Curfman. Financial associations of authors. *N Engl J Med* 346 (2002): 1901–2.

Druss, B. G., S. C. Marcus, M. Olfson et al. Trends in care by nonphysician clinicians in the United States. *N Engl J Med* 348 (2003): 130–37.

Dubé, C., A. Rostom, G. Lewin et al. The use of aspirin for primary prevention of colorectal cancer: A systematic review prepared for the U.S. Preventive Services Task Force. *Ann Intern Med* 146 (2007): 365–75.

Eastham, J. A., E. Riedel, P. T. Scardino et al. Variation of serum prostate-specific-antigen levels. *JAMA* 289 (2003): 2695–700.

Edmond, S. L., and D. T. Felson. Prevalence of back symptoms in elders. *J Rheumatol* 27 (2000): 220–25.

Eisenberg, D. M., D. E. Post, R. B. Davis et al. Addition of choice of complementary therapies to usual care for acute low back pain. *Spine* 32 (2007): 151–58.

Elmer, P. J., E. Obarzanek, W. M. Vollmer et al. Effects of comprehensive lifestyle modification on diet, weight, physical fitness, and blood pressure control: 18-month results of a randomized trial. *Ann Intern Med* 144 (2006): 485–95.

Elmore, J. G., and G. Gigerenzer. Benign breast disease — the risks of communicating risk. *N Engl J Med* 353 (2005): 297–99.

Elmore, J. G., C. Wells, C. H. Lee et al. Variability in radiologists' interpretations of mammograms. *N Engl J Med* 331 (1994): 1493–99.

Elmore, J. G., M. B. Barton, V. M. Moceri et al. Ten-year risk of false positive screening mammograms and clinical breast examinations. *N Engl J Med* 338 (1998): 1089–96.

Engelhart, M. J., M. I. Geerlings, A. Ruitenberg et al. Dietary intake of antioxidants and risk of Alzheimer Disease. *JAMA* 287 (2002): 3223–29.

Erichsen, J. E. *Railway and Other Injuries of the Nervous System*. London: Walton and Maberly, 1866.

Ernst, E. The risk-benefit profile of commonly used herbal therapies: Ginkgo, St. John's wort, ginseng, Echinacea, saw palmetto, and kava. *Ann Intern Med* 136 (2002): 42–53.

Estruch, R., M. A. Martinez-González, D. Corella et al. Effects of a Mediterranean-style diet on cardiovascular risk factors. *Ann Intern Med* 145 (2006): 1–11.

Ettinger, B., D. M. Black, B. H. Mitlak et al. Reduction of vertebral fracture risk in postmenopausal women with osteoporosis treated with raloxifene. *JAMA* 282 (1999): 637–45.

Fagerlin, A., B. J. Zikmund-Fisher, and P. A. Ubel. How making a risk estimate can change the feel of that risk: Shifting attitudes toward breast cancer risk in a general public survey. *Patient Education and Counseling* 57 (2005): 294–99.

Fagerlin, A., D. Rovner, S. Stableford et al. Patient education materials about the treatment of early-stage prostate cancer: A critical review. *Ann Intern Med* 140 (2004): 721–28.

Fairfield, K. M., and R. H. Fletcher. Vitamins for chronic disease prevention in adults. *JAMA* 287 (2002): 3116–26.

Farmer, J. A. Learning from the cerivastatin experience. *Lancet* 358 (2001): 1383–85.

Fawzi, W., and M. J. Stampfer. A role for multivitamins in infection? *Ann Intern Med* 138 (2003): 430–31.

Felson, D. T., and T. E. McAlindon. Glucosamine and chondroitin for osteoarthritis: To recommend or not to recommend? *Arthritis Care Res* 13 (2000): 179–82.

Fernández-de-las-Peñas, C., C. Alonso-Blanco, M. L. Cuadrado et al. Are manual therapies effective in reducing pain from tension-type headache? *Clin J Pain* 22 (2006): 278–85.

Ferreira-González, I., J. W. Busse, D. Heels-Ansdell et al. Problems with use of composite end points in cardiovascular trials: Systematic review of randomized controlled trials. *BMJ* 334 (2007): 786–90.

Ferrie, J. E., J. Head, M. J. Shipley et al. Injustice at work and incidence of psychiatric morbidity: The Whitehall II study. *J Occup Environ Med* 63 (2006): 443–50.

Ferrie, J. E., M. J. Shipley, M. G. Marmot, S. A. Stansfeld, and G. Davey Smith. An uncertain future: The health effects of threats to employment security in white-collar men and women. *Am J Public Health* 88 (1998): 1030–36.

Feskanich, D., W. Willett, and G. Colditz. Walking and leisure-time activity and risk of hip fracture in postmenopausal women. *JAMA* 288 (2002): 2300–306.

Finkler, K. *Experiencing the New Genetics*. Philadelphia: University of Pennsylvania Press, 2000.

Fischoff, B., and S. Wesseley. Managing patients with inexplicable health problems. *BMJ* 326 (2003): 595–97.

Fisher, B., C. Redmond, E. R. Fisher et al. Ten-year results of a randomized clinical trial comparing radical mastectomy and total mastectomy with or without radiation. *N Engl J Med* 312 (1985): 674–81.

Fisher, B., J. H. Jeong, S. Anderson et al. Twenty-five-year follow-up of a randomized trial comparing radical mastectomy, total mastectomy, and total mastectomy followed by irradiation. *N Engl J Med* 347 (2002a): 567–75.

Fisher, B., S. Anderson, J. Bryant et al. Twenty-year follow-up of a randomized trial comparing total mastectomy, lumpectomy, and lumpectomy plus irradiation for the treatment of invasive breast cancer. *N Engl J Med* 347 (2002b): 1233–41.

Fisher, E. S., D. E. Wennberg, T. A. Stukel et al. The implications of regional variations in Medicare spending, part 1: The content, quality, and accessibility of care. *Ann Intern Med* 138 (2003a): 273–87.

———. The implications of regional variations in Medicare spending, part 2: Health outcomes and satisfaction with care. *Ann Intern Med* 138 (2003b): 288–98.

Fitzpatrick, R. Social status and mortality. *Ann Intern Med* 134 (2001): 1001–3.

Flegal, K. M., B. I. Graubard, D. F. Williamson, and M. H. Gail. Excess deaths associated with underweight, overweight and obesity. *JAMA* 293 (2005): 1861–67.

Fletcher, S., and G. Colditz. Failure of estrogen plus progestin therapy for prevention. *JAMA* 288 (2002): 366–68.

Fletcher, S., and J. G. Elmore. Mammographic screening for breast cancer. *N Engl J Med* 348 (2003): 1672–80.

Foley, D. J., and L. R. White. Dietary intake of antioxidants and risk of Alzheimer Disease. *JAMA* 287 (2002): 3261–63.

Fonsecca, R., L. C. Hartmann, I. V. Petersen et al. Ductal carcinoma in situ of the breast. *Ann Intern Med* 127 (1997): 1013–22.

Fontanarosa, P. B., A. Flanagin, and C. D. DeAngelis. Reporting conflicts of interest, financial aspects of research and role of sponsors in funded studies. *JAMA* 294 (2005): 110–11.

Fontanarosa, P. B., D. Rennie, and C. D. DeAngelis. The need for regulation of dietary supplements—lessons from ephedra. *JAMA* 289 (2003): 1568–70.

Ford, E. S., W. H. Giles, and W. H. Dietz. Prevalence of the metabolic syndrome among U.S. adults. *JAMA* 287 (2002): 356–59.

Ford, I., H. Murray, C. J. Packard et al. Long-term follow-up of the West of Scotland Coronary Prevention Study. *N Engl J Med* 357 (2007): 1477–86.

Forseth, K. O., G. Husby, J. T. Gran, and O. Førre. Prognostic factors for the development of fibromyalgia in women with self-reported musculoskeletal pain: A prospective study. *J Rheumatol* 26 (1999): 2458–67.

Foster, N. E., E. Thomas, P. Barlas et al. Acupuncture as an adjunct to exercise-based physiotherapy for osteoarthritis of the knee: Randomised controlled trial. *BMJ* 335 (2007): 436.

Foucault, M. *The Birth of the Clinic: An Archaeology of Medical Perception.* London: Tavistock, 1973.

Fox, C. S., S. Coady, P. D. Sorlie et al. Trends in cardiovascular complications of diabetes. *JAMA* 292 (2004): 2495–99.

Fraenkel, L., B. Gulanski, and D. R. Wittink. Preference for hip protectors among older adults at high risk for osteoporotic fractures. *J Rheumatol* 33 (2006): 2064–68.

Fransen, M., S. McConnell, and M. Bell. Therapeutic exercise for people with osteoarthritis of the hip or knee: A systematic review. *J Rheumatol* 29 (2002): 1737–45.

Fraser, C. G., C. M. Matthew, N. A. Mowat et al. Immunochemical testing of individuals positive for guaiac faecal occult blood test in a screening programme for colorectal cancer: An observational study. *Lancet Oncology* 7 (2006): 127–31.

Frazier, A. L., G. A. Colditz, C. S. Fuchs, and K. M. Kuntz. Cost-effectiveness of screening for colorectal cancer in the general population. *JAMA* 284 (2000): 1954–61.

Freemantle, N. Commentary: Is NICE delivering the goods? *BMJ* 329 (2004): 1003–4.

Freemantle, N., M. Calvert, J. Woods, J. Eastaugh, and C. Griffin. Composite outcomes in randomized trials. *JAMA* 289 (2003): 2554–59.

Friedberg, F., D. W. Leung, and J. Quick. Do support groups help people with chronic fatigue syndrome and fibromyalgia? A comparison of active and inactive members. *J Rheumatol* 32 (2005): 2416–20.

Friedman, H. S. Coronary bypass graft surgery: Reexamining the assumptions. *J Gen Intern Med* 5 (1990): 80–83.

Frost, H., and S. Stewart-Brown. Acupressure for low back pain. *BMJ* 332 (2006): 680–81.

Furlan, A. D., L. Brosseau, M. Imamura, and E. Irvin. Massage for low-back pain: A systematic review within the framework of the Cochrane Collaboration Back Review Group. *Spine* 27 (2002): 1896–1910.

Furlan, A. J. Carotid-artery stenting — case open or closed? *N Engl J Med* 355 (2006): 1726–29.

Gabbay, J., and A. le May. Evidence-based guidelines or collectively constructed "mindlines?" Ethnographic study of knowledge management in primary care. *BMJ* 329 (2004): 1013–16.

Gadamer, H. G. *The Enigma of Health: The Art of Healing in a Scientific Age*. Stanford: Stanford University Press, 1996.

Gagnier, J. J., M. W. van Tulder, B. Berman, and C. Bombardier. Herbal medicine for low back pain: A Cochrane review. *Spine* 32 (2007): 82–92.

Gami, A. S., B. J. Witt, D. E. Howard et al. Metabolic syndrome and risk of incident cardiovascular events and death. *J Am Col Cardiol* 49 (2007): 403–14.

Garro, L. C. Chronic illness and the construction of narratives. In *Pain as Human Experience: An Anthropological Perspective*, edited by M. J. D. Good, P. E. Brodwin, B. J. Good, and A. Kleinman, 100–137. Berkeley: University of California Press, 1992.

Gerstein, H. C. Glycosylated hemoglobin: Finally ready for prime time as a cardiovascular risk factor. *Ann Intern Med* 141 (2004): 475–76.

Gevitz, N. Sectarian medicine. *JAMA* 257 (1987): 1636–40.

Gibson, J. N. A., I. C. Grant, and G. Waddell. The Cochrane review of surgery for lumbar disc prolapse and degenerative lumbar spondylosis. *Spine* 24 (1999): 1820–32.

Gillespie, L. D., W. J. Gillespie, R. Cumming et al. Review: multiple risk factor modification reduces falls in elderly persons. Cochrane Database of Systematic Reviews, issue 1. Cochrane Library, Oxford: Update Software, 1998.

Gillies, C. L., K. R. Abrams, P. C. Lambert et al. Pharmacological and lifestyle interventions to prevent or delay type 2 diabetes in people with impaired glucose tolerance: Systematic review and meta-analysis. *BMJ* 334 (2007): 299–304.

Glickman, S. W., F. S. Ou, E. R. DeLong et al. Pay for performance, quality of care, and outcomes in acute myocardial infarction. *JAMA* 297 (2007): 2373–80.

Gøetzsche, P. C. Believability of relative risks and odds ratios in abstracts: Cross-sectional study. *BMJ* 333 (2006): 231–34.

Gøetzsche, P. C., and O. Olsen. Is screening for breast cancer with mammography justifiable? *Lancet* 355 (2000): 129–34.

Goldacre, M. J., S. E. Roberts, and D. Yeates. Mortality after admission to hospital with fractured neck of femur: Database study. *BMJ* 325 (2002): 868–69.

Goldberg, R. J., J. M. Gore, J. S. Alpert, and J. E. Dalen. Recent changes in attack and survival rates of acute myocardial infarction (1975–81). *JAMA* 255 (1986): 2774–79.

Gomez-Marin, O., A. R. Folsom, T. E. Kottke et al. Improvement in the long-term survival among patients hospitalized with acute myocardial infarction (1970–80). *N Engl J Med* 21 (1987): 1354–59.

Goodman, S. N. The mammography dilemma: A crisis for evidence-based medicine? *Ann Intern Med* 137 (2002): 363–65.

Graat, J. M., E. G. Schouten, and F. J. Kok. Effect of daily vitamin E and multivitamin-mineral supplementation on acute respiratory tract infections in elderly persons. *JAMA* 288 (2002): 715–21.

Gradishar, W. J., and V. G. Kaklamani. Adjuvant therapy of breast cancer in the elderly: Does one size fit all? *JAMA* 293 (2005): 1118–20.

Graham, D. J., D. Compen, R. Hui et al. Risk of acute myocardial infarction and sudden cardiac death in patients treated with cyclo-oxygenase 2 selective and non-selective non-steroidal anti-inflammatory drugs: Nested case-control study. *Lancet* 365 (2005): 475–81.

Greenhalgh, S. *Under the Medical Gaze: Facts and Fictions of Chronic Pain*. Berkeley: University of California Press, 2001.

Greenspan, S. L., E. R. Myers, L. A. Maitland et al. Fall severity and bone mineral density as risk factors for hip fracture in ambulatory elderly. *JAMA* 271 (1994): 128–33.

Greenspan, S. L., R. D. Emkey, H. G. Bone et al. Significant differential effects of alendronate, estrogen, or combination therapy on the rate of bone loss after discontinuation of treatment of postmenopausal osteoporosis. *Ann Intern Med* 137 (2002): 875–83.

Gregg, E. W., J. A. Cauley, K. Stone et al. Relationship of changes in physical activity and mortality among older women. *JAMA* 289 (2003a): 2379–86.

Gregg, E. W., R. B. Gerzoff, T. J. Thompson, and D. F. Williamson. Intentional weight loss and death in overweight and obese U.S. adults 35 years of age and older. *Ann Intern Med* 138 (2003): 383–89.

Gregg, E. W., Y. J. Cheng, B. L. Cadwell et al. Secular trends in cardiovascular disease risk factors according to body mass index in U.S. adults. *JAMA* 293 (2005): 1868–74.

Grodstein, F., T. B. Clarkson, and J. E. Manson. Understanding the divergent data on postmenopausal hormone therapy. *N Engl J Med* 348 (2003): 645–50.

Gross, A. R., J. L. Hoving, T. A. Haines et al. A Cochrane review of manipulation and mobilization for mechanical neck disorders. *Spine* 29 (2004): 1541–48.

Gross, C. P., G. J. McAvay, H. Krumholz et al. The effect of age and chronic illness on life expectancy after a diagnosis of colorectal cancer: Implications for screening. *Ann Intern Med* 145 (2006): 646–53.

Gross, C. P., M. S. Andersen, H. M. Krumholz et al. Relation between Medicare screening reimbursement and stage at diagnosis for older patients with colon cancer. *JAMA* 296 (2006): 2815–22.

Grundy, S. M., J. L. Cleeman, C. N. Merz et al. Implications of recent clinical trials for the National Cholesterol Education Program Adult Treatment Panel III guidelines. *Circulation* 110 (2004): 227–39.

Guastello, S. J., E. A. Johnson, and M. L. Rieke. Nonlinear dynamics of motivational flow. *Nonlinear Dynamics, Psychology, and Life Sciences* 3 (1999): 259–73.

Gureje, O., M. von Korff, G. E. Simon, and R. Gater. Persistent pain and well-being: A World Health Organization study in primary care. *JAMA* 280 (1998): 147–151.

Gurwitz, J. H., T. S. Field, L. R. Harrold et al. Incidence and preventability of adverse drug events among older persons in the ambulatory setting. *JAMA* 289 (2003): 1107–16.

Hacking, I. *The Social Construction of What?* Cambridge: Harvard University Press, 2000.

Hacohen, M. *Karl Popper: The Formative Years, 1902–1945.* Cambridge: Cambridge University Press, 2000.

Hadler, N. M. Legal ramifications of the medical definition of back disease. *Ann Intern Med* 89 (1978): 992–99.

———. There's the Forest: The object lesson of NSAID gastropathy. *J Rheumatol* 17 (1990): 280–82.

———. Knee pain is the malady — not osteoarthritis. *Ann Intern Med* 116 (1992): 598–99.

———. *Occupational Musculoskeletal Disorders.* New York: Raven Press, 1993.

———. The injured worker and the internist. *Ann Intern Med* 120 (1994): 163–64.

———. If you have to prove you are ill, you can't get well: The object lesson of fibromyalgia. *Spine* 21 (1996): 2397–400.

———. Workers' Compensation and chronic regional musculoskeletal pain. *British Journal of Rheumatology* 37 (1998): 815–18.

———. *Occupational Musculoskeletal Disorders.* 2nd ed. Philadelphia: Lippincott Williams & Wilkins, 1999.

———. Laboring for longevity. *J Occup Environ Med* 41 (1999): 617–21.

———. Chiropractic. *Rheumatic Diseases Clinics of North America* 26 (2000): 97–102.

———. Back pain. In *Oxford Textbook of Geriatric Medicine.* 2nd ed. Edited by J. G. Evans, T. F. Williams, B. L. Beattie, J. P. Michel, and G. K. Wilcock. Oxford: Oxford University Press, 2000: 559–65.

———. Rheumatology and the health of the workforce. *Arthritis Rheum* 44 (2001): 1971–74.

———. Point of View on the paper by Coulter et al. *Spine* 27 (2002): 297–98.

———. MRI for regional back pain: Need for less imaging, more understanding. *JAMA* 289 (2003): 2863–65.

———. A ripe old age. *Arch Intern Med* 163 (2003b): 1261–62.

———. The semiotics of backache. *Spine* 29 (2004): 1289.

———. *Occupational Musculoskeletal Disorders.* 3rd ed. Philadelphia: Lippincott Williams & Wilkins, 2005.

———. The health assurance-disease insurance plan: Harnessing reason to the benefits of employees. *J Occup Environ Med* 47 (2005a): 655–57.

Hadler, N. M., and D. B. Gillings. On the design of the phase III drug trial. *Arthritis Rheum* 26 (1983): 1354–61.

Hadler, N. M., and J. P. Evans. Commentary on "The Kin in the Gene." *Current Anthropology* 42 (2001): 252–53.

Hadler, N. M., and S. Greenhalgh. Labeling woefulness: The social construction of fibro-myalgia. *Spine* 30 (2005): 1–4.

Hadler, N. M., P. Curtis, D. B. Gillings, and S. Stinnett. A benefit of spinal manipulation as adjunctive therapy for acute low back pain: A stratified controlled trial. *Spine* 12 (1987): 703–6.

Hadler, N. M., R. C. Tait, and J. T. Chibnall. Back pain in the work place. *JAMA* 297 (2007): 1594–96.

Hagen, E. M., E. Svensen, H. R. Eriksen et al. Comorbid subjective health complaints in low back pain. *Spine* 31 (2006): 1491–95.

Hagen, K. B., G. Hilde, G. Jamtvedt, and M. F. Winnem. The Cochrane review of advice to stay active as a single treatment for low back pain and sciatica. *Spine* 27 (2002): 1736–41.

Haller, C. A., and N. L. Benowitz. Adverse cardiovascular and central nervous system events associated with dietary supplements containing ephedra alkaloids. *N Engl J Med* 343 (2000): 1833–38.

Halligan, P., and M. Aylward, eds. *The Power of Belief: Psychosocial Influence on Illness, Disability and Medicine.* Oxford: Oxford University Press, 2006.

Halton, T. L., W. C. Willet, S. Liu et al. Low-carbohydrate-diet score and the risk of coronary heart disease in women. *N Engl J Med* 355 (2006): 1991–2002.

Hambrecht, R., C. Walther, S. Mobius-Windler et al. Percutaneous coronary angioplasty compared with exercise training in patients with stable coronary artery disease: A randomized trial. *Circulation* 109 (2004): 1371–78.

Hanebuth, D., M. Meinel, and J. E. Fischer. Health-related quality of life, psychosocial work conditions, and absenteeism in an industrial sample of blue- and white-collar employees: A comparison of potential predictors. *J Occup Environ Med* 48 (2006): 28–37.

Hanley, D. F., and E. R. Miller. *Annus horribilis* for vitamin E. *Ann Intern Med* 143 (2005): 143–45.

Hannan, E. L., J. Magaziner, J. J. Wang et al. Mortality and locomotion 6 months after hospitalization for hip fracture. *JAMA* 285 (2001): 2736–42.

Hannan, E. L., M. J. Racz, G. Walford et al. Long-term outcomes of coronary-artery bypass grafting versus stent implantation. *N Engl J Med* 352 (2005): 2174–83.

Harkness, E. F., G. J. Macfarlane, E. S. Nahit, A. J. Silman, and J. McBeth. Risk factors for new-onset low back pain amongst cohorts of newly employed workers. *Rheumatology* 42 (2003): 959–68.

Harris, R., and K. N. Lohr. Screening for prostate cancer: An update of the evidence for the U.S. Preventive Services Task Force. *Ann Intern Med* 137 (2002): 917–29.

Harris, S. T., N. B. Watts, H. K. Genant et al. Effects of risedronate treatment on vertebral and nonvertebral fractures in women with postmenopausal osteoporosis. *JAMA* 282 (1999): 1344–52.

Hartmann, L. C., T. A. Sellers, M. H. Frost et al. Benign breast disease and risk of breast cancer. *N Engl J Med* 353 (2005): 229–37.

Hassett, A. L., J. D. Cone, S. J. Patella, and L. H. Sigal. The role of catastrophizing in the pain and depression of women with fibromyalgia syndrome. *Arthritis Rheum* 43 (2000): 2493–500.

Hays, J., J. K. Ockene, R. L. Brunner et al. Effects of estrogen plus progestin on health-related quality of life. *N Engl J Med* 348 (2003): 1839–54.

Hayward, R. A., T. P. Hofer, and S. Vijan. Narrative review: Lack of evidence for recom-

mended low-density lipoprotein treatment targets: A solvable problem. *Ann Intern Med*
145 (2006): 520 – 30.

Hazemeijer, I., and J. J. Rasker. Fibromyalgia and the therapeutic domain. *Rheumatology*
42 (2003): 507 – 15.

Head, J., M. Kivimäki, P. Martikainen, J. Vahtera, J. E. Ferrie, and M. G. Marmot. Influence of change in psychosocial work characteristics on sickness absence: The Whitehall
II study. *Journal of Epidemiology and Community Health* 60 (2006): 55 – 61.

Healy, B., et al. Conflict of interest guidelines for a multicentre clinical trial of treatment
after coronary-artery bypass-graft surgery. *N Engl J Med* 320 (1989): 949 – 51.

Heaney, R. P., and R. R. Recker. Combination and sequential therapy of osteoporosis.
N Engl J Med 353 (2005): 624 – 25.

Heart Outcomes Prevention Evaluation Study Investigators (HOPE). Vitamin E supplementation and cardiovascular events in high-risk patients. *N Engl J Med* 342 (2000):
154 – 60.

Hedley, A. A., C. L. Ogden, C. L. Johnson et al. Prevalence of overweight and obesity
among U.S. children, adolescents and adults, 1999 – 2002. *JAMA* 291 (2004): 2847 – 50.

Hemingway, H., A. M. Crook, G. Feder et al. Underuse of coronary revascularization
procedures in patients considered appropriate candidates for revascularization. *N Engl
J Med* 344 (2001): 645 – 54.

Hemingway, H., M. J. Shipley, S. Stansfeld, and M. Marmot. Sickness absence from back
pain, psychosocial work characteristics and employment grade among office workers.
Scandinavian Journal of Work, Environment and Health 23 (1997): 121 – 29.

Henderson, R. A., S. J. Pocock, T. C. Clayton et al. Seven-year outcome in the RITA-2
trial: Coronary angioplasty versus medical therapy. *J Am Coll Cardio* 42 (2003):
1161 – 70.

Heos, A. W., D. E. Grobbee, J. Lubsen et al. Diuretics, ß-blockers, and the risk for sudden
cardiac death in hypertensive patients. *Ann Intern Med* 123 (1995): 481 – 87.

Herman, J. Reflections on playing God engendered by a chat with L. *Perspectives in Biology and Medicine* 36 (1993): 592 – 95.

Herman, W. H., T. J. Hoerger, M. Brandle et al. The cost-effectiveness of lifestyle modification of metformin in preventing type 2 diabetes in adults with impaired glucose
tolerance. *Ann Intern Med* 142 (2005): 323 – 32.

Hertzman-Miller, R. R., H. Morgenstern, E. L. Hurwitz et al. Comparing the satisfaction
of low back pain patients randomized to receive medical or chiropractic care: Results
from the UCLA low-back pain study. *Am J Public Health* 92 (2002): 1628 – 33.

Hippisley-Cox, J., and C. Coupland. Risk of myocardial infarction in patients taking
cyclo-oxygenase-2 inhibitors or conventional non-steroidal anti-inflammatory drugs.
BMJ 330 (2005): 1366 – 73.

Hlatky, M. A. Evidence-based use of cardiac procedures and devices. *N Engl J Med* 350
(2004): 2126 – 28.

———. Patient preferences and clinical guidelines. *JAMA* 273 (1995): 1219 – 20.

Hlatky, M. A., D. Boothroyd, E. Vittinghoff et al. Quality-of-life and depressive symptoms in postmenopausal women after receiving hormone therapy. *JAMA* 287 (2002):
591 – 97.

Hochman, J. S., and P. G. Steg. Does preventive PCI work? *N Engl J Med* 356 (2007):
1572 – 74.

Hochman, J. S., G. A. Lamas, C. E. Buller et al. Coronary intervention for persistent occlusion after myocardial infarction. *N Engl J Med* 355 (2006): 2395 – 407.

Hoffman, R. M. Limiting prostate cancer screening. *Ann Intern Med* 144 (2006): 338 – 40.

Hoffman, R. M., M. J. Barry, J. L. Stanford et al. Health outcomes in older men with localized prostate cancer: Results from the prostate cancer outcomes study. *Am J Med* 119 (2006): 418 – 25.

Hollon, M. F. Direct-to-consumer advertising. *JAMA* 293 (2005): 2030 – 33.

Holmberg, L., A. Bill-Axelson, F. Helgesen et al. A randomized trial comparing radical prostatectomy with watchful waiting in early prostate cancer. *N Engl J Med* 347 (2002): 781 – 89.

Holmes, O. W. *Medical Essays: 1842 – 1882.* Boston: Houghton Mifflin, 1899: 39 – 40.

Hoogendoorn, W. E., M. N. M. van Poppel, P. M. Bongers et al. Systematic review of psychosocial factors at work and private life as risk factors for back pain. *Spine* 25 (2000): 2114 – 25.

Hoving, J. L., A. R. Gross, D. Gasner et al. A critical appraisal of review articles on the effectiveness of conservative treatment for neck pain. *Spine* 26 (2001): 196 – 205.

Howard, B. V., L. Van Horn, J. Hsia et al. Low-fat dietary pattern and risk of cardiovascular disease. *JAMA* 295 (2006): 655 – 66.

Hu, F. B., L. Bronner, W. C. Willett et al. Fish and omega-3 fatty acid intake and risk of coronary heart disease in women. *JAMA* 287 (2002): 1815 – 21.

Hu, F. B., M. J. Stampfer, E. B. Rimm et al. A prospective study of egg consumption and risk of cardiovascular disease in men and women. *JAMA* 281 (1999): 1387 – 94.

Huang, H. Y., B. Caballero, S. Chang et al. The efficacy and safety of multivitamin and mineral supplement use to prevent cancer and chronic disease in adults: A systematic review for a National Institutes of Health State-of-the-Science Conference. *Ann Intern Med* 145 (2006): 372 – 85.

Huang, X., H. Chen, W. C. Miller et al. Lower low-density lipoprotein cholesterol levels are associated with Parkinson's disease. *Movement Disorders* 22 (2007): 377 – 81.

Hueb, W., P. R. Soares, B. J. Gersh et al. The medicine, angioplasty, or surgery study (MASS-II): A randomized, controlled clinical trial of three therapeutic strategies for multivessel coronary artery disease: One year results. *J Am Coll Cardiol* 43 (2004): 1743 – 51.

Hughes, G., C. Martinez, E. Myon et al. The impact of a diagnosis of fibromyalgia on health care resource use by primary care patients in the UK. *Arthritis Rheum* 54 (2006): 17 – 83.

Humphrey, L. L., G. K. S. Chan, and H. C. Sox. Postmenopausal hormone replacement therapy and the primary prevention of cardiovascular disease. *Ann Intern Med* 137 (2002): 273 – 84.

Humphrey, L. L., M. Helfand, B. K. S. Chan, and S. H. Woolf. Breast cancer screening: A summary of the evidence for the U.S. Preventive Services Task Force. *Ann Intern Med* 137 (2002): 347 – 60.

Hunt, I. M., A. J. Silman, S. Benjamin et al. The prevalence and associated features of chronic widespread pain in the community using the "Manchester" definition of chronic widespread pain. *Rheumatology* 38 (1999): 275 – 79.

Hurwitz, E. L., H. Morgenstern, G. J. Kominski et al. A randomized trial of chiropractic and medical care for patients with low back pain. *Spine* 31 (2006): 611–21.

IJzelenberg, W., and A. Burdorf. Risk factors for musculoskeletal symptoms and ensuing health care use and sick leave. *Spine* 30 (2005): 1550–56.

Illich, I. *Medical Nemesis: The Expropriation of Health*. New York: Pantheon, 1976.

Imperiale, T. F. Aspirin and the prevention of colorectal cancer. *N Engl J Med* 348 (2003): 879–80.

Imperiale, T. F., D. F. Ransohoff, S. H. Itzkowitz et al. Fecal DNA versus fecal occult blood screening for colorectal-cancer screening in an average-risk population. *N Engl J Med* 351 (2004): 2704–14.

Imperiale, T. F., D. R. Wagner, C. Y. Lin et al. Results of screening colonoscopy among persons 40 to 49 years of age. *N Engl J Med* 346 (2002): 1781–85.

Irnich, D., N. Beharens, H. Molzen et al. Randomized trial of acupuncture compared with conventional massage and "sham" laser acupuncture for treatment of chronic neck pain. *BMJ* 322 (2001): 1574–78.

Irwig, L., K. McCaffery, G. Salkeld, and P. Bossuyt. Informed choice for screening: Implications for evaluation. *BMJ* 332 (2006): 1148–50.

Jackson, R. D., A. Z. LaCroix, M. Gass et al. Calcium plus vitamin D supplementation and the risk of fractures. *N Engl J Med* 354 (2006): 669–83.

Jackson, S. A., A. Tenenhouse, L. Robertson et al. Vertebral fracture definition from population-based data: Preliminary results from the Canadian Multicenter Osteoporosis Study (CaMos). *Osteoporosis International* 11 (2000): 680–87.

Jarvik, J. G., W. Hollingworth, P. J. Heagerty et al. Three-year incidence of low back pain in an initially asymptomatic cohort. *Spine* 30 (2005): 1541–48.

Jellema, P., D. A. W. M. van der Windt, H. E. van der Horst et al. Should treatment of (sub)acute low back pain be aimed at psychosocial prognostic factors? Cluster randomized clinical trial in general practice. *BMJ* 331 (2005): 84–87.

Jemal, A., E. Ward, Y. Hao, and M. Thun. Trends in the leading causes of death in the United States, 1970–2002. *JAMA* 294 (2005): 1255–59.

Jha, P., M. Flather, E. Lonn et al. The antioxidant vitamins and cardiovascular disease: A critical review of epidemiologic and clinical trial data. *Ann Intern Med* 123 (1995): 860–72.

Johansson, J. E., O. Andrén, S. O. Andersson et al. Natural history of early, localized prostate cancer. *JAMA* 291 (2004): 2713–17.

Johnston, J. M., D. P. Landsittel, N. A. Nelson et al. Stressful psychosocial work environment increases risk for back pain among retail material handlers. *American Journal of Industrial Medicine* 43 (2003): 179–87.

Johnstone, R. T. *Occupational Diseases: Diagnosis, Medicolegal Aspects and Treatment*. Philadelphia: Saunders, 1941.

Joines, J. D., and N. M. Hadler. Back pain. In *Hospital Medicine*. 2nd ed. Edited by R. M. Wachter, L. Goldman, and H. Hollander, 1153–62. Philadelphia: Lippincott Williams & Wilkins, 2005.

Jonas, W. B., T. J. Kaptchuk, and K. Linde. A critical overview of homeopathy. *Ann Intern Med* 138 (2003): 393–99.

Jørgensen, A. W., J. Hilden, and P. C. Gøetzsche. Cochrane reviews compared with industry supported meta-analyses and other meta-analyses of the same drugs: Systematic review. *BMJ* 332 (2006): 782–86.

Jørgensen, K. J., and P. C. Gøetzsche. Content of invitations for publicly funded screening mammography. *BMJ* 332 (2006): 538–41.

Julius, S., S. K. Nesbitt, B. M. Egan et al. Feasibility of treating prehypertension with an angiotensin-receptor blocker. *N Engl J Med* 354 (2006): 1685–97.

Jüni, P., A. W. S. Rutjes, and P. A. Dieppe. Are selective COX 2 inhibitors superior to traditional non steroidal anti-inflammatory drugs? *BMJ* 324 (2002): 1287–88.

Kadam, U. T., E. Thomas, and P. R. Croft. Is chronic widespread pain a predictor of all-cause morbidity? A 3 year prospective population-based study in family practice. *J Rheumatol* 32 (2005): 1341–48.

Kahn, R., E. Ferrannini, J. Buse, and M. Stern. The metabolic syndrome: Time for a critical appraisal. *Diabetes Care* 28 (2005): 2289–304.

Kahn, S. E., S. M. Haffner, M. A. Heise et al. Glycemic durability of rosiglitazone, metformin, or glyburide monotherapy. *N Engl J Med* 355 (2006): 2427–43.

Kaila-Kangas, L., I. Keskimäki, V. Notkola et al. How consistently distributed are the socioeconomic differences in severe back morbidity by age and gender? A population based study of hospitalization among Finnish employees. *J Occup Environ Med* 63 (2006): 278–82.

Kaila-Kangas, L., M. Kivimäki, H. Riihimäki, R. Luukkonen, J. Kirjonen, and P. Leino-Arjas. Psychosocial factors at work as predictors of hospitalization for back disorders: A 28-year follow-up of industrial employees. *Spine* 29 (2004): 1823–30.

Kalb, P. E., and K. G. Koehler. Legal issues in scientific research. *JAMA* 287 (2002): 85–91.

Kanjilal, S., E. W. Gregg, Y. J. Cheng et al. Socioeconomic status and trends in disparities in 4 major risk factors for cardiovascular disease among U.S. adults, 1971–2002. *Arch Intern Med* 166 (2006): 2348–55.

Kannus, P., J. Parkkari, S. Koskinen et al. Fall-induced injuries and deaths among older adults. *JAMA* 281 (1999): 1895–99.

Kannus, P., J. Parkkari, S. Niemi et al. Prevention of hip fracture in elderly people with use of a hip protector. *N Engl J Med* 343 (2000): 1506–13.

Kaplan, G. A. Going back to understand the future: Socioeconomic position and survival after myocardial infarction. *Ann Intern Med* 144 (2006): 137–39.

Kaplan, J. B., and T. Bennett. Use of race and ethnicity in biomedical publication. *JAMA* 289 (2003): 2709–16.

Kaptchuk, T. J. The placebo effect in alternative medicine: Can the performance of a healing ritual have clinical significance? *Ann Intern Med* 136 (2002): 817–25.

Kaptchuk, T. J., and D. M. Eisenberg. The persuasive appeal of alternative medicine. *Ann Intern Med* 129 (1998): 1061–65.

Kaptchuk, T. J., W. B. Stason, R. B. Davis et al. Sham device v. inert pill: Randomized controlled trial of two placebo treatments. *BMJ* 332 (2006): 391–97.

Kaptoge, S., K. S. Benevolenskaya, A. K. Bhalla et al. Low BMD is less predictive than reported falls for future limb fractures in women across Europe: Results from the European Prospective Osteoporosis Study. *Bone* 36 (2005): 387–98.

Karasek, R. A., and T. Theorell. *Healthy Work: Stress, Productivity, and the Reconstruction of Working Life*. New York: Basic Books, 1990.

Kato, K., P. F. Sullivan, B. Evengård, and N. L. Pedersen. Importance of genetic influences on chronic widespread pain. *Arthritis Rheum* 54 (2006): 1682–86.

Katz, J. N. Patient preferences and health disparities. *JAMA* 286 (2001): 1506–8.

Kaufman, M. Homeopathy in America: The rise and fall and persistence of a medical heresy. In *Other Healers: Unorthodox Medicine in America*, edited by N. Gevitz, 99–123. Baltimore: Johns Hopkins University Press, 1988.

Kawachi, I., and L. F. Berkman, eds. *Neighborhoods and Health*. Oxford: Oxford University Press, 2003.

Kawachi, I., B. P. Kennedy, and R. G. Wilkinson, eds. *Income Inequality and Health*. Vol. 1 of *The Society and Population Health Reader*. New York: New Press, 1999.

Kearney, P. M., C. Baigent, J. Godwin et al. Do selective cyclo-oxygenase-2 inhibitors and traditional non-steroidal anti-inflammatory drugs increase the risk of atherothrombosis? Meta-analysis of randomized trials. *BMJ* 332 (2006): 1302–8.

Kelch, R. P. Maintaining the public trust in clinical research. *N Engl J Med* 346 (2002): 285–87.

Keller, T., and T. Chappell. The rise and fall of Erichsen's disease (railway spine). *Spine* 21 (1996): 1597–601.

Kersh, B. C., L. A. Bradley, G. S. Alarcón et al. Psychosocial and health status variables independently predict health care seeking in fibromyalgia. *Arthritis Care Res* 45 (2001): 362–71.

Kesselheim, A. S., and J. Avorn. The role of litigation in defining drug risks. *JAMA* 297 (2007): 308–11.

King, S. B. Why have stents replaced balloons? Underwhelming evidence. *Ann Intern Med* 138 (2003): 842–43.

Kivimäki, M., J. E. Ferrie, E. Brunner et al. Justice at work and reduced risk of coronary heart disease among employees. *Arch Intern Med* 165 (2005): 2245–51.

Kjaergard, L. L., and B. Als-Nielsen. Associations between competing interests and authors' conclusions: Epidemiological study of randomized clinical trials published in the *BMJ*. *BMJ* 325 (2002): 249–52.

Klauokalani, D., K. J. Sherman, and D. C. Cherkin. Acupuncture for chronic low back pain: Diagnosis and treatment patterns among acupuncturists evaluating the same patient. *Southern Medical Journal* 94 (2001): 486–92.

Knoops, K. T. B., L. C. P. G. M. de Groot, D. Kromhour et al. Mediterranean diet, lifestyle factors and 10-year mortality in elderly European men and women. *JAMA* 292 (2004): 1433–39.

Koes, B. W. Surgery versus intensive rehabilitation programmes for chronic low back pain. *BMJ* 330 (2005): 1220–21.

Koes, B. W., W. J. Assendelft, G. J. van der Heijden, and L. M. Bouter. Spinal manipulation for low back pain: An updated systematic review of randomized clinical trials. *Spine* 21 (1996): 2860–71.

Kohli, P., and P. Greenland. Role of the metabolic syndrome in risk assessment for coronary heart disease. *JAMA* 295 (2006): 819–21.

Kopec, J. A., B. Goel, P. S. Bunting et al. Screening with prostate specific antigen and metastatic prostate cancer risk: A population based case-control study. *Journal of Urology* 174 (2005): 495–99.

Korn, D. Conflicts of interest in biomedical research. *JAMA* 284 (2000): 2234–37.

Kostis, J. B., A. C. Wilson, R. S. Freudenberger et al. Long-term effect of diuretic-based therapy on fatal outcomes in subjects with isolated systolic hypertension with and without diabetes. *American Journal of Cardiology* 95 (2005): 29 – 35.

Kubzansky, L. D., I. Kawachi, and D. Sparrow. Socioeconomic status, hostility, and risk factor clustering in the normative aging study: Any help from the concept of allostatic load? *Annals of Behavioral Medicine* 21 (1999): 330 – 38.

Kuhn, T. *The Structure of Scientific Revolutions.* 2nd ed. Chicago: University of Chicago Press, 1970.

Kumana, C. R., B. M. Y. Cheung, and I. J. Lauder. Gauging the impact of statins using number needed to treat. *JAMA* 282 (1999): 1899 – 1901.

Lagerqvist, B., S. K. James, U. Stenestrand et al. Long-term outcomes with drug-eluting stents versus bare-metal stents in Sweden. *N Engl J Med* 356 (2007): 1009 – 19.

Laine, C. In the clinic: Type 2 diabetes. *Ann Intern Med* 146 (2007): ITC 1 – 16.

Lakka, H. M., D. E. Laaksonen, T. A. Lakka et al. The metabolic syndrome and total and cardiovascular disease mortality in middle-aged men. *JAMA* 288 (2002): 2709 – 16.

Lakka, T. A., J. M. Venäläinen, R. Rauramaa et al. Relation of leisure-time physical activity and cardiorespiratory fitness to the risk of acute myocardial infarction in men. *N Engl J Med* 330 (1994): 1549 – 54.

Lantz, P. M., J. S. House, J. M. Lepkowski et al. Socioeconomic factors, health behaviors, and mortality. *JAMA* 279 (1998): 1703 – 8.

Lasser, K. E., P. D. Allen, S. J. Woolhandler et al. Timing of new black box warnings and withdrawals for prescription medications. *JAMA* 287 (2002): 2215 – 20.

Lauer, M. S., and E. J. Topol. Clinical trials — multiple treatments, multiple end points, and multiple lessons. *JAMA* 289 (2003): 2575 – 77.

Law, M. R., N. J. Wald, J. K. Morris, R. E. Jordan. Value of low dose combination treatment with blood pressure lowering drugs: Analysis of 354 randomized trials. *BMJ* 326 (2003): 1427 – 35.

Lee, I. M., N. R. Cook, J. M. Gaziano et al. Vitamin E in the primary prevention of cardiovascular disease and cancer: The Women's Health Study: A randomized controlled trial. *JAMA* 294 (2005): 56 – 65.

Leeb, B. F., H. Schweitzer, K. Montag, and J. S. Smolen. A meta-analysis of chondroitin sulfate in the treatment of osteoarthritis. *J Rheumatol* 27 (2000): 205 – 11.

Legakos, S. W. The challenge of subgroup analyses — reporting without distorting. *N Engl J Med* 354 (2006): 1667 – 69.

Leipzig, R. M., R. G. Cumming, and M. E. Tinetti. Drugs and falls in older people: a systematic review and meta-analysis: II. Cardiac and analgesic drugs. *J Am Geriatr Soc* 47 (1999): 40 – 50.

Lerman, C., B. Trock, B. K. Rimer et al. Psychological and behavioral implications of abnormal mammograms. *Ann Intern Med* 114 (1991): 657 – 61.

Lerner, B. H. Fighting the war on breast cancer: Debates over early detection, 1945 to the present. *Ann Intern Med* 129 (1998): 74 – 78.

Lesser, L. I., C. B. Ebbeling, M. Goozner et al. Relationship between funding source and conclusion among nutrition-related scientific articles. *PLoS Medicine* 4, no. 1 (2007): e5.

Lévesque, L. E., J. M. Brophy, and B. Zhang. The risk for myocardial infarction with cyclooxygenase-2 inhibitors: A population study of elderly adults. *Ann Intern Med* 142 (2005): 481 – 89.

Levin, A. The Cochrane collaboration. *Ann Intern Med* 135 (2001): 309–12.

Levin, T. R., W. Zhao, C. Conell et al. Complications of colonoscopy in an integrated health care delivery system. *Ann Intern Med* 145 (2006): 880–86.

Levy, D., and T. J. Thom. Death rates from coronary disease — progress and a puzzling paradox. *N Engl J Med* 339 (1998): 915–17.

Lexchin, J., L. A. Bero, B. Djulbegovic, and O. Clark. Pharmaceutical industry sponsorship and research outcome and quality: Systematic review. *BMJ* 326 (2003): 1167–77.

Li, X., M. A. M. Gignac, and A. H. Anis. Workplace, psychosocial factors, and depressive symptoms among working people with arthritis: A longitudinal study. *J Rheumatol* 33 (2006): 1849–55.

Li, Z., M. Maglione, W. Tu et al. Meta-analysis: Pharmacologic treatment of obesity. *Ann Intern Med* 142 (2005): 532–46.

Li-Chen, L., C. H. Kuo, L. H. Lee et al. Treatment of low back pain by acupressure and physical therapy: Randomized controlled trial. *BMJ* 332 (2006): 696–700.

Lichtenstein, A. H., and R. M. Russell. Essential nutrients: Food or supplements? *JAMA* 294 (2005): 351–58.

Lieberman, D. Colonoscopy: As good as gold? *Ann Intern Med* 141 (2004): 401–3.

Lieberman, D. A., and D. G. Weiss for the Veterans Affairs Cooperative Study Group. One-time screening for colorectal cancer with combined fecal occult-blood testing and examination of the distal colon. *N Engl J Med* 345 (2001): 555–60.

Lieberman, D. A., D. G. Weiss, J. H. Bond et al. Use of colonoscopy to screen asymptomatic adults for colorectal cancer. *N Engl J Med* 342 (2000): 162–68.

Lin, O. S., R. A. Kozarek, D. B. Schembre et al. Screening colonoscopy in very elderly patients. *JAMA* 295 (2006): 2357–65.

Lind, B. K., W. E. Lafferty, P. T. Tyree et al. The role of alternative medical providers for the outpatient treatment of insured patients with back pain. *Spine* 30 (2005): 1454–59.

Linde, K., A. Streng, S. Jürgens et al. Acupuncture for patients with migraine. *JAMA* 293 (2005): 2118–25.

Linde, K., and C. D. Mulrow. St. John's wort for depression: Cochrane review. Cochrane Library, Oxford: Update Software, 1998.

Lindsay, R., S. L. Silverman, C. Cooper et al. Risk of new vertebral fracture in the year following a fracture. *JAMA* 285 (2001): 320–23.

Linton, S. J. A review of psychological risk factors in back and neck pain. *Spine* 25 (2000): 1148–56.

Lips, P. Hypervitaminosis A and fractures. *N Engl J Med* 348 (2003): 347–49.

Lipsky, P. E., S. B. Abramson, F. C. Breedveld et al. Analysis of the effect of COX-2 specific inhibitors and recommendations for their use in clinical practice. *J Rheumatol* 27 (2000): 1338–40.

Litwin, M. S., and D. C. Miller. Treating older men with prostate cancer. *JAMA* 296 (2006): 2733–34.

London, J. *The People of the Abyss.* New York: McMillan, 1903.

Lonn, E., S. Yusuf, M. J. Arnold et al. Homocysteine lowering with folic acid and B vitamins in vascular disease. *N Engl J Med* 354 (2006): 1567–77.

Lötters, F., R. L. Franche, S. Hogg-Johnson, A. Burdorf, and J. D. Pole. The prognostic value of depressive symptoms, fear-avoidance, and self-efficacy for duration of lost-time benefits in workers with musculoskeletal disorders. *J Occup Environ Med* 63 (2006): 794–801.

Lucire, Y. *Constructing RSI: Belief and Desire.* Sydney: UNSW Press, 2003.

———. New drugs, new problems. *Australian Journal of Forensic Sciences* 37 (2005): 9–25.

Lund, T., M. Labriola, K. B. Christensen et al. Psychosocial work environment exposures as risk factors for long-term sickness absence among Danish employees: Results from DWECS/DREAM. *J Occup Environ Med* 47 (2005): 1141–47.

Lurie, P., C. M. Almeida, N. Stine et al. Financial conflict of interest disclosure and voting patterns at Food and Drug Administration drug advisory committee meetings. *JAMA* 295 (2006): 1921–28.

Lu-Yao, G., P. C. Albertsen, J. L. Stanford et al. Natural experiment examining impact of aggressive screening and treatment on prostate cancer mortality in two fixed cohorts from Seattle area and Connecticut. *BMJ* 325 (2002): 740–43.

Lynch, H. T., and A. de la Chapelle. Hereditary colorectal cancer. *N Engl J Med* 348 (2003): 919–32.

Macfarlane, G. J., E. Thomas, A. C. Papageorgiou et al. The natural history of chronic pain in the community: A better prognosis than in the clinic? *J Rheumatol* 23 (1996): 1617–20.

Macfarlane, G. J., S. Morris, I. M. Hunt et al. Chronic widespread pain in the community: The influence of psychological symptoms and mental disorder on healthcare seeking behavior. *J Rheumatol* 26 (1999): 413–19.

MacLean, C. H., S. J. Newberry, W. A. Mojica et al. Effects of omega-3 fatty acids on cancer risk. *JAMA* 295 (2006): 403–15.

Maggard, M. D., L. R. Shugarman, M. Suttorp et al. Meta-analysis: Surgical treatment of obesity. *Ann Intern Med* 142 (2005): 547–59.

Mahoney, E. M., C. T. Jurkovitz, H. Chu et al. Cost and cost-effectiveness of an early invasive vs. conservative strategy for the treatment of unstable angina and non-ST-segment elevation myocardial infarction. *JAMA* 288 (2002): 1851–58.

Main, C. J., and A. C. Williams. Musculoskeletal pain. *BMJ* 325 (2002): 534–37.

Maisel, W. H. Unanswered questions—drug-eluting stents and the risk of late thrombosis. *N Engl J Med* 356 (2007): 981–84.

Mallen, C. D., G. Peat, E. Thomas, and P. R. Croft. Is chronic pain in adulthood related to childhood factors? A population-based case-control study of young adults. *J Rheumatol* 33 (2006): 2286–90.

Mallett, S., and M. Clarke. How many Cochrane reviews are needed to cover existing evidence on the effects of health care interventions? *ACP Journal Club* 139 (July–August 2003): A11–A12.

Malmivaara, A., B. W. Koes, L. M. Bouter, and M. W. van Tulder. Applicability and clinical relevance of results in randomized controlled trials. *Spine* 31 (2006): 1405–9.

Mandel, J. S., J. H. Bond, T. R. Church et al. Reducing mortality from colorectal cancer by screening for fecal occult blood. *N Engl J Med* 328 (1993): 1365–71.

Mandel, J. S., T. R. Church, J. H. Bond et al. The effect of fecal occult-blood screening on the incidence of colorectal cancer. *N Engl J Med* 343 (2000): 1603–7.

Mandelblatt, J., S. Saha, S. Teutsch et al. The cost-effectiveness of screening mammography beyond age 65 years: A systematic review for the U.S. Preventive Services Task Force. *Ann Intern Med* 139 (2003): 835–42.

Manheimer, E., K. Linde, L. Lao, L. M. Bouter, and B. M. Berman. Meta-analysis: Acupuncture for osteoarthritis of the knee. *Ann Intern Med* 146 (2007): 868 – 77.

Mann, C. C., and M. L. Plummer. *The Aspirin Wars.* New York: Knopf, 1991.

Manuel, D. G., K. Kwong, P. Tanuseputro et al. Effectiveness and efficiency of different guidelines on statin treatment for preventing deaths from coronary heart disease: Modeling study. *BMJ* 332 (2006): 1419 – 23.

March, L. M., I. D. Cameron, R. G. Cumming et al. Mortality and morbidity after hip fracture: Can evidence-based clinical pathways make a difference? *J Rheumatol* 27 (2000): 2227 – 31.

Marcus, A. J., M. J. Broekman, and D. J. Pinsky. COX inhibitors and thrombophilia. *N Engl J Med* 347 (2002): 1025 – 26.

Marcus, D. M., and A. P. Grollman. Botanical medicines — the need for new regulations. *N Engl J Med* 347 (2002): 2073 – 76.

Mark, D. B., and M. F. Newman. Protecting the brain in coronary artery bypass graft surgery. *JAMA* 287 (2002): 1448 – 50.

Mark, D. H. Deaths attributable to obesity. *JAMA* 293 (2005): 1918 – 20.

Marmot, M. *The Status Syndrome: How Social Standing Affects Our Health and Longevity.* New York: Henry Holt & Co., 2004.

Marmot, M., and R. H. Wilkinson, eds. *Social Determinants of Health.* Oxford: Oxford University Press, 1999.

Marra, C. A., J. M. Esdaile, H. Sun, and A. H. Anis. The cost of COX inhibitors: How selective should we be? *J Rheumatol* 27 (2000): 2731 – 33.

Martimo, K. P., J. Verbeek, J. Karppinen et al. Manual material handling advice and assistive devices for preventing and treating back pain in workers. *Cochrane Database of Systematic Reviews*, issue 3 (2007). Article no.: CD005958. DOI: 10.1002/14651858. CD005958.pub2.

Mas, J. L., G. Chatellier, B. Beyssen et al. Endarterectomy versus stenting in patients with symptomatic severe carotid stenosis. *N Engl J Med* 355 (2006): 1660 – 71.

Masud, T., and R. M. Francis. The increasing use of peripheral bone densitometry. *BMJ* 321 (2000): 306 – 8.

McAlindon, T. E., M. P. LaValley, J. P. Gulin, and D. T. Felson. Glucosamine and chondroitin for treatment of osteoarthritis: A systematic quality assessment and meta-analysis. *JAMA* 283 (2000): 1469 – 75.

McCally, M., A. Haines, O. Fein et al. Poverty and ill health: Physicians can, and should, make a difference. *Ann Intern Med* 129 (1998): 726 – 33.

McClung, M. R. Osteopenia: To treat or not to treat? *Ann Intern Med* 142 (2005): 796 – 97.

McClung, M. R., P. Geusens, P. D. Miller et al. Effect of risedronate on the risk of hip fracture in elderly women. *N Engl J Med* 344 (2001): 333 – 40.

McDonald, C. J. Medical heuristics: The silent adjudicators of clinical practice. *Ann Intern Med* 124 (1996): 56 – 62.

McGettigan, P., and D. Henry. Cardiovascular risk and inhibition of cyclooxygenase. *JAMA* 296 (2006): 1633 – 44.

McGlynn, E. A., S. M. Asch, J. Adams et al. The quality of health care delivered to adults in the United States. *N Engl J Med* 348 (2003): 2635 – 45.

McGovern, P. G., J. S. Pankow, E. Shahar et al. Recent trends in acute coronary heart disease. *N Engl J Med* 334 (1996): 884 – 90.

McLeod, R. S., and members of the Canadian Task Force on Preventive Health Care. Screening strategies for colorectal cancer: A systematic review of the evidence. *Canadian Journal of Gastroenterology* 136 (2001): 647–60.

McMahon, J. A., T. J. Green, C. M. Skeaff et al. A controlled trial of homocysteine lowering and cognitive performance. *N Engl J Med* 354 (2006): 2764–72.

McNaughton-Collins, M., F. J. Fowler, J. F. Caubet et al. Psychological effects of a suspicious prostate cancer screening test followed by a benign biopsy result. *Am J Med* 117 (2004): 719–25.

McTigue, K. M., J. M. Garrett, and B. M. Popkin. The natural history of the development of diabetes in a cohort of young U.S. adults between 1981 and 1998. *Ann Intern Med* 136 (2002): 857–64.

McWhinney, I. R., R. M. Epstein, and T. R. Freeman. Rethinking somatization. *Ann Intern Med* 126 (1997): 747–50.

Meador, C. K. The art and science of nondisease. *N Engl J Med* 272 (1965): 92–95.

———. The last well person. *N Engl J Med* 330 (1994): 440–41.

Meeker, W. C., and S. Haldeman. Chiropractic: A profession at the crossroads of mainstream and alternative medicine. *Ann Intern Med* 136 (2002): 216–27.

Mehta, S. R., C. P. Cannon, K. A. A. Fox et al. Routine vs. selective invasive strategies in patients with acute coronary syndromes: A collaborative meta-analysis of randomized trials. *JAMA* 293 (2005): 2908–17.

Meier, P., R. Zbinden, M. Togni et al. Coronary collateral function long after drug-eluting stent implantation. *J Am Coll Cardiol* 49 (2007): 15–20.

Melander, H., J. Ahlqvist-Rastad, G. Meijer, and B. Beermann. Evidence b(i)ased medicine-selective reporting from studies sponsored by pharmaceutical industry: Review of studies in new drug applications. *BMJ* 326 (2003): 1171–76.

Metzl, J. M. If direct-to-consumer advertisements come to Europe: Lessons from the USA. *Lancet* 369 (2007): 704–6.

Michaëlsson, K., H. Lithell, B. Vessby, and H. Melhus. Serum retinol levels and the risk of fracture. *N Engl J Med* 348 (2003): 287–94.

Miech, R. A., S. K. Kumanyika, N. Stettler et al. Trends in the association of poverty with overweight among U.S. adolescents, 1971–2004. *JAMA* 295 (2006): 2385–93.

Miettinen, O. S., C. I. Henschke, M. W. Pasmantier et al. Does mammography save lives? *Can Med Assoc J* 166 (2002): 1187–88.

Miettinen, O. S., C. T. Henschke, M. W. Pasmantier et al. Mammographic screening: No reliable supporting evidence? *Lancet* 359 (2002): 404–6.

Mikkelsson, M., J. Kaprio, J. J. Salminen et al. Widespread pain among 11-year-old Finnish twin pairs. *Arthritis Rheum* 44 (2001): 481–85.

Miller, A. B., C. J. Baines, T. To, and C. Wall. Canadian National Breast Screening Study: 1. Breast cancer detection and death rates among women aged 40 to 49 years. *Can Med Assoc J* 147 (1992a): 1459–76.

———. Canadian National Breast Screening Study: 2. Breast cancer detection and death rates among women aged 50 to 59 years. *Can Med Assoc J.* 147 (1992b): 1477–88.

Miller, A. B., T. To, C. J. Baines, and C. Wall. Canadian National Breast Screening Study—2: 13-year results of a randomized trial in women aged 50–59 years. *J Natl Cancer Inst* 92 (2000): 1490–99.

————. The Canadian National Breast Screening Study — 1: Breast cancer mortality after 11 to 16 years of follow-up. *Ann Intern Med* 137 (2002): 305 – 12.

Miller, D. *Popper Selections*. Princeton: Princeton University Press, 1985.

Miller, E. R., R. Pastor-Barriuso, D. Dalal et al. Meta-analysis: High dosage vitamin E supplementation may increase all-cause mortality. *Ann Intern Med* 142 (2005): 37 – 46.

Miller, F. G., D. L. Rosenstein, E. G. DeRenzo. Professional integrity in clinical research. *JAMA* 280 (1998): 1449 – 54.

Mills, J. L. Data torturing. *N Engl J Med* 329 (1993): 1196 – 99.

Minkler, M., E. Fuller-Thompson, J. M. Guralnik. Gradient of disability across the socio-economic spectrum in the United States. *N Engl J Med* 355 (2006): 695 – 703.

Mishkel, G. J., A. L. Moore, S. Markwell et al. Long-term outcomes after management of restenosis or thrombosis of drug-eluting stents. *J Am Coll Cardiol* 49 (2007): 181 – 84.

Mitchell, H. L., A. J. Carr, and D. L. Scott. The management of knee pain in primary care: Factors associated with consulting the GP and referrals to secondary care. *J Rheumatol* 45 (2006): 771 – 76.

Mitka, M. Critics say drug-eluting stents overused. *JAMA* 296 (2006): 2077.

————. Does the metabolic syndrome really exist? *JAMA* 294 (2005): 2010 – 13.

Mittleman, M. A. A 39-year-old woman with hypercholesterolemia. *JAMA* 296 (2006): 319 – 26.

Mixter, W. J., and J. S. Barr. Rupture of the intervertebral disc with involvement of the spinal canal. *N Engl J Med* 211 (1934): 210 – 15.

Mohren, D. C. L., G. M. H. Swaen, L. G. P. M. van Amelsvoort et al. Job insecurity as a risk factor for common infections and health complaints. *J Occup Environ Med* 45 (2003): 123 – 29.

Møller, H., and E. Davies. Over-diagnosis in breast cancer screening. *BMJ* 332 (2006): 691 – 92.

Morin, K., H. Rakatansky, F. A. Riddick et al. Managing conflicts of interest in the conduct of clinical trials. *JAMA* 287 (2002): 78 – 84.

Morris, A. M. Medicare policy and colorectal cancer screening. *JAMA* 296 (2006): 2855 – 56.

Morris, M. C., D. A. Evans, J. L. Bienias et al. Dietary intake of antioxidant nutrients and the risk of incident Alzheimer Disease in a biracial community study. *JAMA* 287 (2002): 3230 – 37.

Morrow, M., and S. J. Schnitt. Treatment selection in ductal carcinoma in situ. *JAMA* 283 (2000): 453 – 55.

Mortality Morbidity Weekly Report (CDC) 43 (1994): 586.

Moseley, J. B., K. O'Malley, N. J. Petersen et al. A controlled trial of arthroscopic surgery for osteoarthritis of the knee. *N Engl J Med* 347 (2002): 81 – 88.

Moses, H., E. Braunwald, J. B. Martin, and S. O. Thier. Collaborating with industry — choices for the academic medical center. *N Engl J Med* 347 (2002): 1371 – 75.

Mozaffarian, D., and E. B. Rimm. Risk intake, contaminants, and human health. *JAMA* 296 (2006): 1885 – 99.

Mozaffarian, D., M. B. Katan, A. Ascherio et al. Trans fatty acids and cardiovascular disease. *N Engl J Med* 354 (2006): 1601 – 13.

Mukherjee, D., S. E. Nissen, and E. J. Topol. Risk of cardiovascular events associated with selective COX-2 inhibitors. *JAMA* 286 (2001): 954–59.

Mulrow, C., and M. Pignone. An editorial update: Should she take aspirin? *Ann Intern Med* 142 (2005): 942–43.

Multiple Risk Factor Intervention Trial Research Group. Multiple Risk Factor Intervention Trial: Risk factor changes and mortality. *JAMA* 248 (1982): 182–87.

Musgrave, D. S., M. T. Vogt, M. C. Nevitt, and J. A. Cauley. Back problems among post-menopausal women taking estrogen replacement therapy. *Spine* 26 (2001): 1606–12.

Muss, H. B., S. Woolf, D. Berry et al. Adjuvant chemotherapy in older and younger women with lymph node–positive breast cancer. *JAMA* 293 (2005): 1073–81.

Mysliwiec, P. A., M. L. Brown, C. N. Klabunde, D. F. Ransohoff. Are physicians doing too much colonoscopy? A national survey of colorectal surveillance after polypectomy. *Ann Intern Med* 141 (2004): 264–71.

Nabel, E. G. Conflict of interest — or conflict of priorities? *N Engl J Med* 355 (2006): 2365–67.

Nadel, M. R., J. A. Shapiro, C. N. Klabunde et al. A national survey of primary care physicians' methods for screening for fecal occult blood. *Ann Intern Med* 142 (2005): 86–94.

Nathan, D. M. Rosiglitazone and cardiotoxicity: Weighing the evidence. *N Engl J Med* 357 (2007): 64–66.

———. Thiazolidinediones for initial treatment of type 2 diabetes? *N Engl J Med* 355 (2006): 2477–80.

National Cholesterol Education Program (NCEP). Executive Summary of the Third Report on Detection, Evaluation and Treatment of High Blood Cholesterol in Adults. *JAMA* 285 (2001): 2486–97.

National Cholesterol Education Program — Adult Treatment Panel III (NCEP-ATP III). Third report of the National Cholesterol Education Program Expert Panel on Detection, Evaluation and Treatment of High Blood Cholesterol in Adults. *Circulation* 106 (2002): 3143.

National Institutes of Health. Osteoporosis prevention, diagnosis and therapy. *NIH Consensus Statement* 17 (2000): 1–45.

———. Third Report of the National Cholesterol Education Program Expert Panel on Detection, Evaluation, and Treatment of High Blood Cholesterol in Adults (Adult Treatment Panel III). NIH Publication 01-3670. Bethesda, Md.: National Institutes of Health, 2001.

National Institutes of Health Consensus Development Panel on Osteoporosis, Prevention Diagnosis and Therapy. Osteoporosis prevention, diagnosis and therapy. *JAMA* 285 (2001): 785–95.

National Institutes of Health State-of-the-Science Panel. National Institutes of Health State-of-the-Science Conference statement: Management of menopause-related symptoms. *Ann Intern Med* 142 (2005): 1003–12.

National Task Force on the Prevention and Treatment of Obesity. Weight cycling. *JAMA* 272 (1994): 1196–202.

Natvig, B., D. Bruusgaard, and W. Eriksen. Localized low back pain and low back pain as part of widespread musculoskeletal pain: Two different disorders? A cross-sectional population study. *Journal of Rehabilitation Medicine* 33 (2001): 21–25.

Neer, R. M., C. D. Arnaud, J. R. Zanchetta et al. Effect of parathyroid hormone (1-34) on fractures and bone mineral density in postmenopausal women with osteoporosis. *N Engl J Med* 344 (2001): 1434–41.

Neerinckx, J., B. van Houdenhove, R. Lysens et al. Attributions in chronic fatigue syndrome and fibromyalgia syndrome in tertiary care. *J Rheumatol* 27 (2000): 1051–55.

Nelemans, P. J., R. A. deBie, H. C. W. deVet, and F. Sturmans. Injection therapy for subacute and chronic benign low back pain. *Spine* 26 (2001): 501–15.

Nelson, H. D., L. L. Humphrey, P. Nygren et al. Postmenopausal hormone replacement therapy. *JAMA* 288 (2002): 872–81.

Nelson, H. D., M. Helfand, S. H. Woolf, and J. D. Allan. Screening for postmenopausal osteoporosis: A review of the evidence for the U.S. Preventive Services Task Force. *Ann Intern Med* 137 (2002): 529–41.

Nelson, M. R., D. Liew, M. Bertram, and T. Vos. Epidemiological modeling of routine use of low dose aspirin for the primary prevention of coronary heart disease and stroke in those aged ≥70. *BMJ* 330 (2005): 306–12.

Nevitt, M. C., B. Ettinger, D. M. Black et al. The association of radiographically detected vertebral fractures with back pain and function: A prospective study. *Ann Intern Med* 128 (1998): 793–800.

Newman, K. S. *No Shame in My Game: The Working Poor in the Inner City*. New York: A. A. Knopf and the Russell Sage Foundation, 1999.

Newman, M. F., J. L. Kirchner, B. Phillips-Bute et al. Longitudinal assessment of neurocognitive function after coronary-artery bypass surgery. *N Engl J Med* 344 (2001): 395–402.

Nicassio, P. M., M. H. Weisman, C. Schuman, C. W. Young. The role of generalized pain and pain behavior in tender point scores in fibromyalgia. *J Rheumatol* 27 (2000): 1056–62.

Nielsen, M. L., R. Rugulies, K. B. Christensen, L. Smith-Hansen, and T. S. Kristensen. Psychosocial work environment predictors of short and long spells of registered sickness absence during a 2-year follow up. *J Occup Environ Med* 48 (2006): 591–98.

Nissen, S. E., and K. Wolski. Effect of rosiglitazone on the risk of myocardial infarction and death from cardiovascular causes. *N Engl J Med* 356 (2007): 2457–71.

Nolan, C. M. Credibility, cookbook medicine, and common sense: Guidelines and the college. *Ann Intern Med* 120 (1994): 966–67.

Nolte, E., and M. McKee. Measuring the health of nations: Analysis of mortality amenable to health care. *BMJ* 327 (2003): 1129–33.

North American Symptomatic Carotid Endarterectomy Trial Collaborators. Beneficial effect of carotid endarterectomy in symptomatic patients with high-grade carotid stenosis. *N Engl J Med* 325 (1991): 445–53.

Nuovo, J. Reporting number needed to treat and absolute risk reduction in randomized controlled trials. *JAMA* 287 (2002): 2813–14.

Nussmeier, N. A., A. A. Whelton, M. T. Brown et al. Complications of the COX-2 inhibitors parecoxib and valdecoxib after cardiac surgery. *N Engl J Med* 352 (2005): 1081–91.

Ogden, C. L., M. D. Carroll, L. R. Curtin et al. Prevalence of overweight and obesity in the United States, 1999–2004. *JAMA* 295 (2006): 1549–55.

Oh, K., F. B. Hu, J. E. Manson et al. Dietary fat intake and risk of coronary heart disease in women: 20 years of follow-up of the Nurses' Health Study. *American Journal of Epidemiology* 161 (2005): 672–79.

Okie, S. Raising the safety bar — the FDA's coxib meeting. *N Engl J Med* 352 (2005): 1283 – 87.

Olsen, A. H., S. H. Njor, I. Vejborg et al. Breast cancer mortality in Copenhagen after introduction of mammography screening: Cohort study. *BMJ* 330 (2005): 220 – 22.

Olsen, O., and P. C. Gøetzsche. Cochrane review on screening for breast cancer with mammography. *Lancet* 358 (2001): 1340 – 42.

O'Reilly, D., M. Rosato, and C. Patterson. Self-reported health and mortality: Ecological analysis based on electoral wards across the United Kingdom. *BMJ* 331 (2005): 38 – 39.

Orwoll, E., M. Ettinger, S. Weiss et al. Alendronate for the treatment of osteoporosis in men. *N Engl J Med* 343 (2000): 604 – 10.

Page, D. L., and J. F. Simpson. Ductal carcinoma in situ — the focus for prevention, screening and breast conservation in breast cancer. *N Engl J Med* 340 (1999): 1499 – 500.

Page, D. L., and R. A. Jensen. Ductal carcinoma in situ of the breast. *JAMA* 275 (1996): 948 – 49.

Palumbo, F. B., and C. D. Mullins. The development of direct-to-consumer prescription drug advertising regulation. *Food and Drug Law Journal* 57 (2002): 423 – 43.

Pamuk, E., D. Makuc, K. Heck et al. *Socioeconomic Status and Health Chartbook: Health, United States, 1998.* Hyattsville, Md.: National Center for Health Statistics, 1998.

Park, Y., D. J. Hunter, D. Siegelman et al. Dietary fiber intake and risk of colorectal cancer. *JAMA* 294 (2005): 2849 – 57.

Parker, M. J., L. D. Gillespie, and W. J. Gillespie. Hip protectors for preventing hip fractures in the elderly: Cochrane review. Cochrane Library, Oxford: Update Software, 1 May 1999.

Parker, M. J., W. J. Gillespie, and L. D. Gillespie. Effectiveness of hip protectors for preventing hip fractures in elderly people: Systematic review. *BMJ* 332 (2006): 571 – 74.

Passamani, E., K. B. Davis, M. J. Gillespie, T. Killip, and the CASS Principal Investigators and their Associates. A randomized trial of coronary artery bypass surgery: Survival of patients with a low ejection fraction. *N Engl J Med* 312 (1985): 1665 – 71.

Pasternak, R. C. The ALLHAT lipid lowering trial — less is less. *JAMA* 288 (2002): 3042 – 44.

Patrono, C., L. A. Garcia Rodriguez, R. Landolfi, and C. Baigent. Lo-dose aspirin for the prevention of atherothrombosis. *N Engl J Med* 353 (2005): 2373 – 83.

Payer, L. *Disease Mongers: How Doctors, Drug Companies, and Insurers Are Making You Feel Sick.* New York: Holt, 1992.

———. *Medicine & Culture: Varieties of Treatment in the United States, England, West Germany, and France.* New York: Holt, 1988.

Pearson, S. K., and M. D. Rawlins. Quality, innovation and value for money: NICE and the British National Health Service. *JAMA* 294 (2005): 2618 – 22.

Pedula, K. L., A. L. Coleman, T. A. Hillier et al. Visual acuity, contrast sensitivity, and mortality in older women: Study of osteoporotic fractures. *J Am Geriatr Soc* 54 (2006): 1871 – 77.

Pell, S., and W. E. Fayerweather. Trends in the incidence of myocardial infarction and in associated mortality and morbidity in a large employed population, 1957 – 1983. *N Engl J Med* 16 (1985): 1005 – 11.

Pendleton, A., N. Arden, M. Dougados et al. EULAR recommendations for the management of knee osteoarthritis: Report of a task force of the Standing Committee for International Clinical Studies Including Therapeutic Trials (ESCISIT). *Ann Rheum Dis* 59 (2000): 936–44.

Perry, H. M., B. R. Davis, T. R. Price et al. Effect of treating isolated systolic hypertension on the risk of developing various types and subtypes of stroke. *JAMA* 284 (2000): 465–71.

Persell, S. D., and D. W. Baker. Studying interventions to prevent the progression from prehypertension to hypertension: Does TROPHY win the prize? *American Journal of Hypertension* 19 (2006): 1095–97.

Petitti, D. B. Some surprises, some answers, and more questions about hormone therapy. *JAMA* 294 (2005): 245–46.

Pfisterer, M. Long-term outcome in elderly patients with chronic angina managed invasively versus by optimized medical therapy: Four-year follow-up on the randomized Trial of Invasive versus Medical Therapy in Elderly Patients (TIME). *Circulation* 110 (2004): 1213–18.

Pfisterer, M., P. Buser, S. Osswald et al. Outcome of elderly patients with chronic symptomatic coronary artery disease with an invasive vs. optimized medical treatment strategy. *JAMA* 289 (2003): 1117–23.

Phillips, K. A., G. Glendon, and J. A. Knight. Putting the risk of breast cancer in perspective. *N Engl J Med* (340) 1999: 141–44.

Phillips, P. S., R. H. Haas, S. Bannykh et al. Statin-associated myopathy with normal creatine kinase levels. *Ann Intern Med* 137 (2002): 581–85.

Picirillo, J. F., R. M. Tierney, I. Costas et al. Prognostic importance of comorbidity in a hospital-based cancer registry. *JAMA* 291 (2004): 2441–47.

Pignone, M., S. Earnshaw, J. A. Tice, and M. J. Pletcher. Aspirin, statins, or both drugs for the primary prevention of coronary heart disease events in men: A cost-utility analysis. *Ann Intern Med* 144 (2006): 326–36.

Pignone, M., S. Saha, T. Heorger, and J. Mandelblatt. Cost-effectiveness analyses of colorectal cancer screening: A systematic review for the U.S. Preventive Services Task Force. *Ann Intern Med* 137 (2002): 96–104.

Pincus, T., A. K. Burton, S. Vogel, and A. P. Field. A systematic review of psychological factors as predictors of chronicity/disability in prospective cohorts of low back pain. *Spine* 27 (2002): E109–E120.

Pisano, E. D., C. Gatsonis, E. Hendrick et al. Diagnostic performance of digital versus film mammography for breast-cancer screening. *N Engl J Med* 353 (2005): 1–11.

Podolsky, D. K. Going the distance — the case for true colorectal-cancer screening. *N Engl J Med* 343 (2000): 207–8.

Pogach, L., M. Engelgau, and D. Aron. Measuring progress toward achieving Hemoglobin A1c goals in diabetes care. *JAMA* 297 (2007): 520–22.

Popescu, I., M. S. Vaughan-Sarrazin, and G. E. Rosenthal. Certificate of need regulations and use of coronary revascularization after acute myocardial infarction. *JAMA* 295 (2006): 2141–47.

Popper, K. *Conjectures and Refutations: The Growth of Scientific Knowledge.* London: Routledge, 2000.

Porthouse, J., S. Cockayne, C. King et al. Randomized controlled trial of calcium and supplementation with cholecalciferol (vitamin D_3) for prevention of fractures in primary care. *BMJ* 330 (2005): 1003–9.

Poynter, J. N., S. B. Gruber, P. D. R. Higgins et al. Statins and the risk of colorectal cancer. *N Engl J Med* 352 (2005): 2184–92.

PREMIER Collaborative Research Group. Effects of comprehensive lifestyle modification on blood pressure control. *JAMA* 289 (2003): 2083–93.

Prentice, R. L., T. R. Chlebowski, R. Patterson et al. Low-rat dietary pattern and risk of invasive breast cancer. *JAMA* 295 (2006): 629–42.

Price, J. R., and J. Couper. (1998) Cognitive behaviour therapy for adults with chronic fatigue syndrome: Cohcrane review. Cochrane Library, Oxford: Update Software, 24 August 1998.

Prince, R. L., A. Devine, S. S. Dhaliwal, and I. M. Dick. Effects of calcium supplementation on clinical fracture and bone structure. *Arch Intern Med* 166 (2006): 869–75.

Psaty, B. M., and C. D. Furberg. The record on rosiglitazone and the risk of myocardial infarction. *N Engl J Med* 357 (2007): 67–69.

Psaty, B. M., and D. Rennie. Clinical trial investigators and their prescribing patterns. *JAMA* 295 (2006): 2787–90.

Psaty, B. M., N. S. Weiss, and C. D. Furberg. Recent trials in hypertension: Compelling science or commercial speech? *JAMA* 295 (2006): 1704–6.

Psaty, B. M., N. S. Weiss, C. D. Furberg et al. Surrogate end points, health outcomes, and the drug-approval process for the treatment of risk factors for cardiovascular disease. *JAMA* 282 (1999): 786–90.

Psaty, B. M., T. Lumley, C. D. Furberg et al. Health outcomes associated with various anti-hypertensive therapies used as first-line agents. *JAMA* 289 (2003): 2534–44.

Qaseem, A., V. Snow, K. Sherif et al. Screening mammography for women 40 to 49 years of age: A clinical practice guideline from the American College of Physicians. *Ann Intern Med* 146 (2007): 511–15.

Quandt, S. A., D. E. Thompson, D. L. Schneider et al. Effect of alendronate on vertebral fracture risk in women with bone mineral density T scores of –1.6 to –2.5 at the femoral neck: The Fracture Intervention Trial. *Mayo Clinic Proceedings* 80 (2005): 343–49.

Quandt, S. A., H. Chen, J. G. Grzywacz et al. Use of complementary and alternative medicine by persons with arthritis: Results of the National Health Interview Survey. *Arthritis Rheum* (*Arthritis Care Res*) 53 (2005b): 748–55.

Raisz, L. G. Screening for osteoporosis. *N Engl J Med* 353 (2005): 164–71.

Randomized Intervention Treatment of Angina (RITA-2) trial participants. Coronary angioplasty versus medical therapy for angina: The second Randomized Intervention Treatment of Angina (RITA-2). *Lancet* 350 (1997): 461–68.

Ransohoff, D. F. Bias as a threat to the validity of cancer molecular-marker research. *Nature Reviews Cancer* 5 (2005a): 142–49.

———. Have we oversold colonoscopy? *Gastroenterology* 129 (2005b): 1815.

———. Lessons from controversy: Ovarian cancer screening and serum proteomics. *J Natl Cancer Inst* 97 (2005): 315–19.

Ransohoff, D. F., and R. S. Sandler. Screening for colorectal cancer. *N Engl J Med* 346 (2002): 40–44.

Ransohoff, D. F., M. M. Collins, and F. J. Fowler. Why is prostate cancer screening so common when the evidence is so uncertain? A system without negative feedback. *Am J Med* 113 (2002): 663–67.

Rapp, S. R., M. A. Espeland, S. A. Shumaker et al. Effect of estrogen plus progestin on global cognitive function in postmenopausal women. *JAMA* 289 (2003): 2663–72.

Ratcliffe, J., K. J. Thomas, H. MacPherson, and J. Brazier. A randomized controlled trial of acupuncture care for persistent low back pain: Cost effectiveness analysis. *BMJ* 333 (2006): 629–72.

Ray, W. A., C. M. Stein, J. R. Daugherty et al. COX-2 selective non-steroidal anti-inflammatory drugs and risk of serious coronary heart disease. *Lancet* 360 (2002): 1071–73.

Reaven, G. M. Importance of identifying the overweight patient who will benefit the most by losing weight. *Ann Intern Med* 138 (2003): 420–23.

RECORD Trial Group. Oral vitamin D3 and calcium for secondary prevention of low-trauma fractures in elderly people: A randomized placebo-controlled trial. *Lancet* 365 (2005): 1621–28.

Regula, J., M. Rupinski, E. Kraszewska et al. Colonoscopy in colorectal-cancer screening for detection of advanced neoplasia. *N Engl J Med* 355 (2006): 1863–72.

Reichenbach, S., R. Sterchi, M. Scherer et al. Meta-analysis: Chondroitin for osteoarthritis of the knee or hip. *Ann Intern Med* 146 (2007): 580–90.

Reissman, D. B., P. Orris, R. Lacey, and D. E. Hartman. Downsizing, role demands, and job stress. *J Occup Environ Med* 41 (1999): 289–93.

Rekola, K. E., S. Levoska, J. Takala, and S. Keinänen-Kiukaanniemi. Patients with neck and shoulder complaints and multisite musculoskeletal symptoms — a prospective study. *J Rheumatol* 24 (1997): 2424–28.

Relman, A. S. Dealing with conflicts of interest. *N Engl J Med* 310 (1984): 1182–83.

———. Defending professional independence. *JAMA* 289 (2003): 2418–20.

———. Economic incentives in clinical investigation. *N Engl J Med* 320 (1989): 933–34.

———. Financial associations of authors. *N Engl J Med* 347 (2002): 1043.

———. New "Information for Authors" — and readers. *N Engl J Med* 323 (1990): 56.

———. Separating continuing medical education from pharmaceutical marketing. *JAMA* 285 (2001): 2009–12.

Rennie, D., and H. S. Luft. Pharmacoeconomic analyses: Making them transparent, making them credible. *JAMA* 283 (2000): 2158–60.

Rex, D. K., C. S. Cutler, G. T. Lemmel et al. Colonoscopic miss rates of adenomas determined by back-to-back colonoscopies. *Gastroenterology* 112 (1997): 24–28.

Rey, R. *The History of Pain*. Cambridge, Mass.: Harvard University Press, 1995.

Ridker, P. M., and J. Torres. Reported outcomes in major cardiovascular clinical trials funded by for-profit and not-for-profit organizations: 2000–2005. *JAMA* 295 (2006): 2270–74.

Ridker, P. M., N. R. Cook, I. M. Lee et al. A randomized trial of low-dose aspirin in the primary prevention of cardiovascular disease in women. *N Engl J Med* 352 (2005): 1293–304.

Riggs, B. L., and L. C. Hartmann. Selective estrogen-receptor modulators — mechanisms of action and application to clinical practice. *N Engl J Med* 348 (2003): 618–29.

Rimm, E. B., A. Ascherio, E. Giovannucci et al. Vegetable, fruit and cereal fiber intake and risk of coronary heart disease among men. *JAMA* 275 (1996): 447–51.

Rivero-Arias, O., H. Campbell, A. Gray et al. Surgical stabilization of the spine compared with a programme of intensive rehabilitation for the management of patients with chronic low back pain: Cost utility analysis based on a randomized controlled trial. *BMJ* 330 (2005): 1239 – 43.

Roche, J. J. W., R. T. Wenn, O. Sahota, and C. G. Moran. Effect of comorbidities and post-operative complications on mortality after hip fracture in elderly people: Prospective observational cohort study. *BMJ* 331 (2005): 1374 – 79.

Romano, P. S. Improving the quality of hospital care in America. *N Engl J Med* 353 (2005): 302 – 4.

Roos, H., M. Laurén, T. Adalberth et al. Knee osteoarthritis after meniscectomy. *Arthritis Rheum* 41 (1998): 687 – 93.

Rosa, L., E. Rosa, L. Sarner, and S. Barrett. A close look at therapeutic touch. *JAMA* 279 (1998): 1005 – 10.

Rosamond, W. D., L. E. Chambless, A. R. Folsom et al. Trends in the incidence of myocardial infarction and in mortality due to coronary heart disease, 1987 – 1994. *N Engl J Med* 339 (1998): 861 – 67.

Rosen, C. J. Postmenopausal osteoporosis. *N Engl J Med* 353 (2005): 595 – 603.

———. The rosiglitazone story: Lessons from an FDA Advisory Committee meeting. *N Engl J Med* 357 (2007): 844 – 46.

Rosenberg, I. H., and D. C. Mulrow. Trials that matter: Should we routinely measure homocysteine levels and "treat" mild hyperhomocysteinemia? *Ann Intern Med* 145 (2006): 226 – 27.

Rosenthal, M. B., E. R. Berndt, J. M. Donohue et al. Promotion of prescription drugs to consumers. *N Engl J Med* 346 (2002): 498 – 505.

Rosenzweig, A. Circulating endothelial progenitors — cells as biomarkers. *N Engl J Med* 353 (2005): 1055 – 57.

Rostom, A., C. Dubé, G. Lewin et al. Non steroidal anti-inflammatory drugs and cyclooxygenase-2 inhibitors for primary prevention of colorectal cancer: A systematic review prepared for the U.S. Preventive Services Task Force. *Ann Intern Med* 146 (2007): 376 – 89.

Rothman, K. *Causal Inference*. Cambridge: Epidemiology Resources, 1988.

Rubenstein, L. Z. Hip protectors — a breakthrough in fracture prevention. *N Engl J Med* 343 (2000): 1562 – 63.

Rubenstein, L. Z., K. R. Josephson, P. R. Trueblood et al. Effects of a group exercise program on strength mobility and falls among fall-prone elderly men. *Journal of Gerontology* 55A (2000): M317 – 21.

Salkeld, G., I. D. Cameron, R. G. Cumming et al. Quality of life related to fear of falling and hip fracture in older women: A time trade-off study. *BMJ* 320 (2000): 241 – 46.

Salpeter, S. R., P. Gregor, T. M. Ormiston et al. Meta-analysis: Cardiovascular events associated with nonsteroidal anti-inflammatory drugs. *Am J Med* 119 (2006): 552 – 59.

Santen, R. J., R. Mansel. Benign breast disorders. *N Engl J Med* 353 (2005): 275 – 85.

Sapolsky, R. M. The influence of social hierarchy on primate health. *Science* 308 (2005): 648 – 52.

Satariano, W. A., and D. R. Ragland. The effect of comorbidity on 3-year survival of women with primary breast cancer. *Ann Intern Med* 120 (1994): 104 – 10.

Scarry, E. *The Body in Pain: The Making and Unmaking of the World*. New York: Oxford University Press, 1985.

Scharf, H. P., U. Mansmann, K. Streitberger et al. Acupuncture and knee osteoarthritis. *Ann Intern Med* 145 (2006): 12–20.

Schneider, L. S. Estrogen and dementia: Insights from the Women's Health Initiative Memory Study. *JAMA* 291 (2004): 3005–6.

Schoenbaum, S. C. Toward fewer procedures and better outcomes. *JAMA* 269 (1993): 794–96.

Schoenfeld, P., B. Cash, A. Flood et al. Colonoscopic screening of average-risk women for colorectal neoplasia. *N Engl J Med* 352 (2005): 2061–68.

Scholten, R. J., W. L. Devillé, W. Opstelten et al. The accuracy of physical diagnostic tests for assessing meniscal lesions of the knee: A meta analysis. *Journal of Family Practice* 50 (2001): 938–44.

Schousboe, J. T., J. A. Nyman, R. L. Kane, and K. E. Ensrud. Cost-effectiveness of alendronate therapy for osteopenic postmenopausal women. *Ann Intern Med* 142 (2005): 734–41.

Schroeder, S. A. We can do better: Improving the health of the American people. *N Engl J Med* 357 (2007): 1221–28.

Schroter, S., J. Morris, S. Chaudhry et al. Does the type of competing interest statement affect readers' perceptions of the credibility of research? Randomized trial. *BMJ* 328 (2004): 742–43.

Schulman, K. A., D. M. Seils, J. W. Timbie et al. A national survey of provisions in clinical trial agreements between medical schools and industry sponsors. *N Engl J Med* 347 (2002): 1335–41.

Schunkert, H. Pharmacotherapy for prehypertension — mission accomplished. *N Engl J Med* 354 (2006): 1742–44.

Schwartz, L. M., and S. Woloshin. News media coverage of screening mammography for women in their 40s and tamoxifen for primary prevention of breast cancer. *JAMA* 287 (2002): 3136–42.

———. Participation in mammography screening. *BMJ* 335 (2007): 731–32.

Schwartz, L. M., S. Woloshin, F. J. Fowler, and H. G. Welch. Enthusiasm for cancer screening in the United States. *JAMA* 291 (2004): 71–78.

Seigel, D. Clinical trials, epidemiology, and public confidence. *Statistics in Medicine* 22 (2003): 3419–25.

Selvin, E., S. Marinopoulos, G. Berkenblit et al. Meta-analysis: Glycosylated hemoglobin and cardiovascular disease in diabetes mellitus. *Ann Intern Med* 141 (2004): 421–31.

Shah, R. V., T. J. Albert, V. Bruegel-Sanchez et al. Industry support and correlation to study outcome for papers published in *Spine*. *Spine* 30 (2005): 1099–104.

Sharp, P. C., R. Michielutte, R. Freimanis et al. Reported pain following mammography screening. *Arch Intern Med* 163 (2003): 833–36.

Sharpe M. The report of the Chief Medical Officer's CFS/ME working group: What does it say and will it help? *Clin Med JRCPL* 2 (2002): 427–29.

Sheetz, M. J., and G. L. King. Molecular understanding of hyperglycemia's adverse effects for diabetic complications. *JAMA* 288 (2002): 2579–88.

Shepherd, J., S. M. Cobbe, I. Ford et al. Prevention of coronary heart disease with pravastatin in men with hypercholesterolemia. *N Engl J Med* 333 (1995): 1301–7.

Shishehbor, M. H., D. Litaker, C. E. Pothier, and M. S. Lauer. Association of socioeconomic status with functional capacity, heart rate recovery, and all-cause mortality. *JAMA* 295 (2006): 784–92.

Showalter, E. *Hystories: Hysterical Epidemics and Modern Culture*. New York: Columbia University Press, 1996.

Shuchman, M. Debating the risks of drug-eluting stents. *N Engl J Med* 356 (2007): 325–28.

Shumaker, S. A., C. Legault, L. Kuller et al. Conjugated equine estrogens and incidence of probable dementia and mild cognitive impairment in postmenopausal women. *JAMA* 291 (2004): 2947–58.

Shumaker, S. A., C. Legault, S. R. Rapp et al. Estrogen plus progestin and the incidence of dementia and mild cognitive impairment in postmenopausal women. *JAMA* 289 (2003): 2651–62.

Silverman, S. L., W. Shen, M. E. Minshall et al. Prevalence of depressive symptoms in postmenopausal women with low bone mineral density and/or prevalent vertebral fracture: Results for the Multiple Outcomes of Raloxifene Evaluation (MORE) study. *J Rheumatol* 34 (2007): 140–44.

Silverstein, F. E., G. Faich, J. L. Goldstein et al. Gastrointestinal toxicity with celecoxib vs. nonsteroidal anti-inflammatory drugs for osteoarthritis and rheumatoid arthritis: The CLASS Study: A randomized controlled trial. *JAMA* 284 (2000): 1247–55.

Simon, G. E., M. VonKorff, M. Piccinelli, C. Fullerton, and J. Ormel. An international study of the relation between somatic symptoms and depression. *N Engl J Med* 341 (1999): 1329–35.

Simon, J. B., and R. Fletcher. Should all people over the age of 50 have regular fecal occult blood tests? (Simon, con); If it works, why not do it? (Fletcher, pro). *N Engl J Med* 338 (1998): 1151–55.

Simpson, S. H., D. T. Eurich, S. R. Majumdar et al. A meta-analysis of the association between adherence to drug therapy and mortality. *BMJ* 333 (2006): 14–20.

Singh, H., D. Turner, L. Xue et al. Risk of developing colorectal cancer following a negative colonoscopy examination. *JAMA* 295 (2006): 2366–73.

Singh, S., H. Sun, and A. Anis. Cost-effectiveness of hip protectors in the prevention of osteoporosis related hip fractures in elderly nursing home residents. *J Rheumatol* 31 (2004): 1607–13.

Singleton, S. Data sources and performance measurement. *BMJ* 335 (2007): 730.

Sloan, R. P., E. Bagiella, L. VandeCreek et al. Should physicians prescribe religious activities? *N Engl J Med* 342 (2000): 1913–16.

Smidt, N., D. A. van der Windt, W. J. Assendelft et al. Corticosteroid injections, physiotherapy or wait-and-see policy for lateral epicondylitis: A randomized controlled trial. *Lancet* 359 (2002): 657–62.

Smith, B. L. Approaches to breast-cancer staging. *N Engl J Med* 342 (2000): 580–81.

Smith, I. E., and G. M. Ross. Breast radiotherapy after lumpectomy — no longer always necessary. *N Engl J Med* 351 (2004): 1021–23.

Smith, R. In search of "non-disease." *BMJ* 324 (2002): 83–85.

Smith-Bindman, R., P. W. Chu, D. L. Miglioretti et al. Comparison of screening mammography in the United States and the United Kingdom. *JAMA* 290 (2003): 2129–37.

Snyder, C., and G. Anderson. Do quality improvement organizations improve the quality of hospital care for Medicare beneficiaries? *JAMA* 293 (2005): 2900–907.

Solomon, C. G., and R. G. Dluhy. Rethinking postmenopausal hormone therapy. *N Engl J Med* 348 (2003): 579–80.

Solomon, D. H., J. Avorn, T. Stürmer et al. Cardiovascular outcomes in new users of coxibs and nonsteroidal anti-inflammatory drugs. *Arthritis Rheum* 54 (2006): 1378–89.

Solomon, S. D., J. J. V. McMurray, M. A. Pfeffer et al. Cardiovascular risk associated with celecoxib in a clinical trial for colorectal adenoma prevention. *N Engl J Med* 352 (2005): 1071–80.

Sonnenberg, A., F. Delcò, and J. M. Inadomi. Cost-effectiveness of colonoscopy in screening for colorectal cancer. *Ann Intern Med* 133 (2000): 547–49.

Sornay-Rendu, E., C. Allard, F. Munoz et al. Disc space narrowing as a new risk factor for vertebral fracture. *Arthritis Rheum* 54 (2006): 1262–69.

Sox, H. An editorial update: Should benefits of radical prostatectomy affect the decision to screen for early prostate cancer? *Ann Intern Med* 143 (2005): 232–33.

———. Practice guidelines: 1994. *Am J Med* 97 (1994): 205–7.

———. Screening mammography for younger women: Back to basics. *Ann Intern Med* 137 (2002): 361–62.

Spaulding, C., J. Daeman, E. Boersma et al. A pooled analysis of data comparing sirolimus-eluting stents with bare-metal stents. *N Engl J Med* 356 (2007): 989–97.

Spitzer, W. O., F. LeBlanc, M. Dupuis et al. Scientific approach to the assessment and management of activity-related spinal disorders. *Spine* 12, suppl. 7 (1987): S1–S59.

Stadtmauer, E. A., A. O'Neill, L. J. Goldstein et al. Conventional-dose chemotherapy compared with high-dose chemotherapy plus autologous hematopoietic stem-cell transplantation for metastatic breast cancer. *N Engl J Med* 342 (2000): 1069–76.

Starr, P. *The Social Transformation of American Medicine*. New York: Basic Books, 1982.

Steinbrook, R. Financial conflicts of interest and the Food and Drug Administration's advisory committees. *N Engl J Med* 352 (2005): 116–18.

———. Guidance for guidelines. *N Engl J Med* 356 (2007): 331–33.

Steineck, G., F. Helgesen, J. Adolfsson et al. Quality of life after radical prostatectomy or watchful waiting. *N Engl J Med* 347 (2002): 790–96.

Stelfox, H. T., G. Chua, K. O'Rourke, and A. S. Detsky. Conflict of interest in the debate over calcium channel antagonists. *N Engl J Med* 338 (1998): 101–6.

Stone, G. W., J. W. Moses, S. G. Ellis et al. Safety and efficacy of sirolimus- and paclitaxel-eluting coronary stents. *N Engl J Med* 356 (2007): 998–1008.

Stone, J., W. Wojcik, D. Durrance et al. What should we say to patients with symptoms unexplained by disease? The "number needed to offend." *BMJ* 325 (2002): 1449–50.

Strand, V., and M. C. Hochberg. The risk of cardiovascular thrombotic events with selective cyclooxygenase-2 inhibitors. *Arthritis Rheum* 47 (2002): 349–55.

Stratton, I. M., A. I. Adler, A. W. Neil et al. Association of glycaemia with macrovascular and microvascular complications of type 2 diabetes (UKPDS 35): Prospective observational study. *BMJ* 321 (2000): 405–12.

Straus, S. E. Herbal medicines—what's in the bottle? *N Engl J Med* 347 (2002): 1997–98.

Sullivan, P. F., B. Evengård, A. Jacks, and N. L. Pedersen. Twin analyses of chronic fatigue in a Swedish national sample. *Psychol Med* 35 (2005): 1327–36.

Sullivan, P. F., W. Smith, and D. Buchwald. Latent class analysis of symptoms associated with chronic fatigue syndrome and fibromyalgia. *Psychol Med* 32 (2002): 881–88.

Sutkowski, P. A., W. B. Kannel, and R. B. D'Agostino. Changes in risk factors and the decline in mortality from cardiovascular disease. *N Engl J Med* 322 (1990): 1635–41.

Swingler, G. H., J. Volmink, and J. P. A. Ioannidis. Number of published systematic reviews and global burden of disease: Database analysis. *BMJ* 327 (2003): 1083–84.

Tait, R. C., J. T. Chibnall, E. M. Andresen, and N. M. Hadler. Disability determination: Validity with occupational low back pain. *Journal of Pain* 7 (2006): 951–57.

———. Management of occupational back injuries: Differences among African Americans and Caucasians. *Journal of Pain* 112 (2004): 389–96.

Taylor, P. Making decisions about mammography. *BMJ* 330 (2005): 915–16.

Taylor, R., and J. Giles. Cash interests taint drug advice. *Nature* 437 (2005): 1070–71.

Temple, R. Are surrogate markers adequate to assess cardiovascular disease drugs? *JAMA* 282 (1999): 790–95.

Thomas, K. J., H. MacPherson, L. Thorpe et al. Randomized controlled trial of a short course of traditional acupuncture compared with usual care for persistent non-specific low back pain. *BMJ* 333 (2006): 623–29.

Thompson, I. M., D. K. Pauler, P. J. Goodman et al. Prevalence of prostate cancer among men with a prostate-specific antigen level < or = 4.0 ng per milliliter. *N Engl J Med* 350 (2004): 2239–46.

Thompson, P. D., P. Clarkson, and R. H. Karas. Statin-associated myopathy. *JAMA* 289 (2003): 1681–90.

Thornton, H., and M. Dixon-Woods. Prostate specific antigen testing for prostate cancer. *BMJ* 325 (2002): 725–26.

Thurfjell, E. Breast density and the risk of breast cancer. *N Engl J Med* 347 (2002): 866.

Tirosh, A., I. Shai, D. Tekes-Manova et al. Normal fasting plasma glucose levels and type 2 diabetes in young men. *N Engl J Med* 353 (2005): 1454–62.

Tomes, N. Patient empowerment and the dilemmas of late-modern medicalization. *Lancet* 369 (2007): 698–700.

Towler, B., L. Irwig, P. Glasziou et al. A systematic review of the effects of screening for colorectal cancer using the faecal occult blood test, Hemoccult. *BMJ* 317 (1998): 559–65.

Trichopoulou, A., P. Orfanos, T. Norat et al. Modified Mediterranean diet and survival: EPIC-elderly prospective cohort study. *BMJ* 330 (2005): 991–98.

Trichopoulou, A., T. Costacou, C. Bamia, and D. Trichopoulos. Adherence to a Mediterranean diet and survival in a Greek population. *N Engl J Med* 348 (2003): 2599–608.

Trinh, K., N. Graham, A. Gross et al. Acupuncture for neck disorders. *Spine* 32 (2007): 236–43.

Trivedi, D. P., R. Doll, and K. T. Khaw. Effect of four monthly oral vitamin D_3 (cholecalciferol) supplementation on fractures and mortality in men and women living in the community: Randomized double blind controlled trial. *BMJ* 326 (2003): 469.

Tunstall-Pedoe, H., J. Connaghan, M. Woodward et al. Pattern of declining blood pressure across replicate population surveys of the WHO MONICA project, mid-1980s to mid-1990s, and the mole of medication. *BMJ* 332 (2006): 629–35.

Tuomilehto, J. Primary prevention of type 2 diabetes: Lifestyle intervention works and saves money, but what should be done with smokers? *Ann Intern Med* 142 (2005): 381–82.

Tuomilehto, J., D. Rastenyte, W. H. Birkenhäger et al. Effects of calcium-channel blockade in older patients with diabetes and systolic hypertension. *N Engl J Med* 340 (1999): 677–84.

Tuomilehto, J., J. Lindström, J. G. Eriksson et al. Prevention of type 2 diabetes mellitus by changes in lifestyle among subjects with impaired glucose tolerance. *N Engl J Med* 344 (2001): 1343–50.

Turk, D. Clinical effectiveness and cost-effectiveness of treatments for patients with chronic pain. *Clin J Pain* 18 (2002): 355–65.

Turner, R. B. Echinacea for the common cold: Can alternative medicine be evidence-based medicine? *Ann Intern Med* 137 (2002): 1001–2.

Turner, R. B., R. Bauer, K. Woelkart et al. An evaluation of *Echinacea angustifolia* in experimental rhinovirus infections. *N Engl J Med* 353 (2005): 341–48.

UK Prospective Diabetes Study Group. Intensive blood-glucose control with sulphony-lureas or insulin compared with conventional treatment and risk of complications in patients with type 2 diabetes (UKPDS 33). *Lancet* 352 (1998a): 837–53.

———. Tight blood pressure control and risk of macrovascular and microvascular complications in type 2 diabetes: UKPDS 38. *BMJ* 317 (1998b): 703–13.

University Group Diabetes Program (UGDP). A study of the effects of hypoglycemic agents on vascular complications in patients with adult-onset diabetes. *Diabetes* 25 (1976): 1129–53.

Urwin, M., D. Symmons, T. Allison et al. Estimating the burden or musculoskeletal disorders in the community: The comparative prevalence of symptoms at different anatomical sites, and the relation to social deprivation. *Ann Rheum Dis* 57 (1998): 649–55.

U.S. Preventive Services Task Force. Hormone therapy for the prevention of chronic conditions in postmenopausal women: Recommendations from the U.S. Preventive Services Task Force. *Ann Intern Med* 142 (2005): 855–60.

———. Postmenopausal hormone replacement therapy for primary prevention of chronic conditions: Recommendations and rationale. *Ann Intern Med* 137 (2002): 834–39.

———. Routine aspirin or nonsteroidal anti-inflammatory drugs for the primary prevention of colorectal cancer. *Ann Intern Med* 146 (2007): 361–64.

———. Screening for breast cancer: Recommendations and rationale. *Ann Intern Med* 137 (2002): 344–46.

———. Screening for colorectal cancer: Recommendation and rationale. *Ann Intern Med* 137 (2002): 129–41.

Vahtera, J., M. Kivimäkl, and J. Pentti. Effect of organisational downsizing on health of employees. *Lancet* 350 (1997): 1124–28.

Van Dam, R. M., and F. B. Hu. Coffee consumption and risk of type 2 diabetes. *JAMA* 294 (2005): 97–104.

Vandenbroucke, J. P., and A. J. M. de Craen. Alternative medicine: A "mirror image" for scientific reasoning in conventional medicine. *Ann Intern Med* 135 (2001): 507–13.

Van de Werf, F. Drug-eluting stents in acute myocardial infarction. *N Engl J Med* 355 (2006): 1169–70.

Van de Werf, F., J. M. Gore, A. Avezum et al. Access to catheterization facilities in patients admitted with acute coronary syndrome: Multinational registry study. *BMJ* 330 (2005): 441–47.

Van Dijk, D., M. Spoor, R. Hijman et al. Cognitive and cardiac outcomes 5 years after off-pump vs. on-pump coronary artery bypass graft surgery. *JAMA* 297 (2007): 701–8.

Van Dijk, G. M., J. Dekker, C. Veenhof et al. Course of functional status and pain in osteoarthritis of the hip or knee: A systematic review of the literature. *Arthritis Rheum* (*Arthritis Care Res*) 55 (2006): 779–85.

Van Leeuwen, R., S. Boekhoorn, J. R. Vingerling et al. Dietary intake of antioxidants and risk of age-related macular degeneration. *JAMA* 294 (2005): 3101–7.

Van Tulder, M. W., A. Malmivaara, R. Esmail, and B. Koes. Exercise therapy for low back pain. *Spine* 25 (2000): 2784–96.

Van Tulder, M. W., B. W. Koes, and L. M. Bouter. Conservative treatment of acute and chronic low back pain: A systematic review of randomized controlled trials of the most common interventions. *Spine* 22 (1997): 2128–56.

Van Tulder, M. W., D. C. Cherkin, B. Berman et al. The effectiveness of acupuncture in the management of acute and chronic low back pain: A systematic review within the framework of the Cochrane Collaboration Back Review Group. *Spine* 24 (1999): 1113–23.

Van Tulder, M. W., R. J. P. M. Scholten, B. W. Koes, and R. A. Deyo. Nonsteroidal anti-inflammatory drugs for low back pain. *Spine* 25 (2000): 2501–13.

Varnauskas, E., and the European Coronary Surgery Study Group. Twelve-year follow-up of survival in the randomized European coronary surgery study. *N Engl J Med* 319 (1988): 332–37.

Vastag, B. Study concludes that moderate PSA levels are unrelated to prostate cancer outcomes. *JAMA* 287 (2002): 969–70.

Vercoulen, J. H. M. M., C. M. A. Swanink, J. F. M. Fennis et al. Prognosis in chronic fatigue syndrome: A prospective study on the natural course. *Journal of Neurology, Neurosurgery, and Psychiatry* 60 (1996): 489–94.

Verghese, J., R. B. Lipton, M. J. Katz et al. Leisure activities and the risk of dementia in the elderly. *N Engl J Med* 348 (2003): 2508–16.

Veronesi, U., N. Cascinelli, L. Mariani et al. Twenty-year follow-up of a randomized study comparing breast-conserving surgery with radical mastectomy for early breast cancer. *N Engl J Med* 347 (2002): 1227–32.

Veterans Administration Coronary Artery Bypass Surgery Cooperative Study Group. Eleven-year survival in the Veterans Administration randomized trial of coronary bypass surgery for stable angina. *N Engl J Med* 311 (1984): 1333–39.

Vickers, A. J., P. Fisher, C. Smith et al. Homoeopathy for delayed onset muscle soreness: A randomized double blind placebo controlled trial. *British Journal of Sports Medicine* 31 (1997): 304–7.

Viner, R., and M. Hotopf. Childhood predictors of self reported chronic fatigue syndrome/myalgic encephalomyelitis in adults: National birth cohort study. *BMJ* 329 (2004): 941–43.

Wallace, R. B. Bone health in nursing home residents. *JAMA* 284 (2000): 1018–19.

Walsh, J. M. E., and J. P. Terdiman. Colorectal cancer screening. *JAMA* 289 (2003): 1288–96.

Walsh, P. C. Surgery and the reduction of mortality from prostate cancer. *N Engl J Med* 347 (2002): 839–40.

Walter, L. C., D. Bertenthal, K. Lindquist, and B. R. Konety. PSA screening among elderly men with limited life expectancies. *JAMA* 296 (2006): 2336–42.

Wardle, J., N. H. Brodersen, T. J. Cole et al. Development of adiposity in adolescence:

Five-year longitudinal study of an ethnically and socioeconomically diverse sample of young people in Britain. *BMJ* 332 (2006): 1130–35.

Wardwell, W. I. Chiropractors: Evolution to acceptance. In *Other Healers: Unorthodox Medicine in America*, edited by N. Gevitz, 157–91. Baltimore: Johns Hopkins University Press, 1988.

Wassertheil-Smoller, S., B. Psaty, P. Greenland et al. Association between cardiovascular outcomes and antihypertensive drug treatment in older women. *JAMA* 292 (2004): 2849–59.

Wassertheil-Smoller, S., S. L. Hendrix, M. Limacher et al. Effect of estrogen plus progestin on stroke in postmenopausal women. *JAMA* 289 (2003): 2673–84.

Waxman, H. J. The lessons of Vioxx — drug safety and sales. *N Engl J Med* 352 (2005): 2576–78.

Wazana, A. Physicians and the pharmaceutical industry: Is a gift ever a gift? *JAMA* 283 (2000): 373–80.

Weinberger, M. H. More novel effects of diet on blood pressure and lipids. *JAMA* 294 (2005): 2497–98.

Weinsier, R. L., and C. L. Krumdieck CL. Dairy foods and bone health: Examination of the evidence. *American Journal of Clinical Nutrition* 72 (2000): 681–89.

Weinstein, J. N., J. D. Lurie, P. R. Olson et al. United States' trends and regional variations in lumbar spine surgery: 1992–2003. *Spine* 31 (2006): 2707–14.

Weinstein, J. N., T. D. Tosteson, J. D. Lurie et al. Surgical vs. nonoperative treatment for lumbar disk herniation. *JAMA* 296 (2006a): 2441–50.

Welch, H. G., S. Woloshin, and L. M. Schwartz. Skin biopsy rates and incidence of melanoma: Population-based ecological study. *BMJ* 331 (2005): 481–85.

Wessel, T. R., C. B. Arant, M. B. Olson et al. Relationship of physical fitness vs. body mass index with coronary artery disease and cardiovascular events in women. *JAMA* 292 (2004): 1179–87.

Whelton, P. K., L. J. Appel, M. A. Espeland et al. Sodium reduction and weight loss in the treatment of hypertension in older persons. *JAMA* 279 (1998): 839–46.

Whitaker, R. Anatomy of an epidemic: Psychiatric drugs and the astonishing rise of mental illness in America. *Ethical Human Psychology and Psychiatry* 7 (2005): 23–35.

———. *Mad in America: Bad Science, Bad Medicine, and the Enduring Mistreatment of the Mentally Ill*. New York: Perseus, 2002.

White, K. P., T. Ostbye, M. Harth et al. Perspectives on posttraumatic fibromyalgia: A random survey of Canadian general practitioners, orthopedists, physiatrists, and rheumatologists. *J Rheumatol* 27 (2000): 790–96.

White, P., G. Lewith, P. Prescott, and J. Conway. Acupuncture versus placebo for the treatment of chronic mechanical neck pain. *Ann Intern Med* 141 (2004): 911–19.

Whiting, P., A. M. Bagnall, A. J. Sowden et al. Interventions for the treatment and management of chronic fatigue syndrome: A systematic review. *JAMA* 286 (2001): 1360–68.

Wilkes, M. S., B. H. Doblin, and M. F. Shapiro. Pharmaceutical advertisements in leading medical journals: Experts' assessments. *Ann Intern Med* 116 (1992): 912–19.

Wilkinson, R. G. *The Impact of Inequality: How to Make Sick Societies Healthier*. New York: New Press, 2005.

———. *Unhealthy Societies: The Afflictions of Inequality*. London: Routledge, 1996.

Willett, W. C., M. J. Stampfer, J. E. Manson et al. Coffee consumption and coronary heart disease in women: A ten-year follow-up. *JAMA* 275 (1996): 458–62.

Williams, D. A., M. A. Cary, K. H. Groner et al. Improving physical functional status in patients with fibromyalgia: A brief cognitive behavioral intervention. *J Rheumatol* 29 (2002): 1280–86.

Williams, S. C., S. P. Schmaltz, D. J. Morton et al. Quality of care in U.S. hospitals as reflected by standardized measures, 2002–2004. *N Engl J Med* 353 (2005): 255–64.

Wilson, A., I. Hickie, A. Lloyd et al. Longitudinal study of outcome of chronic fatigue syndrome. *BMJ* 308 (1994): 756–59.

Wilt, T. J., A. Ishani, G. Stark et al. Saw palmetto extracts for treatment of benign prostatic hyperplasia: A systematic review. *JAMA* 280 (1998): 1604–9.

Winkelmayer, W. C., M. J. Stampfer, W. C. Willett, and G. C. Curhan. Habitual caffeine intake and the risk of hypertension in women. *JAMA* 294 (2005): 2330–35.

Winkleby, M., C. Cubbin, and D. Ahn. Low individual socioeconomic status, neighborhood socioeconomic status and adult mortality. *Am J Public Health* 96 (2006): 2145–53.

Winzenberg, T., K. Shaw, J. Fryer, and G. Jones. Effects of calcium supplementation on bone density in healthy children: Meta-analysis of randomized controlled trials. *BMJ* 333 (2006): 775–81.

Wolfe, F., and J. J. Rasker. The symptom intensity scale, fibromyalgia, and the meaning of fibromyalgia-like symptoms. *J Rheumatol* 33 (2006): 2291–99.

Wolfe, S. M. Direct-to-consumer advertising—education or emotion promotion? *N Engl J Med* 346 (2002): 524–26.

Wolk, A., J. E. Manson, M. J. Stampfer et al. Long-term intake of dietary fiber and decreased risk of coronary heart disease among women. *JAMA* 281 (1999): 1998–2004.

Wolsko, P. M., D. M. Eisenberg, R. B. Davis et al. Patterns and perceptions of care for treatment of back and neck pain. *Spine* 28 (2003): 292–98.

Woo, S. B., J. W. Hellstein, and J. R. Kalmar. Systematic review: Bisphosphonates and osteonecrosis of the jaws. *Ann Intern Med* 144 (2006): 753–61.

Woods, F., A. Z. LaCroix, S. L. Gray et al. Frailty: Emergence and consequences in women aged 65 and older in the Women's Health Initiative Observational Study. *J Am Geriatr Soc* 53 (2005): 1321–30.

Woodson, G. Dual X-ray absorptiometry T-score concordance and discordance between the hip and spine measurement sites. *Journal of Clinical Densitometry* 3 (2000): 319–24.

Woolf, S. H., and R. S. Lawrence. Preserving scientific debate and patient choice: Lessons for the consensus panel on mammography screening. *JAMA* 278 (1997): 2105–8.

Woolhead, G. M., J. L. Donovan, and P. A. Dieppe. Outcomes of total knee replacement: A qualitative study. *Rheumatology* 44 (2005): 1032–37.

Wootton, D. *Bad Medicine: Doctors Doing Harm since Hippocrates*. Oxford: Oxford University Press, 2006.

Wright, J. P., and P. Potter, eds. *Psyche and Soma: Physicians and Metaphysicians on the Mind-Body Problem from Antiquity to Enlightenment*. Oxford: Oxford University Press, 2000.

Writing Group for the Women's Health Initiative Investigators. Risks and benefits of estrogen plus progestin in healthy postmenopausal women. *JAMA* 288 (2002): 321–23.

Wynne-Jones, G., G. J. Macfarlane, A. J. Silman, and G. T. Jones. Does physical trauma lead to an increase in the risk of new onset widespread pain? *Ann Rheum Dis* 65 (2006): 391–93.

Yadav, J. S., M. H. Wholey, R. E. Kuntz et al. Protected carotid-artery stenting in patients with symptomatic severe carotid stenosis. *N Engl J Med* 351 (2004): 1493–501.

Zackrisson, S., I. Andersson, L. Janzon et al. Rate of over-diagnosis of breast cancer 15 years after end of the Malmö mammographic screening trial: Follow-up study. *BMJ* 332 (2006): 689–91.

Zahl, P. H., B. H. Strand, and J. Mæhlen. Incidence of breast cancer in Norway and Sweden during introduction of nationwide screening: Prospective cohort study. *BMJ* 328 (2004): 921–24.

Zeller, J. L. Artificial spinal disk superior to fusion for treating degenerative disk disease. *JAMA* 296 (2006): 3665–67.

Zochling, J., L. M. March, J. Lapsley et al. Use of complementary medicine for osteoarthritis — a prospective study. *Ann Rheum Dis* 63 (2004): 549–54.

about the author

Nortin M. Hadler, M.D., F.A.C.P., F.A.C.R., F.A.C.O.E.M. (A.B. Yale University, M.D. Harvard Medical School) trained at the Massachusetts General Hospital, the National Institutes of Health in Bethesda, and the Clinical Research Centre in London, England, before joining the faculty of the Departments of Medicine and Microbiology/Immunology of the University of North Carolina at Chapel Hill in 1973. He was promoted to professor of medicine and microbiology in 1985 in the School of Medicine of the University of North Carolina and serves as attending rheumatologist at the University of North Carolina Hospitals.

Over 200 papers and thirteen books bear witness to his scholarship. He is a student of the various approaches that nations take to the challenge of applying disability- and compensation-insurance schemes to such predicaments as back pain and arm pain. He has dissected the fashion in which medicine turns disputative and thereby iatrogenic in the process of disability determination, whether for back or arm pain or a more global illness narrative such as "fibromyalgia." He is widely regarded for his critical assessment of the limitations of certainty regarding medical and surgical management of the regional musculoskeletal disorders. Finally, he is spearheading an initiative to replace the current American "health-care delivery system" with a rational iteration.

Dr. Hadler has lectured widely, garnered multiple awards, and served visiting professorships in England, France, Israel, and Japan. He has been elected to membership in the American Society for Clinical Investigation and the National Academy of Social Insurance and to fellowship in the American College of Physicians, American College of Rheumatology, and the American College of Occupational and Environmental Medicine. He is certified by the American Boards of Medicine, Rheumatology, Geriatrics, and Allergy and Immunology.

index

American Urological Association, 95
Amitriptyline, 195
Analgesics, 114
Angina, 19–32; causes of, 19; coping with, 30–32; crescendo, 23; definition of, 19, 32; diagnosis of, 32; role of plaque in, 20–24; supplementary readings on, 239–42; symptoms of, 19, 32; vs. transient ischemic attack, 29–30
Angina treatments, 19–30; angioplasty, 25–28; clinical trials of, 21–26, 28; coronary artery bypass graft, 22–24; ligation, 21–22; pericardial poudrage, 21; placebo effect in, 21, 28; recommendations on, 31–32
Angioplasty: clinical trials of, 25–26, 28; vs. coronary artery bypass grafts, 17, 25, 26; costs of, 27; definition of, 17, 25; forms of, 26; outcomes of, 25–27; supplementary readings on, 238–42; symptoms after, 28; timing of, 26–27
Angiotensin-converting enzyme (ACE) inhibitors, 54
Animal magnetism, 197
Animal models, 124
Annals of Internal Medicine, 51, 92
Antidepressants, 278
Antifreeze, 125
Antihypertensive agents: clinical trials of, 52–54, 55; decision making about, 55; supplementary readings on, 256–57
Antihypertensive and Lipid-Lowering Treatment to Prevent Heart Attack Trial—Lipid-Lowering Treatment (ALLHAT-LLT), 40, 54, 55, 244, 256–57
Anti-inflammatories: mechanism of, 125; NSAIDs as, 124, 125
Antimalarials, 122
Antioxidants, 63, 206–7, 307
Antipyretics, 122, 197
Arab world, 196
Arm pain: alternative therapies for, 195; in workforce, 174
Artificial discs, 282–83

Artificial diseases, 12
Aspirin: acetaminophen competing with, 124; for colorectal cancer, 73–75, 262; development of, 123–24; hazards of, 37; for heart attacks, 17, 32, 37; marketing of, 123–24; mechanism of, 125; vs. NSAIDs, 125; sales of, 124; for transient ischemic attacks, 30
AstraZeneca LP, 54
Atherosclerosis: and angina, 19; definition of, 20; lipid metabolism and, 41–42; plaques in, 16–17, 20
Athletes, bone mineral density of, 167
Australia, breast cancer trial in, 92, 270
Avicenna, 201

Baby-boom generation, 10
Backache, 111–22; adverse work context and, 180, 185–87; alternative therapies for, 207, 210; causes of, 116, 177–78; as compensable injury, 174–80, 183–85; coping with, 111–12, 114, 173; in elderly, 157–58; ergonomics and, 178, 179, 183–85; history of theories about, 174–77; ineffectiveness of treatments for, 115–16; prevalence of, 111; regional, 111–12; supplementary readings on, 279–89; truths about, 113–16; vignette of, 117; in workforce, 173–80, 185–87. *See also* Regional musculoskeletal disorders
Back belts, 187
Back sprain, 177
Bad days, 135–36. *See also* Syndrome of Being Out-of-Sorts
Balance, in elderly, 159
Bankruptcy, 214
Bark, tree, 122, 196
Barr, Joseph, 176
Baycol, 38
Bayer aspirin, 123
Behavior modification: for hypertension, 53. *See also* Diet; Lifestyle
Belief, in alternative medicine, 193–95, 211–12, 309–10
Benefit/risk ratio: for alternative medicine,

92, 267–68; prostate cancer screening in, 97

Cancer: deaths from, 65; soft-tissue, 68–69. *See also specific types*

Candesartan, 54

Cannon, Walter Bradford, 41

Cardiology, 15–32; angina treatments in, 19–32; history of diseases in, 18–19; peer review in, 15–17; profitability of, 15; supplementary readings on, 236–44; symptoms in, 19, 26–27; Type II Medical Malpractice in, 20, 31

Cardiology, interventional: angioplasty in, 17, 25–26; clinical trials of, 25–26, 28; costs of, 27; vs. neuroradiology, 29–30; peer review in, 15; profitability of, 15; rise of, 24–25; stents in, 16–17, 25, 26; supplementary readings on, 236–44

Cardiovascular surgery: for angina, 21–24; clinical trials of, 21–26, 28; coronary artery bypass graft, 16–17, 22–24; costs of, 27; vs. neurosurgery, 29–30; profitability of, 15; sham, 21–22, 28; supplementary readings on, 236–44

Carnegie, Andrew, 123

Carotenoids, 206

Carotid endarterectomy, 30, 243–44

Carter, Jimmy, 181

Case-control studies, 97. *See also* Clinical trials

Case Western Reserve University, 132

Catalona, William, 97, 273

Catastrophizing, 147, 292

Catheterization, development of, 25. *See also* Cardiology, interventional

Cayenne, 305–6

Celebrex: clinical trials of, 126, 128–29; and colorectal cancer, 74–75; as COXIB, 122; development of, 126; marketing of, 127–28, 129; supplementary readings on, 284–85; withdrawal from market, 130–31

Centers for Disease Control (CDC): on body mass index, 45; on cholesterol screening, 41

Cervical cancer, 69

Charef-Ed-Din, 201

Charity, 175–76

Chemistry, Prussian, 122–24

Chemotherapy, for breast cancer, 82, 264–65

Chest pain. *See* Angina

Childhood: ear infections in, 13; tonsillectomy in, 13; vulnerability in, 146–47

Chincona tree, 122

Chinese medicine, 196

Chiropractic medicine, 199–201, 208–10; clinical trials of, 208–10; history of, 199–200; supplementary readings on, 304–5; techniques of, 200–201

Cholera, 198

Cholesterol, 33–41; costs associated with, 37–38; and life expectancy, 33–34; in Metabolic Syndrome, 42–43; metabolism of, 41–42; negative labeling of, 39; relative vs. absolute risk reduction in, 37; screening for, 40–41; supplementary readings on, 244–48; treatments for, 34–41

Chondroitin, 114, 283

Christian Science, 198

Chronic Fatigue Syndrome (CFS), 138, 146

Cigna, 227

Civil service, 186

Civil War, American, 198

Class, socioeconomic. *See* Socioeconomic status

CLASS trial, 128–29, 284, 286

Cleveland Clinic, 131–32

Clinical trials, 13–14; of alternative therapies, 195, 208–10; of breast cancer screening, 77–79, 89–93; of breast cancer treatments, 80–83; in cardiology, 21–26, 28; case-control, 97–98; of cholesterol treatments, 34–36, 40; of colorectal cancer screening, 71; conflicts of interests in, 58, 126, 133; of COXIBs, 126, 128–30; data dredging in, 58, 259–60; data torturing in, 35, 237; development of methods of, 13–14; for devices, 132–33, 282–83; of diabetes treatments, 48–51; on diet, 58–64; of fibromyalgia treatments, 144; of hormone replacement therapy, 162–64; of hypertension treatments, 52–54, 55; meta-analyses of, 246–47; in neurology, 29–30; noise in, 35–36; observational method in, 13; of osteopenia interventions, 162–64, 166–67; peer review in, 15–17; pharmaceutical sponsors of, 58, 126, 133; phase IV, 38–39n, 132; in private sector, 126, 133; of prostate cancer screening, 97–102; randomized controlled, 34–36, 268–69; relative vs. absolute risk reduction in, 37, 247; socioeconomic status in, 232–33; statistical significance in, 35–36; of vitamin supplements, 206–7. *See also* Observational studies; Supplementary readings

Clinton, Bill, 184

Cochrane, Archibald, 233

Cochrane Collaboration, 14, 91, 233–35

Cochrane Library, 280–81

Codfish vertebrae, 157

Coffee, 258

Cognitive defects: after coronary artery bypass graft, 22–23; vitamin E and, 206–7

Cognitive dissonance, 33

Cohen, Wilbur, 216

Colchicine, 202

Cold, common, 178

Colectomies, 67–68

Collagen, 155, 161

Collaterals, 20–21

Colles fractures, 159–60

Colonic obstruction, 69–70

Colonoscopy, 71–73; costs of, 67; recommendations on, 72–73, 75–76; reliability of, 72; risks of, 71; supplementary readings on, 260–63; virtual, 76, 262

Colorectal cancer, 65–76; deaths from, 65; development of, 69–70, 84; dwell time for, 69; natural history of, 68–70; NSAIDs and, 73–75, 130; prevention of, 73–75

Colorectal cancer screening, 66–76; age and, 66; by colonoscopy, 67, 71–73, 75–76;

costs of, 67; efficiency of, 66–67, 75; by fecal occult blood testing, 70–73, 75–76; recommendations on, 72–73, 75–76; sigmoidoscopy in, 72, 73; supplementary readings on, 260–63

Colostomy, 70

Common sense, 4

Community, and regional musculoskeletal disorders, 120

Compensable injury, backache as, 174–80, 183–85

Complementary and alternative medicine (CAM), 207. *See also* Alternative medicine

Composite end point, 24

Compression fractures, spinal, 157–58, 159

Computerized tomography (CT), 168

Conflicts of interest: in clinical trials, 58, 126, 133; in FDA, 127; in marketing, 95; supplementary readings on, 285–89

Confounders, 59, 60, 179, 259–60

Congress, U.S.: on breast cancer screening, 91; on ergonomics, 184; and health-care delivery system, 226; and pharmaceutical industry, 131

Connecticut, prostate cancer study in, 100–102, 272

Consortium Health Group, 227

Contracted research organizations (CROs), 126

Co-pays, in reform plan, 223–24

Cope, Oliver, 80, 263

Copeland, Royal S., 125

Coping: with angina, 30–32; with morbidity, 3–5, 107–9, 140, 191–92; on our own, 191–92; with persistent widespread pain, 144–45; with regional musculoskeletal disorders, 111–12, 114, 120–21, 141–42; work situation and, 172–73

Coronary artery bypass grafts (CABGs), 22–25; adverse effects of, 22–23, 25; vs. angioplasty, 17, 25, 26; vs. cholesterol treatment, 34; clinical trials of, 22–24; costs of, 27; development of, 16; number performed in United States, 23; outcomes of, 22–25; supplementary readings on, 237–42; symptoms after, 28

COURAGE Trial, 26, 241

Couric, Katie, 72

COX-1, 125–26

COX-2, 125–26, 127

COXIBs, 122–34; adverse effects of, 130, 131; clinical trials of, 126, 128–30; definition of, 122; development of, 122, 125–26; introduction of, 122; marketing for, 127–29; recommendations on, 128, 134; success of, 127–28; supplementary readings on, 284–85; withdrawal from market, 130–31

Crescendo angina, 23

Cyclooxygenase (COX), 125–26

Cyriax, James, 201, 210

Dairy foods, 294–95

Dark Ages, 196

DASH collaborative research group, 63, 64

Data dredging, 58, 259–60

Data torturing, 35, 237

Datril, 124

Death: from cancer, 65; cause of, 5, 11, 18; inevitability of, 5, 9, 11, 106, 153; medicalization of, 5–6; timing of, 9, 11

Decision making: about cholesterol treatments, 36–37; about hypertension treatments, 55–56; about predicaments, 109; about prostate cancer screening, 95–96, 102–4. *See also* Recommendations

Dementia, vitamin E and, 206–7

Denmark: adverse work context in, 186; breast cancer screening in, 92–93, 270–71

Denosumab, 300

Depression, after coronary artery bypass graft, 22

Descartes, René, 149–50

Devices, testing of, 132–33, 282–83

DEXA scanning, 168, 299

Diabetes: conventional vs. intensive therapy for, 49–51; cutoff for classification of, 47–48; diet and, 63–64; hypertension combined with, 55–56; hypoglycemic

agents for, 48–51; and Metabolic Syndrome, 42, 44, 46–51; screening for, 48; supplementary readings on, 251–55; surrogate measures of outcome, 46–47, 49–51, 251–52; treatments for, 46–51; type 1, 46–47; type 2, 47–51, 63–64; vascular complications of, 46–47, 50

Diabetes Control and Complications Trial (DCCT), 252

Diabetes Prevention Program Research Group, 64

Diabetes Prevention Program (DPP) trial, 253

Diagnoses: offensive, 137–38; uncertainty in, 193

Diet, 57–64; changes to recommendations on, 57, 64; and diabetes, 63–64; and hypertension, 63, 64; Mediterranean, 59, 231–32, 259; and Metabolic Syndrome, 44; observational studies on, 58–62, 257–59; omega-3 in, 57, 59–62; randomized controlled trials on, 58, 62–64; supplementary readings on, 257–60

Dietary Supplement and Health Education Act of 1994, 203

Dietary supplements: adverse effects of, 203–4; in alternative medicine, 203–7; marketing of, 203, 204–5; for osteopenia, 160–61; supplementary readings on, 305–7

Digitalis, 202

Digital mammography, 87, 266–67

Direct-to-consumer (DTC) marketing, 126–28, 205, 288–89

Disability: determination of, 180–83, 215–16; proof of, 147–48, 182; regional musculoskeletal disorders as, 174, 179–83

Discs: artificial, 282–83; loss of, 157; ruptured, 115, 176–77

Disease(s): absence of, vs. wellness, 106, 107–8; graying as, 153; historical trends in, 18–19; in illness-disease paradigm, 139; illness without, 139–42; indeterminate, 140; natural vs. artificial, 12; vs.

predicament, 109; supplementary readings on, 274–78; symptoms as, 139

Disease insurance, 222–23

Disease mongering, 105–9, 274–78

Distant healing, 210

Distress: idioms of, 6, 142; in medicalization, 4

Diuretics, for hypertension, 52–54, 56

Dixon, J. Michael, 93

Dogmatists, 195–96

Dole, Bob, 96

Dowager's hump, 157

Downsizing, and backache, 179–80, 186, 303

Drazen, J. M., 287–88

Drexel University, 197

Drugs. *See* Pharmaceutical drugs

Ductal carcinoma in situ (DCIS), 88–89, 102, 267

Duisberg, Friedrich Carl, Jr., 123

Dwell time, 69

Ear infections, 13

Ecclesiastes, 9

Echinacea, 204

Ecological experiments: on mammography, 92–93; on prostate cancer treatments, 102

Eddy, Mary Baker, 106, 198

Educational institutions: homeopathy in, 197; osteopathy in, 199

Educational status, and longevity, 12

Effectiveness Movement, 219

Effectiveness of care, 218–20, 223–24

Eggs, 258

Egypt, ancient, 195

Eisenhower, Dwight, 181

Elbow pain, 116, 283

Elderly: colorectal cancer screening for, 66; falls among, 159–60; fragility fractures among, 156–60; mild hypertension in, treatment of, 53; prostate cancer screening for, 103; spine disorders in, 157–58; vitamin supplements for, 161. *See also* Octogenarians

Eli Lilly, 169

Elmore, J. G., 92, 266–67

Employment. *See* Workforce

Endarterectomy, 30, 243–44

Envelope, therapeutic: in alternative medicine, 194, 202–10; definition of, 194, 202

Ephedra, 203

Epidemics: heroic medicine in, 198, 199; natural vs. artificial, 12

Epidemiology: of health, 108; life-course, 14, 231–33; observational studies in, 58; proximate-cause, 18, 42, 231–33; supplementary readings on, 231–35; threats to credibility of, 58

Epitonin, 203

Erectile dysfunction, from prostate cancer treatments, 96, 97, 99–100

Ergonomics: and backache, 178, 179, 183–85; physical stress in, 187

Erichsen, John Eric, 174–75, 302–3

Eskimos, 59

Estrogen receptors, 163–64

Estrogen therapy, after menopause, 161. *See also* Hormone replacement therapy

Ethics: in alternative medicine, 210–12; in colorectal cancer screening, 66; of health insurance, 215–17; of reform plan, 225; of sham surgery, 21, 22

Ethnicity. *See* Race/ethnicity

Ethylene glycol, 125

Etidronate, 165–66

European Association for the Study of Diabetes, 44, 249, 250

European medicine, history of, 196–97

European Prospective Osteoporosis Study, 159

Evidence-based medicine (EBM), 13–14; development of, 13–14; in health-care reform, 222–23. *See also* Clinical trials

Evista, 163–64

Exercise, observational studies of, 62–63, 259

Faith healing, 198

Falls, fractures caused by, 159–60

False-positive results, in mammography, 85–86, 266–67

Fatigue: in Chronic Fatigue Syndrome, 138, 146; as symptom in women, 19, 27

Fecal occult blood testing (FOBT), 70–73; clinical trials of, 71; improvements to, 75–76; reliability of, 70–71; supplementary readings on, 260

Federal Food, Drug, and Cosmetic Act of 1938, 125, 126

Federal Trade Commission, 126

Feinstein, Alvan, 81

Fever: antipyretics for, 122, 197; in homeopathy, 197

Fiber, dietary, 75, 258

Fibromyalgia (FM), 143–51; cause of, 143–44, 145–46; definition of, 143; diagnosis of, 138, 143, 146; as meme, 170; proof of, 147–48; supplementary readings on, 291–93; treatment of, 143–44

Finkler, Kaja, 230

Finland: diabetes in, 63–64; Metabolic Syndrome in, 43, 44; regional musculoskeletal disorders among workforce of, 186, 302, 303

Finnish Diabetes Prevention Study Group, 63–64

Fish, 57, 59–62, 258–59

Fisher, Bernard, 80, 83, 88, 263–64

FIT trial, 297

Fletcher, S., 92

Flu, 199

Folic acid, 205, 207

Food and Drug Administration (FDA), U.S.: advertising regulated by, 126–27; advisory panels of, 127, 128–29, 133; application process of, 133; on bisphosphonates, 166; drugs withdrawn after approval by, 39; efficacy vs. safety at, 125, 132–33; establishment of, 124; evidence required by, 13, 125; goals recommended for, 132–33; on herbal therapies, 203, 204; Institute of Medicine and, 132; mission of, 124–25; on neurosurgery, 30, 243; New Initiative of, 132–33; on NSAIDs,

124–31; outside influences on, 127; on stents, 241, 243

Food-drug interactions, 204

Forearm, distal, fragility fractures of, 156, 159–60

Fosamax, 166–67

Foucault, Michel, 139

Fragility fractures, 156–60; bisphosphonates and, 166–67; of distal forearm, 156, 159–60; of hip, 156, 158–59; SERM and, 164–65; of spine, 156–58, 159, 164; supplementary readings on, 293–300

Frailty, in octogenarians, 10–11

Fraud, in FDA mission, 124–25

Friedrich Bayer & Co., 123

Friendly Societies, 215

Functional somatic syndromes, 145–47, 291, 292

Funeral expenses, 215

Furlan, A. J., 243

Gadamer, Hans-George, 107–8, 274

Gastrointestinal symptoms, of Syndrome of Being Out-of-Sorts, 136

Gastropathy, NSAID, 125, 134

Gender: and bone mineralization, 155; and breast cancer, 77

Genetics: in colorectal cancer, 75; of race/ethnicity, 43n

Gerstein, H. C., 51

Ginkgo, 204

Ginseng, 204

Giuliani, Rudy, 96

Gleason score, 103

Glucosamine, 114, 283

Glucose. See Blood sugar

Gøetzsche, P. C., 91–92

Golden hour, 26–27

Goldstein, Joe, 40

Goodman, Steven, 92

Government employees, 186

Government Reform Committee, House, 131

Graham, James, 197, 198

Graham, Sylvester, 106

Graying: as disease, 153; as illness, 153–54
Greek diet, 59, 259
Greek mythology, 195
Groopman, Jerome, 127–28

Hacohen, Malachi, 229
Hahnemann, Samuel, 196–97
Hair, graying of, 153–54
Hands-on modalities of alternative medicine, 207–10
Harvard Medical School, 197
Harvey, William, 149, 196
Health: enigma of, 107–9; epidemiology of, 108; self-rated, adverse work context and, 186–87; social construction of, 1–2. *See also* Wellness
Health-care delivery system, U.S., 213–14; administration in, 216–17, 226; cardiology in, 30–31; costs of, 214–15; effectiveness of care in, 218–20; future of, 214; inefficiency of, 214–15; leadership of, 226; moral hazards of insurance in, 215–17; quality of care in, 217–20; rational, 220–21; self-service in, 226; supplementary readings on, 310; time with patients in, 30–31
Health-care reform, 213–27; administration in, 224–25; costs of, 225; effectiveness of care in, 218–20, 223–24; financing of, 221; moral hazards in, 225; need for, 213–14; Plan A component of, 221–22; Plan B component of, 222–24; quality of care in, 217–20; recommendations on approach to, 214–27; supplementary readings on, 310
Health insurance, 213–27; administration of, 216–17; alternative medicine under, 207, 211–12; effectiveness of care in, 219–20; employer-based, 216–17, 221, 227; marketing by, 95; moral hazards of, 215–17; national schemes for, 27; not-for-profit, 95, 216; origins of, 215–16; proof of illness for, 147–48; in reform plan, 222–24, 227
Health Professionals Follow-up Study, 61–62, 257–58

Health Promotion, Disease Prevention (HPDP), 5–6, 12
Heart attacks: history of, 16, 17, 18; lipid metabolism and, 41–42; plaques in, role of, 16–17, 20–21; primary prevention of, 34, 37, 39–40; relative vs. absolute risk reduction for, 37; secondary prevention of, 34, 37, 40
Heart disease: after menopause, 161; quality of care for, 218. *See also* Cardiology; Heart attacks
Heart valve surgery, 22
Height: in body mass index, 44; loss of, in elderly, 157
Hemoglobin A1c blood test, 51, 54, 253–55
Herbal remedies, 201, 203–5, 305–6. *See also* Dietary supplements
Heroic medicine, 198, 199
High-density lipoprotein (HDL) cholesterol, 33
Hip(s): bisphosphonates and, 167; fragility fractures of, 156, 158–59, 167; replacement surgery for, 116; supplementary readings on, 293–94
Hippocrates, 195
History. *See* Medical histories
Hlatky, Mark, 236–37
Hofmann, Felix, 123
Holmes, Oliver Wendell, 197
Homeopathy: history of, 196–99; supplementary readings on, 304
Homeostasis, 41
Homeowners insurance, 215
Homocysteine, 207
HOPE trial, 206
Hormone replacement therapy (HRT), 161–65; adverse effects of, 162; beneficial effects of, 161; benefit/risk ratio for, 162–64; clinical trials of, 162–64; for osteopenia, 161–65; recommendations on, 163; vs. SERM, 164–65; supplementary readings on, 295–96
Hospital Quality Alliance, 218
HOT trial, 55
House of Representatives, U.S., 131

Kaiser Permanente, 261–62
Kefauver-Harris Amendments (1962), 125, 126
Kellogg, John Harvey, 106, 198
Kidney damage: in type 1 diabetes, 46; in type 2 diabetes, 49–50
Kirksville (Missouri), 199
Knee pain, 115; COXIBs for, 126; supplementary readings on, 283; surgery for, 116, 118, 119, 283; vignettes of, 118–19
Kuhn, Thomas, 230
Kyphosis, 157, 300

Labeling: of cholesterol levels, 39; in fibromyalgia, 143; offensive diagnoses and, 137–38
Lancet (journal), 48
Lassalle, Ferdinand, 176
Lawrence, R. S., 91, 268
Lawsuits: over COXIBs, 131; personal injury, 147; in reform, 242, 245
Lead-time bias, 101
Left Main Disease, 22, 23, 25
Leukemia, 165
Life conditions: and persistent widespread pain, 144–47; and regional musculoskeletal disorders, 112, 114, 121, 141
Life-course epidemiology, 14, 231–33
Life expectancy, 9–12. *See also* Longevity
Lifestyle changes: for hypertension, 53, 56; randomized controlled trials on, 62–64; supplementary readings on, 257–60; for type 2 diabetes, 56. *See also* Diet
Ligation, for angina, 21–22
Limbs, phantom, 149–50
Lipid metabolism, 41–42
Lipitor, 40
Lister, Joseph, 196, 198
Litigation. *See* Lawsuits
Living wills, 31
Lloyd George, David, 215
London, Jack, 175–76
Longevity, 9–12; artificial diseases and, 12; body mass index and, 44–46; cholesterol levels and, 33–34; exercise and, 62–63;

fixed, 10–11; socioeconomic status and, 11–12, 42, 171, 232–33; supplementary readings on, 231–33; work and, 12, 42, 171–72
Los Angeles Times, 144
Lovostatin, 40
Low back pain, 111–12. *See also* Regional musculoskeletal disorders
Low-density lipoprotein (LDL) cholesterol, 33
Low-fat diets, 62
Löwig, Karl, 123
Lumbago, 177
Lumpectomy, 81, 82, 264
Lung cancer: vs. breast cancer, 84–85; deaths from, 65; development of, 84–85

Macular degeneration, 207
Magnetic Institute, 197
Magnetism, 197, 199, 304
Magora, Alexander, 179
Ma Huang, 203
Maigne, Robert, 201
Malaria, 122
Malmö (Sweden) breast cancer trial, 77–79, 90–92, 263, 268–71
Mammography: age and, 78–79, 92; clinical trials of, 77–79, 89–93; digital, 87, 266–67; early detection through, 81, 85–87; false-positive results in, 85–86, 266–67; improvements to, 87; limitations of, 85–87; recommendations on, 90–93; reliability of, 85–87; as rite of passage, 89–93; supplementary readings on, 263–71
Management style, and workforce injury, 180, 185–86
Manchester (England), 290–91
Manipulation, spine, 200–201, 208–10, 308
Manual therapy, 201
Margarine, 57, 61–62
Marketing: of aspirin, 123–24; beneficiaries of, 95; of dietary supplements, 203, 204–5; direct-to-consumer, 126–28, 205,

288–89; FDA regulation of, 126–27; of NSAIDs, 123–24, 127–30; of osteopenia interventions, 166; to physicians, 131; sales representatives in, 131; of statins, 40; supplementary readings on, 277–78, 288–89

Marx, Karl, 176

Massage, therapeutic, 201

Massengill Company, 125

Mastectomy, 79–82, 88, 264

Mather, Cotton, 175

Mayo Clinic, 69–70

McClung, M. R., 297

McGuire, William, 216

McKinley, William, 197

McNeil Pharmaceuticals, 124

MDRD trial, 55

Media coverage: of cardiovascular surgery, 24; of colorectal cancer screening, 72; of dietary recommendations, 57; and health-care reform, 214; of hormone replacement therapy, 162; supplementary readings on, 277–78

Medical histories: dangers of, 275; employment as part of, 172; for persistent widespread pain, 149

Medicalization: of aging, 154, 169–70; coping with morbidity and, 4, 5, 107–9; of death, 5–6; definition of, 4, 106, 230; disease mongering and, 106–9; of menopause, 161; public awareness of, 1; supplementary readings on, 230, 275–78; of Syndrome of Being Out-of-Sorts, 137–51; terminology of, 109

Medical Malpractice, Type II, 1, 20, 31

Medical therapy: for angina, 22–23, 25–26, 28, 31–32; attitudes toward and effectiveness of, 28–29; for cholesterol, 34–41; for hypertension, 52–54, 55; for regional musculoskeletal disorders, 114, 116; for type 2 diabetes, 48–51

Medicare: colorectal cancer screening in, 72; prostate cancer screening in, 101–2; quality of care in, 218; supplementary readings on, 280

Medicine, modern: history of, 195–202; illness-disease paradigm in, 139

Medicine and Culture (Payer), 137–38, 276

Mediterranean diet, 59, 231–32, 259

Memes, 170

Memorial Sloan-Kettering Cancer Center, 204

Meningitis, 199

Meniscectomy, 118, 283

Menopause: medicalization of, 161; and osteoporosis, 161–62, 295

Merck: bisphosphonates of, 166, 168; NSAIDs of, 74, 126–32

Mesmer, Franz Anton, 106, 197, 199

Meta-analyses, 246–47

Metabolic Syndrome, 41–56; blood sugar in, 46–51; body mass index in, 44–46; criteria for, 42–43, 250; debate over existence of, 44, 249; hypertension in, 51–54; incomplete/early stages of, 43–44; prevalence of, 43; prognosis for, 42; supplementary readings on, 248–51; treatments for, 44

Metaphysics, 198

Metastases, 68–69

Metformin, 64

Methuselah, 9

Michigan State University, 199

Microcirculatory disease, 46–47

Miettinen, Olli, 92, 269–70

Miles Laboratory, 124

Miller, David, 229

Mind, symptoms in the, 137–38, 148–51

Mind-body duality, 149–51

Mineralization, of bones, 155–56

Minnesota Colon Cancer Control Study, 71, 260

Missouri, osteopathy in, 199

Mittleman, M. A., 244

Mixers, in chiropractic medicine, 200

Mixter, W. J., 176, 179

Modalities of alternative medicine, 193, 202–12; definition of, 202; hands-on, 207–10; over-the-counter, 202–7

Modeling: with animals, 124; epidemiology's use of, 58
Mood disorders, 278
Moral hazards: of health insurance, 215–17; in reform plan, 225. *See also* Ethics
Moral relativism, death and, 9
Morbidity, coping with, 3–5, 107–9, 140, 191–92
Morbid obesity: body mass index in, 44, 45; redefinition of, 45–46
MORE trial, 296
Motrin, 124
Multiple Risk Factor Intervention Trial (MR FIT), 52–53, 54, 255–56
Muscles, statins damaging, 38
Musculoskeletal disorders, regional. *See* Regional musculoskeletal disorders
Musculoskeletal symptoms, of Syndrome of Being Out-of-Sorts, 136
Myocardial infarction. *See* Heart attacks
Myositis ossificans, 165
Mythology, 195

Napropathy, 200
Naproxen, 128–29
National Academies of Science, 132
National Business Group on Health, 227
National Cancer Institute, 91, 93
National Committee for Quality Assurance, 218
National Health Interview Survey, 207
National Institute for Occupational Safety and Health, 187
National Institute of Medicine, 64
National Institutes of Health (NIH): on bone mineral density screening, 168; on breast cancer screening, 91; on hormone replacement therapy, 162; on Metabolic Syndrome, 42–43; on vitamin supplements, 205
Natural diseases, vs. artificial diseases, 12
Naturopathy, 199, 200, 201
Neck collars, 120
Neck pain: alternative therapies for, 207; diagnosis of, 116; vignette of, 119–20

Neoplasms, 68
Nerve pain, pinched, 115
Neurology, interventional, 29–30, 243–44
Neuropathy, 200
Neuroradiology, 29–30
Neurosurgery, 29–30
Neutriceuticals, 114, 283
New Age social construction, 170
New England Journal of Medicine: advertising in, 205; conflicts of interest in, 287–88; studies published in, 34, 72, 83, 98, 118, 128, 129
New Yorker, 127–28
New York Medical College, 197
New York Times, 130
Nicholson, John, 124
Nissen, Steven, 132, 255
Nitroglycerine, 32
Nociception, 151
Noise, in clinical trials, 35–36
Nonagenarians, 10
Noncompliance, 41
Non–insulin dependent diabetes mellitus (NIDDM). *See* Diabetes: type 2
Nonsteroidal anti-inflammatory drugs. *See* NSAIDs
Nordic Cochrane Centre, 93, 268
North American Spine Society (NASS), 280
North Carolina Memorial Hospital, 213
Northern California Kaiser Permanente, 261–62
Norway, breast cancer screening in, 92–93, 270–71
Novartis, 169
NSAIDs, 122–34; and colorectal cancer, 73–75, 130, 262; definition of, 122; development of, 122–24, 126; FDA on, 124–31; gastrointestinal effects of, 125–26, 129–30, 134; marketing of, 123–24, 127–30; mechanism of action, 125; recommendations on, 128, 134; supplementary readings on, 283–85; uses for, 122; war between, 122

Number Needed to Treat (NNT), 38, 223, 247

Nurses' Health Study, 60–62, 186–87, 257

Obesity: in Metabolic Syndrome, 42–43, 249–51; morbid, 44, 45–46

Observational method, 13

Observational studies: on diet, 58–64, 257–59; flaws in, 58; on osteoporosis, 159; on prostate cancer treatments, 100–101, 102; on regional musculoskeletal disorders in workforce, 186–87. *See also* Clinical trials

Occupational Diseases (Johnstone), 177

Occupational diseases, history of, 176, 181

Occupational Musculoskeletal Disorders (Hadler), 128, 135, 215, 230, 281, 283–84, 301, 302

Occupational neurosis, 176

Octogenarians, 9–12; colorectal cancer screening in, 66; goals of, 189–90; high-functioning, 10–11; proximate cause of death in, 11, 18; recommendations to, 189–90; wellness in, 189. *See also* Elderly

Olsen, O., 91–92

Omega-3, 57, 59–62, 258–59

Ontario (Canada), breast cancer in, 83

Orgasm, medicalization of, 106

Osteomalacia, 161

Osteopathy, 199, 201

Osteopenia, 154–70; age-dependence of, 154–56; bone mineral density and, 166, 167–69; definition of, 156; fragility fractures in, 156–60; social construction of, 169–70; supplementary readings on, 293–300

Osteopenia interventions, 159–67; benefit/risk ratio of, 156, 159–60, 162–64; bisphosphonates as, 165–67, 168, 169; clinical trials of, 162–64, 166–67; dietary supplements as, 160–61; effectiveness of, 156; hormone replacement therapy as, 161–65; marketing of, 166; recommendations on, 163, 164, 167; SERM as, 164–65

Osteoporosis: definition of, 156; fear of, 154; fragility fractures in, 156–60; menopause and, 161–62; observational studies on, 159; vs. osteomalacia, 161; screening for, 154–55

Outcomes: defining, 24; surrogate measures of, 46–47, 49–51, 251–52

Out-of-Sorts. *See* Syndrome of Being Out-of-Sorts

Outsourcing, and backache, 179–80, 186

Over-the-counter modalities of alternative medicine, 202–7

Paget's disease of bone, 165

Paget's disease of the breast, 88

Pain: and mind-body duality, 149–51; as suffering, 151, 293. *See also specific types*

Pall, life under, 144–46

Palmer, Arnold, 96

Palmer, B. J., 200

Palmer, Daniel David (D. D.), 106, 199–200

Pap smears, 69

Paré, Ambroise, 201

Parenting, 146–47

Pascal, Blaise, 150

Pasteur, Louis, 196, 198

Patents, on aspirin, 123–24

Payer, Lynne, 137–38, 140, 276–77

Pay-for-performance programs, 310

Peer review, in cardiology, 15–17

Pentecostal movement, 198

People of the Abyss (London), 175–76

Pericardial poudrage, 21

Persistent widespread pain, 143–51; cause of, 148–49; coping with, 144–45; life conditions and, 144–47; medicalization of, 148–49; as in the mind, 148–51; proof of, 147–48; supplementary readings on, 289–93

Peruvian bark, 122, 196

Pfizer: NSAIDs of, 74, 126, 127, 128–31; statins of, 40

Phantom limbs, 149–50

Pharmaceutical drugs: vs. alternative therapies, 201–2; dietary supplements affecting, 203–4; direct-to-consumer marketing of, 126–28, 205; and goals of octogenarians, 189–90; Phase IV trials of, 38–39n, 132; samples of, 39; withdrawn from market, 39, 130–31. *See also* Medical therapy; *specific drugs*

Pharmaceutical industry: clinical trials sponsored by, 58, 126, 133; Congress and, 131; direct-to-consumer marketing by, 126–28, 205; FDA ties to, 133; origins of, 122–24; sales representatives in, 131

Pharmacia, 126, 128, 129

Pharmacology, experimental, history of, 196–97

Pharyngitis, 13

Phase IV drug trials, 38–39n, 132

Phillips, Kelly-Anne, 83

Philosophy of science, 3, 229–30

Physical therapy, for neck pain, 120

Physicians: drug marketing to, 131; recruit, 126

Pignone, Michael, 66

Pinched nerve pain, 115

Placebo effect: in alternative medicine, 195; in cardiology, 21, 28

Plaques: in angina, 20–24; in heart attacks, 16–17, 20–21; in transient ischemic attacks, 29; treatments for, 19–32

Plato, 195

Pleasure, 150

Poland, colorectal cancer screening in, 261

Popper, Karl, 3, 4, 91, 98, 211, 229–30

Postal Service, U.S., 97

Posture, 157–58

Poverty: and charity, 175–76; definition of, 171; and longevity, 171

Pravachol, 34–41

Pravastatin, 34–41, 244–46

Predicaments, 108–9

Prehypertension, 54

PREMIER trial, 53, 64, 257

Press. *See* Media coverage

Prevention, primary vs. secondary, 34, 37, 39–40, 74

Preventive Services Task Force. *See* U.S. Preventive Services Task Force

Private sector, clinical trials conducted by, 126, 133

Proctor & Gamble, 165–66

Proof, of disability, 147–48, 182

Property insurance, 215

Prostaglandins, 125

Prostate: enlargement of, 99; functions of, 96

Prostate cancer, 96–97; biopsies of, 96, 101, 103; deaths from, 65, 98, 102; development of, 69, 96, 102–3; diagnosis of, 101; early detection of, 96, 101–2; incidence of, 96

Prostate Cancer Prevention Trial, 272

Prostate cancer screening, 95–104; clinical trials of, 97–102; decision making about, 95–96, 102–4; recommendations on, 95, 97, 101, 103–4; supplementary readings on, 271–74

Prostate cancer treatments, 96–97; adverse effects of, 96, 97, 99–100; clinical trials of, 98–102. *See also* Prostatectomy

Prostatectomy, 96–97; adverse effects of, 96, 97, 99–100; clinical trials of, 98–102; decision making about, 103; supplementary readings on, 272–73

Prostate Specific Antigen (PSA), production of, 96, 103

Prostate Specific Antigen (PSA) screening, 95, 96, 97; clinical trials of, 97–102; limitations of, 103; supplementary readings on, 271–74

Prostatism, 99

Proximate-cause epidemiology, 18, 42, 231–33

Proximate cause of death, in octogenarians, 11, 18

Prussia: chemistry in, 122–24; disability determination in, 180–81, 215–16; social legislation in, 176, 180

Psychological stress, 187–88

Psychology, industrial, 187, 303

Psychophysics, 183

Psychosocial context, of work, 185–87, 301–3

Public health, and employment, 172
Purity, of dietary supplements, 203
Putrefaction, 196

Quality Movement, 218–19
Quality of care, 217–20, 310
Quatelet index. *See* Body mass index
Quebec Task Force on Spinal Disorders, 279
Quinine, 122

Race/ethnicity: genetics of, 43n; and Metabolic Syndrome, 43; as social construction, 170; and socioeconomic status, 43
Radiation therapy: for breast cancer, 80–82; for prostate cancer, 97, 102
Radicular pain, 115, 116, 119–20
Radiculopathy, 119–20
Railway spine, 174–75
Raloxifene, 163–64, 296
Randomization errors, 36, 269
Randomized controlled trials (RCT), 34–36; on diet, 58, 62–64; randomization errors in, 36, 269; size of, 269; uses for, 268–69. *See also* Clinical trials
Ransohoff, David, 66
Realignment, in osteopathy, 199
Recommendations: on alternative medicine, 193–94, 201–2, 211–12; on angina treatments, 31–32; on bone mineral density screening, 168–69; on breast cancer screening, 90–93; on cholesterol screening, 41; on colorectal cancer screening, 72–73, 75–76; on diet, changes to, 57, 64; on FDA goals, 132–33; on health-care reform, 214–27; on hormone replacement therapy, 163; on NSAIDs, 128, 134; to octogenarians, 189–90; on osteopenia interventions, 163, 164, 167; on prostate cancer screening, 95, 97, 101, 103–4; on regional musculoskeletal disorders, 120–21; on vitamin supplements, 160–61, 205–7
Recruit physicians, 126
Rectal screening, for prostate cancer, 95, 102

Reform. *See* Health-care reform
Regional musculoskeletal disorders, 112–22; adverse work context and, 180, 185–87; alternative therapies for, 195; causes of, 116, 141, 173, 177–78; in chiropractic medicine, 200–201; as compensable injury, 174–80, 183–85; coping with, 114, 120–21, 141–42, 173; COXIBs for, 126; diagnosis of, 116; as disability, 174, 179–83; ergonomics and, 178, 179, 183–85; forms of, 112; history of theories about, 174–77; importance of, 113–14; ineffectiveness of treatments for, 115–16, 141–42, 182; normality of, 115, 178–79; persistent widespread pain in, 142; prevalence of, 112, 141, 178–79; proof of, 147, 182; recommendations on, 120–21; social construction of, 112–13, 174–79, 183–85; supplementary readings on, 279–89, 301–3; surgery for, 116, 282–83; truths about, 113–16; vignettes of, 117–20; in workforce, 173–80, 185–87
Relative risk reduction, 37, 247
Religion: in alternative medicine, 211, 309–10; in history of medicine, 195–96, 198
Relman, A. S., 286–87, 289
Remodeling, of bones, 155, 165
Research organizations, contracted, 126
Resorption, 155, 165
Retinol, 206
Retirement, 189–90
Retribution, 174
Rheumatoid arthritis (RA): COXIBs for, 126, 128; history of, 18
Rheumatology, medical therapy in, 28–29
Risedronate, 166–67, 296–97
Risk/benefit ratio. *See* Benefit/risk ratio
Risk factors, 5–6; biological, interdependence of, 42; body mass index as, 44–45; cholesterol as, 33–34; for heart disease, 19
Risk reduction, relative vs. absolute, 37, 247
RITA-2 trial, 239, 240

Rite of passage: bone mineral density measurement as, 167; mammography as, 89–93; prostate cancer screening as, 97
Robert Wood Johnson Foundation, 210
Rockefeller, John D., 123
Rogers, Will, 81
Rome, ancient, 195
Rosiglitazone, 255
Rotterdam study, 206–7
Ruptured discs, 115, 176–77

Safety, workplace, 187
Sales representatives, pharmaceutical, 131
Salicin, 122–23
Salicylic acid, 123
Samples, drug, 39
Sandler, Robert, 66
Santayana, George, 135
Saponification, 165
Saw palmetto, 204
Scandinavian Trial, 98–101, 103, 272
Schedules, in disability determination, 181
Schwartz, L. M., 93, 268
Schwarzkopf, Norman, 96
Science, philosophy of, 3, 229–30
Scientific method, 4, 13
Scott-Levin, 127
Screening: criteria justifying, 168. *See also specific types*
Seattle, prostate cancer screening in, 101–2, 272
Sectarian medicine, 198–200
Selective Estrogen-Receptor Modulator (SERM), 164–65
Self-employment, 217
Self-insurance, 216
Self-rated health (SRH), 186–87
Semiotics, 137
Senate, U.S., 91
Sepsis, 196
Sham acupuncture, 195
Sham surgery: in cardiology, 21–22, 28; ethics of, 21, 22
SHEP trial, 55, 256
Shirley Amendment (1912), 124

Shoulder pain, 117–18
Sigmoidoscopy, flexible, 72, 73, 260–61
Silicon breast implants, 61
Similia similibus, theory of, 196
Skeleton. *See* Bones; Osteopenia
Skin cancer screening, 266
Snook, Stover, 183
Social consequences of illness, 3–4
Social construction(s): of aging, 153; of health, 1–2; of human capital, 188; New Age, 170; of osteopenia, 169–70; pervasiveness of, 169–70; of race, 170; refutation of, 169–70; of regional musculoskeletal disorders, 112–13, 174–79, 183–85
Social reformation, 175–76
Social Security disability insurance, 180, 181, 216
Social welfare, 175–76, 180–81
Socioeconomic status (SES): and exercise, 63; and longevity, 11–12, 42, 171, 232–33; and race/ethnicity, 43; supplementary readings on, 231–33, 300–301
Sodium salicylate, 123
Soft-tissue cancer, 68–69
Somatic syndromes, functional, 145–47, 291, 292
Somatization disorder, 150
Somatoform disorders, 150
Sontag, Susan, 89
Sox, Harold, 92
Spinal cord, 115
Spine: in chiropractic medicine, 200–201, 208–10; degeneration of, 157–58; fragility fractures of, 156–58, 159, 164; manipulation of, 200–201, 208–10, 308; railway, 174–75; ruptured discs in, 115
Spitzer, Walter O., 279–80
St. John's wort, 204
Stability, of elderly, 159
Staging, of cancer, 69
Statins, 34–41; adverse effects of, 38–39; clinical trials of, 34–36, 40; costs of, 37–38; development of, 40; marketing of, 40; noncompliance in use of, 41; personal risk assessment for, 37–39; in

secondary prevention, 34, 40; supplementary readings on, 244–48
Statistical significance, 35–36
Stem-cell transplantation, 82
Stents: in cardiology, 16–17, 25, 26, 240–42; in neurology, 29–30, 243–44; supplementary readings on, 240–44
Sterling Products, 123–24
Still, Andrew Taylor, 106, 199
Stockholm (Sweden), breast cancer trial in, 90, 91
Stomach lining, NSAIDs and, 125–26, 129–30, 134
Stone, Edward, 122
Straights, in chiropractic medicine, 200
Streptomycin, for tuberculosis, 18
Stress, and well-being, 187–88
Strokes: history of, 18; hormone replacement therapy and, 162–63; interventional treatment for, 29–30
Subluxations, 200
Suffering, pain as, 151, 293
Sulfanilamide, 125
Superstition, 196
Supplemental security insurance, 180, 181
Supplementary readings, 229–310; on alternative medicine, 304–10; on breast cancer, 263–71; on cardiology, 236–44; on cholesterol, 244–48; on colorectal cancer, 260–63; on diet, 257–60; on disease mongering, 274–78; on epidemiology, 231–35; on health-care reform, 310; how to use, 1–2; on hypertension, 255–57; on marketing, 277–78, 288–89; on medicalization, 230, 275–78; on Metabolic Syndrome, 248–51; on osteopenia, 293–300; on prostate cancer screening, 271–74; on regional musculoskeletal disorders, 279–89, 301–3; on socioeconomic status, 231–33, 300–301; on Syndrome of Being Out-of-Sorts, 289–93; on type 2 diabetes, 251–55; on workforce, 300–304
Surgery. See specific types
Sweden: breast cancer trials in, 77–79,

90–93, 263, 268–71; prostate cancer study in, 100–101, 272
Sydenham, Thomas, 139, 150
Symptoms: diagnosis of, 192–93; as diseases, 139; focus on, 6; in heart disease, 19, 26–27; medically unexplainable, 140, 145, 146; as in the mind, 137–38, 148–51; treatment of, 193, 196–97. See also Morbidity
Syndrome of Being Out-of-Sorts (SOOS), 135–51; cause of, 137–39; diagnosis of, 137–39; manifestations of, 135–36; medicalization of, 137–51; as medically unexplainable symptoms, 140, 145, 146; mind-body duality and, 149–51; persistent widespread pain in, 142–51; prevalence of, 136; supplementary readings on, 289–93; tolerance for, 136; and well-being, 140
Syndrome X. See Metabolic Syndrome

Tamoxifen, 163
Telegraphist's wrist, 176
Tennis elbow, 116, 283
Teriparatide, 299–300
Thalidomide, 125
Theology, 195–96
Therapeutic massage, 201
Therapeutic ratios, 202
Therapeutic touch, 210, 309
Time: dwell, 69; lead, 101; with patients, 30–31
Timing: of angioplasty, 26–27; of death, 9, 11
Tischauer, Ernest, 183
Today Show, 72
TONE study, 53, 257
Tonsillectomy, 13
Topol, Eric, 131–32
Toronto (Canada), prostate cancer screening in, 97
Trans-fatty acids, 61–62, 258
Transient ischemic attacks (TIAs), 29–30
Treatment, adverse effects of. See Iatrogenicity

Treatment acts: in alternative medicine, 202, 210–12; definition of, 202

Trials. *See* Clinical trials

Triglitazone, 50, 64

TROPHY trial, 54, 257

Truth(s): Popper on, 3, 229; about regional musculoskeletal disorders, 113–16

Tuberculosis, 18

Tumors: benign, 68–69; development of, 69; malignant, 68–69. *See also* Cancer

Tylenol, 124

Uncertainty, 4–5, 140, 193

Union movement, 176

United Health Care, 216–17

United Health Group, 227

United Kingdom: breast cancer screening in, 93; epidemiology in, 231–32; ibuprofen in, 124; persistent widespread pain in, 290–91; poverty in, 175–76; prostate cancer screening in, 95; railway spine in, 174–75; regional musculoskeletal disorders among workforce of, 186; union movement in, 176

United Kingdom Diabetes Study Group, 49

United Kingdom Prospective Diabetes Study (UKPDS), 48–51, 55, 252

United Parcel Service (UPS), 179–80, 185

University of North Carolina, 213

Upjohn, 124

Urinary incontinence, from prostate cancer treatments, 96, 97, 99–100

U.S. Preventive Services Task Force: on bone mineral density screening, 168, 299; on breast cancer screening, 90, 92, 268, 271; on colorectal cancer, 66, 73, 74–75, 262; on hormone replacement therapy, 163

Vaccination, 197

Vacuum phenomenon, 200–201

Vane, Sir John, 125

Veronesi, Umberto, 80, 83, 88

Vertebral fractures (VF), 157, 164, 166, 298, 300

"VERT" Trial, 167

Veterans Administration, 23

Veterans Affairs, Department of, 26, 97–98

Victoria, Queen, 174

VIGOR trial, 128–30, 284

Vioxx: adverse effects of, 131; clinical trials of, 126, 128–30; and colorectal cancer, 74–75; as COXIB, 122; development of, 126; marketing of, 127, 131; supplementary readings on, 284–85; withdrawal from market, 130–31

Virchow, Rudolf, 12

Virtual colonoscopy, 76, 262

Vitalism, 200–201

Vitamin A, 206

Vitamin C, 207

Vitamin D, 160–61, 294–95

Vitamin E, 206–7

Vitamin supplements: lack of need for, 160–61, 205–7; for osteopenia, 160–61; recommendations on, 160–61, 205–7; supplementary readings on, 306–7

Vulnerability, sense of, 146–47

Wall Street Journal, 144

Wal-Mart, 187

Walsh, Patrick, 97, 272

Washington (state), prostate cancer screening in, 101–2

Watchful waiting, with prostate cancer, 98–101

Waxman, Henry, 131

Weight, body: in body mass index, 44; medicalization of, 106; as risk factor, 44, 45, 250–51

Weight loss industry, 45

Welfare, social, 175–76, 180–81

Wellness, 2–4; vs. absence of disease, 106, 107–8; alternative conception of, 193–94; being vs. feeling well, 3, 191; coping with morbidity in, 3, 4, 107–9, 140; focus on symptoms and, 6; in octogenarians, 189; predicaments threatening, 108–9; sense of invincibility in, 2, 106, 140; stress and,

187–88; in Syndrome of Being Out-of-Sorts, 135–36

West of Scotland Study, 34–36, 38, 40, 244, 246

Whitehall studies, 186, 302, 303

Willow tree, 122

Will Rogers Phenomenon, 81

Wills, living, 31

The Wisdom of the Body (Cannon), 41

Wolfe, Sid, 203

Woloshin, S., 93, 268

Women: fatigue as symptom in, 19, 27; hormone replacement therapy for, 161–65

Women's Health Initiative: on diet, 62; on hormone replacement therapy, 162, 163, 164, 295–96

Woolf, S. H., 91, 268

Workers' compensation: for backache, 176–80, 183–85; and catastrophizing, 147; disability determination for, 180–83; during downsizing and outsourcing, 179–80; origins of, 176; supplementary readings on, 279, 301–2

Workforce, 171–90; adverse context for, 180, 185–87; aged, 188–89; backache in, 173–80; disability determination for, 180–83; ergonomics in, 178, 179, 183–85; health insurance through, 216–17, 221, 227; insecurity in, 172; and longevity, 12, 42, 171–72; and public health, 172; retired, 189–90; stress in, 187–88; supplementary readings on, 300–304

Work incapacity, 3–4; determination of, 180–83; and longevity, 12; tasks associated with, 174, 184

Wrist fractures, 156, 159–60

Writer's cramp, 176

X-ray absorptiometry, dual-energy, 168

Yadav, J. S., 243

Zoledronic acid, 169

H. Eugene and Lillian Youngs Lehman Series

Lamar Cecil, *Wilhelm II: Prince and Emperor, 1859–1900* (1989).

Carolyn Merchant, *Ecological Revolutions: Nature, Gender, and Science in New England* (1989).

Gladys Engel Lang and Kurt Lang, *Etched in Memory: The Building and Survival of Artistic Reputation* (1990).

Howard Jones, *Union in Peril: The Crisis over British Intervention in the Civil War* (1992).

Robert L. Dorman, *Revolt of the Provinces: The Regionalist Movement in America* (1993).

Peter N. Stearns, *Meaning Over Memory: Recasting the Teaching of Culture and History* (1993).

Thomas Wolfe, *The Good Child's River*, edited with an introduction by Suzanne Stutman (1994).

Warren A. Nord, *Religion and American Education: Rethinking a National Dilemma* (1995).

David E. Whisnant, *Rascally Signs in Sacred Places: The Politics of Culture in Nicaragua* (1995).

Lamar Cecil, *Wilhelm II: Emperor and Exile, 1900–1941* (1996).

Jonathan Hartlyn, *The Struggle for Democratic Politics in the Dominican Republic* (1998).

Louis A. Pérez Jr., *On Becoming Cuban: Identity, Nationality, and Culture* (1999).

Yaakov Ariel, *Evangelizing the Chosen People: Missions to the Jews in America, 1880–2000* (2000).

Philip F. Gura, *C. F. Martin and His Guitars, 1796–1873* (2003).

Louis A. Pérez Jr., *To Die in Cuba: Suicide and Society* (2005).

Peter Filene, *The Joy of Teaching: A Practical Guide for New College Instructors* (2005).

John Charles Boger and Gary Orfield, eds., *School Resegregation: Must the South Turn Back?* (2005).

Jock Lauterer, *Community Journalism: Relentlessly Local* (2006).

Michael H. Hunt, *The American Ascendancy: How the United States Gained and Wielded Global Dominance* (2007).

Michael Lienesch, *In the Beginning: Fundamentalism, the Scopes Trial, and the Making of the Antievolution Movement* (2007).

Eric L. Muller, *American Inquisition: The Hunt for Japanese American Disloyalty in World War II* (2007).

John McGowan, *American Liberalism: An Interpretation for Our Time* (2007).

Nortin M. Hadler, M.D., *Worried Sick: A Prescription for Health in an Overtreated America* (2008).